PEDIATRIC CRITICAL CARE REVIEW

Edited by

RASHED A. HASAN, MD

*Boston Children's Hospital
Department of Medicine
Harvard University Medical School
Boston, MA*

MICHAEL D. PAPPAS, MD

*Children's Intensive Caring
and Department of Pediatrics
Medical University of Ohio
Toledo, OH*

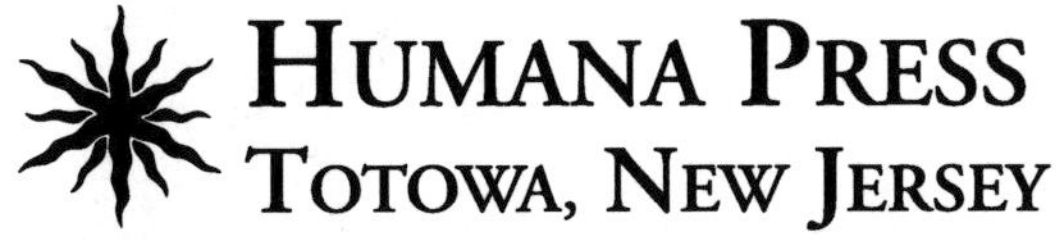

Printed in the United States of America.   10 9 8 7 6 5 4 3 2 1
eISBN: 1-59745-105-3
Library of Congress Cataloging-in-Publication Data
Pediatric critical care review / edited by Rashed A. Hasan, Michael D. Pappas.
       p. ; cm.
   Includes bibliographical references.
   ISBN 1-58829-829-9 (alk. paper)
   1. Pediatric intensive care--Examinations, questions, etc.
   [DNLM: 1. Critical Care--Examination Questions. 2. Child. WS
18.2 P36993 2006] I. Hasan, Rashed A. II. Pappas, Michael D.
   RJ370.P422 2006
   618.92'0028076--dc22
                         2005034068

DEDICATION

This book is dedicated to the happiness, health, and welfare of all children.

PREFACE

Thank you for selecting *Pediatric Critical Care Review*. This study guide is not intended to be a substitute for major textbooks or leading articles in pediatric critical care medicine, nor is it meant to replace bedside clinical medicine where knowledge is integrated with exciting and challenging realities.

It is our hope that students and physicians in training will find the pathophysiological foundation of the case scenarios and questions a useful guide in their learning process. Additionally, we hope that these case scenarios and questions will be interesting and challenging enough for the experienced critical care clinician who would like to sharpen his or her clinical skills, case analyses, and decision-making abilities.

In *Pediatric Critical Care Review*, you will find questions relevant to current clinical practices. We have also included in-depth, detailed explanations and points of reference in the answer section.

We welcome your comments and criticisms regarding *Pediatric Critical Care Review*.

Rashed A. Hasan, MD
Michael D. Pappas, MD

Acknowledgment

We wish to recognize Ms. Julie Hall, who has been instrumental in the development and completion of this book. She has functioned as a transcriber, artist, diplomat, and coordinator, bringing this endeavor to completion. Julie is a true example of hard work and commitment. Thank you, Julie.

CONTENTS

CONTRIBUTORS

The following contributed to the gathering of information for this volume.

KIMBERLY E. FENTON, MD • *Department of Critical Care Medicine, Children's National Medical Center; and The George Washington University School of Medicine, Washington, DC*

VIPUL V. PATEL, MD • *Medical Director, Pediatric Critical Care, Dayton Children's Hospital, Dayton, OH*

ANTHONY D. SLONIM, MD • *Fellowship Director and Pediatric Intensivist, Children's National Medical Center; and the Departments of Internal Medicine and Pediatrics, The George Washington University School of Medicine, Washington, DC*

MARK SORRENTINO, MD • *Director of Medical Sciences, MedImmune Inc.; and Department of Pediatrics, The George Washington University School of Medicine, Washington, DC*

GLENN STRYJEWSKI, MD • *Department of Critical Care Medicine, Children's National Medical Center; and the Department of Pediatrics, The George Washington University School of Medicine, Washington, DC*

COMPANION CD

The Companion CD contains an interactive version of the test questions found in this volume. The Companion CD is compatible with both Mac and PC operating systems that run any web browser over 4.0.

1 Respiratory System

The following chapter will focus on the respiratory system. Pertinent questions, answers, and rationale will be reviewed. Answers for this chapter can be found beginning on page 101.

Key Words: Lungs; airway; ventilator; oxygen; pulmonary.

1. Which of the following is true regarding endotracheal intubation in infants and children?
   a. The presence of a Murphy eye side hole provides absolute protection against obstruction of the endotracheal tube.
   b. Tube obstruction in infants is as high as 30%.
   c. Incidence of obstruction with small tubes is similar to the incidence with large tubes.
   d. The endotracheal tube insertion guide is the channel on the straight blade.
   e. Age is a more reliable determinant of endotracheal tube size than height.

2. The incidence of subglottic stenosis following intubation in children is approximately:
   a. 5%.   c. 15%.
   b. 10%.   d. 20%.

3. Predisposing risk factors for tracheal injury and subglottic stenosis following tracheal intubation include:
   a. General medical condition of the patient.
   b. Seizures.
   c. Head position.
   d. Endotracheal tube material.
   e. All of the above.

4. Which of the following is true of postextubation croup?
   a. Occurs in 50% of children.
   b. Begins within 18 hours, peaks at 48 hours, and resolves by 5 days.
   c. Less prevalent in patients with frequent coughing.
   d. More prevalent in children 1–4 years of age who have undergone neck surgery.
   e. All of the above.

5. Postextubation croup is most closely associated with which of the following?
   a. Failure to lubricate the endotracheal tube prior to insertion.
   b. Failure to use analgesic sprays.
   c. Excess humidification.
   d. History of upper respiratory infection prior to intubation.
   e. Surgery within the neck area.

6. Which of the following is true of tracheostomy?
   a. The highest complication rate occurs in infants.
   b. A mortality rate of up to 3% has been reported.
   c. Complications are higher with emergency tracheostomy compared with tracheostomy following endotracheal intubation.
   d. Airway secretions are increased 24–48 hours following tracheostomy.
   e. All of the above.

7. Acute postoperative complications of tracheostomy include:
   a. Subcutaneous emphysema.
   b. Pneumothorax.
   c. Pneumomediastinum.
   d. Increased airway secretions.
   e. All of the above.

8. Immediate postoperative care of a child with a new tracheostomy includes:
   a. Evaluation of a chest radiograph for tube position.
   b. Evaluation for subcutaneous emphysema.
   c. Monitoring for bleeding.
   d. More frequent suctioning.
   e. All of the above.

From: *Pediatric Critical Care Review*
Edited by: R. A. Hasan and M. D. Pappas © Humana Press Inc., Totowa, NJ

9. Which of the following is true pertaining to tracheostomy tubes?
   a. Must measure 0.5 mm smaller in size than the previously used endotracheal tube.
   b. Initial tracheostomy change may be done by the bedside nurse.
   c. Cuffed tracheostomy tubes are not suitable for infants because of the small diameter of the airway.
   d. All of the above.

10. A 9-year-old boy with a tracheostomy in place for 8 years is emergently transferred to the pediatric intensive care unit (ICU) because copious amounts of fresh blood had been noted coming out of the tracheostomy tube. Regarding the diagnosis and immediate intervention:
   a. A cuffed tracheostomy tube must be passed and the cuff inflated immediately.
   b. Erosion of the thyroid vein is the most likely diagnosis.
   c. The patient should be intubated orally and the tracheostomy tube removed.
   d. Tracheal granuloma is the most likely diagnosis.
   e. All of the above.

11. A 3-year-old with a tracheostomy for two and a half years is being decanulated. Immediately following decannulation, he develops stridor and respiratory distress. Possible etiologies include all of the following except:
   a. Tracheal stenosis or granulation tissue.
   b. An obstructing flap of the posterior tracheal wall.
   c. Fusion of vocal cords.
   d. Temporary laryngeal abductor failure.

12. Which of the following is true regarding use of tracheostomy for a prolonged period of time?
   a. The tracheostomy tube is placed above the narrowest portion of the airway in children.
   b. The tracheostomy stoma frequently needs suture closure.
   c. In infants, the tracheostomy tube is plugged prior to decannulation.
   d. Bronchoscopy is often indicated prior to decannulation.

13. Select whether the following statements are true or false regarding a child with globe injury.
   _____ a. Apply the same principles of treatment for closed head injury.
   _____ b. Avoid succinyl choline because it increase intraocular pressure.

14. Contraindications to nasotracheal intubation include which of the following?
   a. A platelet count of $18,000/mm^3$.
   b. A prothrombin time of 18 seconds.
   c. Fracture of the cribriform plate of the ethmoid bone.
   d. All of the above.

15. Which of the following medication combinations is most appropriate for intubating a 5-year-old with a closed head injury who has a capillary refill of 5 seconds, and fractured right femur because of a crushing injury he sustained 5 hours ago?
   a. Succinylcholine, thiopental, and lidocaine.
   b. Ketamine, succinyl choline, and lidocaine.
   c. Vecuronium, lidocaine, and low-dose thiopental.
   d. Pancuronium, thiopental, and lidocaine.

16. A 2-year-old male with a history of vomiting and diarrhea for 2 days is admitted to the pediatric ICU from the emergency department. He appears very lethargic; pulse 195/min; blood pressure (BP) 60/palpable; and capillary refill is 6 seconds. In preparing for tracheal intubation, which of the following combinations of drugs is best?
   a. Ketamine, vecuronium.
   b. Thiopental, vecuronium.
   c. Thiopental, pancuronium, and lidocaine.
   d. Thiopental, succinyl choline.

17. The relationship between helium and the effect on airway resistance is best described by which of the following?
   a. Helium–oxygen mixtures (HeliOx) have much lower viscosity than oxygen–nitrogen mixtures.
   b. Use of oxyhood is highly recommended in children with croup.
   c. To minimize airway resistance, helium must be mixed with carbon dioxide.
   d. When HeliOx is administered through the ventilator direct volume measurements are necessary.

18. Acute pulmonary edema has been described in children with the relief of airway obstruction with which of the following?
   a. Epiglottis.
   b. Laryngotracheobronchitis.
   c. Laryngospasm.
   d. Obstructed endotracheal tube.
   e. All of the above.

19. Bronchopulmonary dysplasia occurs in association with which of the following conditions in the neonate?
    a. Pulmonary hypoplasia.
    b. Hyaline membrane disease.
    c. Diaphragmatic hernia.
    d. Tracheoesophageal fistula.
    e. All of the above.

20. Risk factors for development of bronchopulmonary dysplasia (BPD) include:
    a. Male sex.
    b. White race.
    c. Birth weight less than 750 g.
    d. All of the above.

21. Factors that promote formation of pulmonary edema include all of the following except:
    a. More negative pleural pressure.
    b. Higher pulmonary blood flow.
    c. Lower plasma protein.
    d. More positive pleural pressure.

22. Infections likely to predispose the preterm infant to BPD include:
    a. Group B streptococcal infection.
    b. Ureaplasma urealyticum.
    c. Respiratory syncytial virus infection soon after birth.
    d. Cytomegalovirus infection.
    e. All of the above.

23. Pulmonary interstitial emphysema promotes which of the following?
    a. Pulmonary edema.
    b. Hyperinflation.
    c. Higher airway resistance.
    d. Pneumoperitoneum, pneumopericardium, and subcutaneous emphysema.
    e. All of the above.

24. The primary event in the development of pulmonary interstitial emphysema is:
    a. Subcutaneous emphysema.
    b. Increased airway resistance.
    c. Impaired lymphatic drainage.
    d. Epithelial necrosis.

25. Physiological changes unique to preterm infants with BPD that places them at higher risk for respiratory failure is least likely to include which of the following?
    a. Low intercostal muscle activity during rapid eye movement sleep.
    b. Disuse atrophy following prolonged mechanical ventilation.
    c. A blunted arousal response to hypoxia.
    d. Absence of the peripheral chemoreceptor response.

26. In infants with BPD, progressive pulmonary hypertension can lead to all of the following except:
    a. Systemic to pulmonary anastomoses with intrapulmonary shunting.
    b. Increased right ventricular preload.
    c. Restriction of right coronary blood flow to diastole.
    d. Subendocardial ischemia.
    e. Restriction of blood flow through the right coronary artery to systole.

27. Which of the following is the most essential drug for infants with BPD?
    a. Oxygen.
    b. Morphine.
    c. Acetylcholine.
    d. Caffeine.

28. Side effects of aerosolized β_2-agonist include all of the following except:
    a. Tachycardia.
    b. Hypokalemia.
    c. Impaired mucociliary clearance.
    d. Tremor.
    e. Arrhythmia.

29. Which of the following statements is least accurate regarding use of bronchodilators and anti-inflammatory medications in infants with BPD?
    a. Methylxanthines increase chemoreceptor sensitivity to CO_2.
    b. Cromolyn Na+, like methylxanthine, has anti-inflammatory effects.
    c. Combination of ipratropium bromide and β_2-agonist appears to have an antagonistic effect.
    d. Improved mucociliary function is a recognized effect of β_2-agonists.

30. Side effects of methylxanthines include all of the following except:
    a. Hyperglycemia.
    b. Hypokalemia.
    c. Hypothermia.
    d. Agitation and seizures.

31. Which one of the following is the least likely effect of diuretics when used in patients with BPD?
    a. Improved pulmonary mechanics.
    b. Improved survival.
    c. Decreased pulmonary vascular resistance.
    d. Improved lymphatic drainage from lungs.

32. Which of the following is true regarding use of furosemide in BPD?
    a. Chloride depletion induced by furosemide has been associated with poor outcome.
    b. The hypokalemic metabolic alkalosis induced by furosemide can decrease minute ventilation leading to elevation of PCO_2.
    c. Furosemide is associated with renal calcification.
    d. All of the above.

33. Advantages of tracheostomy for infants with bronchopulmonary dysplasia include:
    a. A stable, chronic access to airway.
    b. A decrease in work of breathing
    c. More freedom of mobility and physical therapy.
    d. Pleasant oral stimulation, such as nippling.
    e. All of the above.

34. Factors that contribute to decreased respiratory muscle capacity include:
    a. Respiratory acidosis.
    b. Hyperinflation.
    c. Disuse atrophy.
    d. All of the above.

35. In infants with BPD, factors that may adversely lead to elevation of CO_2 include all of the following except:
    a. Agitation with patient ventilator asynchrony.
    b. Fever.
    c. Hyperalimentation with 68% carbohydrate.
    d. Tracheostomy.

36. Increased dead space contributes significantly to work of breathing. In a setting of increased dead space, a small increase in CO_2 production may require significant increases in minute ventilation for adequate CO_2 elimination. The ratio of dead space to tidal volume can be improved by:
    a. Allowing patient's spontaneous respiratory rate to have a higher contribution to the total ventilatory support.
    b. Use of pulmonary vasodilators.
    c. Tracheostomy.
    d. A and C only.
    e. A, B, and C.

37. In infancy, congenital anomalies are the most common cause of death. The second most common cause of death in infancy is the result of disorders in:
    a. The cardiovascular system.
    b. The respiratory system.
    c. The central nervous system.
    d. The gastrointestinal system.
    e. The cardiovascular system.

38. Whenever lung disease leads to respiratory failure, the most common mechanism responsible for abnormal gas exchange is:
    a. Ventilation–perfusion mismatch.
    b. Diffusion defect.
    c. Alveolar hypoventilation.
    d. Shunt.

39. A newborn diagnosed with a left-sided diaphragmatic hernia at the 22nd week of gestation underwent complete repair on the first day of life. He is on mechanical ventilation and recovering from surgery. In the ensuing several months, it is expected that:
    a. Progressive branching of airways will occur.
    b. Progressive regression of airways will occur.
    c. Airway branching will occur albeit very slowly over the next few years.
    d. Postnatal branching of airways will not occur and left lung hypoplasia is irreversible.
    e. The airway branching will continue in the left lung, but growth of the distal airway will lag behind the proximal airway in the first 5 years of life.

40. Developmental changes in lungs that predispose the infant to respiratory failure include all of the following except:
    a. Bronchial cartilage is incomplete and continues to increase in number for several months.
    b. Growth of the distal airway lags behind growth of the proximal airway in the first 5 years of life.
    c. The smaller alveolar size and number predisposes the infant to airway collapse.
    d. Absence of pores of Kohn.
    e. The presence of canals of Lambert.

41. Match the following with their correct associated description:

> | a. Pores of Kohn. | c. Both. |
> |---|---|
> | b. Canals of Lambert. | d. Neither. |

____ Appear in the second year of life.
____ Do not appear until the frontal sinuses start forming.

42. A 4-year-old (20 kg) child is breathing at a rate of 20 breaths per minute. The concentration of CO_2 in the alveolar gas is estimated to be 40 torr, whereas the concentration of CO_2 in the exhaled gas is estimated to be 30 torr. Assuming that the spontaneous tidal volume is 5 mL/kg, the total volume of the anatomic dead space is:
    a. 100 mL.   d. 400 mL.
    b. 200 mL.   e. 500 mL.
    c. 300 mL.

43. A 3-month-old with bronchiolitis is on mechanical ventilation for respiratory failure. The arterial PCO_2 is 55 mmHg, whereas the end tidal CO_2 on capnography that is attached to the end of the endotracheal tube is 35 mmHg. The infant is being ventilated with a tidal volume of approx 50 mL at a rate of 35 breaths per minute. The physiological dead space in this patient is:
    a. 235 mL.   d. 725 mL.
    b. 345 mL.   e. 125 mL.
    c. 636 mL.

44. The physiological dead space in this infant is:
    a. Normal.
    b. Slightly increased.
    c. Slightly decreased.
    d. Cannot be determined from this data.

45. Infants have a very compliant chest wall and a reduced elastic recoil. Both of these factors lead to higher intrapleural pressure with subsequent collapse of airways and alveoli in dependent lung regions. However, functional residual capacity is maintained by:
    a. Expiratory braking.
    b. Grunting constantly.
    c. Increasing closing capacity.
    d. Increasing closing volume.

46. Regarding expiratory braking in infants, all of the following are true except:
    a. It is decreased during active sleep in premature infants.
    b. It is increased during active sleep in premature infants.
    c. Absence of expiratory braking in premature infants during active sleep exacerbates loss of O_2 stores during apnea.
    d. Abolished by anesthesia.

47. Regarding respiratory physiology, which one of the following statements is least accurate?
    a. With laminar flow, resistance to flow is proportional to viscosity.
    b. With turbulent flow, resistance to flow is proportional to density.
    c. Specific compliance is the same for adults and children, but specific conductance is higher in children.
    d. Peripheral airway resistance in children less than 5 years old is fourfold higher than in older children or adults.

48. The diagrams below schematically represent two compartment lung units. If inflation were interrupted prematurely in these examples:

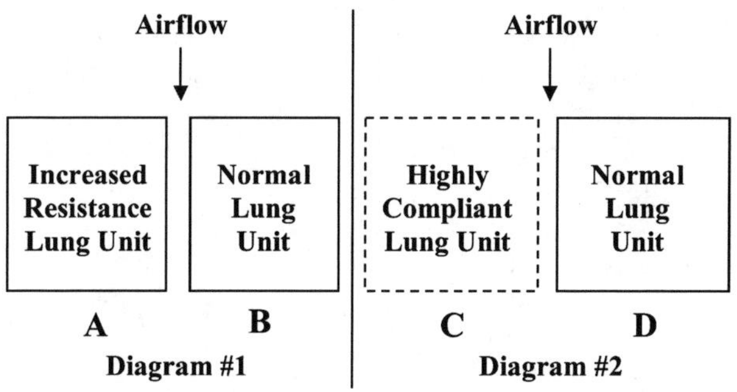

    a. Units A and C will have higher volumes of gas.
    b. Units D and B will contain higher volumes of gas.
    c. Units A and C are considered fast units.
    d. The pressure within C will be higher than in D.

49. Regarding developmental changes of pulmonary blood flow and lung development, all of the following are true except:
    a. Pulmonary blood flow plays a significant role in the growth of lungs.
    b. Diaphragmatic hernias adversely affect airway and alveolar development, but not pulmonary vascular development.
    c. In the newborn, muscular arteries end at the level of terminal bronchioles.
    d. The onset of congestive heart failure from left to right shunt occurs earlier in the premature than the full-term infant.

50. With regard to pulmonary circulation in infants and children, which one of the following statements is least accurate?
    a. The hypoxic pulmonary vasoconstriction response is more dramatic in infants than in the older child.
    b. During hypoxic pulmonary vasoconstriction, driving pressure increases much more than flow in the whole lung.
    c. Regional hypoxic pulmonary vasoconstriction increases pulmonary vascular resistance dramatically.
    d. Newborns who live at high altitudes have persistent right ventricular hypertrophy.

51. Examples of "shunt" include which of the following?
    a. Cyanotic congenital heart disease.
    b. Bronchial circulation.
    c. Thebesian circulation.
    d. Blood flow through completely atelectatic lung segments.
    e. All of the above.

52. The alveolar air equation, $PaO_2 = PIO_2 - PaCO_2/R$, does not make which one of the following assumptions?
    a. There is no inert gas exchange.
    b. There is no difference in inspired and expired gas volume.
    c. Normally, more O_2 is consumed than CO_2 is produced.
    d. Normally, the amount of O_2 consumed and CO_2 produced are the same.

53. Regarding the oxygen cascade and oxygen transport, all of the following statements are true except:
    a. If the percentage of shunt (QS/QT) is close to zero, the response to increasing FiO_2 is linear.
    b. An increase in FiO_2 will have a negligible effect on PaO_2 with a QS/QT of 50%.
    c. If cardiac output falls while O_2 consumption (VO_2) remains constant, then mixed venous content must fall.
    d. If VO_2 rises for a constant cardiac output, mixed venous O_2 content will increase.

54. The normal newborn exhibits a lower PaO_2 than an adult. The mechanism that contributes least to this phenomenon is:
    a. A right-to-left shunt through the foramen ovale.
    b. A right-to-left shunt through the patent ductus arteriosus.

    c. Shunting caused by atelectatic areas of the lungs.
    d. Low ventilation/perfusion (V/Q) segments.

55. The alveolar capillary membrane is the physical barrier that separates alveolar gas from pulmonary capillary blood and thus acts as a gaseous diffusion barrier and a fluid transfer barrier. All of the following statements describing this barrier are true except:
    a. Diffusion block is rarely, if ever, the sole cause of significant hypoxemia.
    b. Diffusion is measured by diffusing capacity.
    c. In practice, diffusing capacity is measured by using the diffusing capacity for carbon monoxide instead of oxygen.
    d. Transfer factor refers to diffusing capacity in relation to alveolar ventilation.
    e. Transfer factor increases with age.

56. The type of hemoglobin (Hb) and the position of the O_2–Hb dissociation curve play a significant role in O_2 delivery (DO_2) to tissues. All of the following statements are true regarding this topic except:
    a. 2,3-Diphosphoglycerate (DPG) lowers the affinity of Hb for O_2 by binding to the β-chain of Hb.
    b. The interaction of 2,3-DPG and the γ-chain does not lower O_2–Hb affinity as much as the interaction of DPG with the β-chain.
    c. Hb-S has a lower P_{50} than Hb-A.
    d. The iron in Hb-F is more resistant to oxidation than the iron in Hb-A.

57. Newborns are particularly susceptible to methamoglobinemia following exposure to nitrates because:
    a. Of their smaller size.
    b. Iron in Hb-F is less readily oxidized.
    c. Of exposure to city water at such an early age.
    d. Of the relative deficiency in the enzyme methemoglobin reductase.

58. Regarding DO_2 to and VO_2 by tissues, which of the following least accurately describes these two processes?
    a. A normal DO_2 with a resultant normal mixed venous O_2 content does not guarantee adequate tissue oxygenation.
    b. In the newborn, if environmental temperature drops from 33°C to 31°C, O_2 consumption doubles.

c. The normal O_2 extraction is 0.25.

d. Resting VO_2 in a 1-week-old is approximately half of that for an adult based on kilograms of body weight.

e. Electron transfer requires a minimum of 1 mmHg of O_2 for the mitochondria to properly utilize O_2.

59. Mixed venous PO_2 is least dependent on which of the following factors?

a. DO_2.

b. Circulatory distribution.

c. Inferior vena cava pressure.

d. P_{50}.

e. VO_2.

60. Which of the following options is not true with regard to neural and humoral control of respirations?

a. Carotid bodies respond to falling PaO_2 in an exponential fashion.

b. Peripheral chemoreceptors respond to falling SaO_2 in an exponential fashion.

c. Central chemoreceptors respond to increasing $PaCO_2$ in a linear fashion.

d. Hypoxia increases the slope of the minute ventilation curve in response to increasing CO_2.

61. There are a number of pulmonary receptors that modulate breathing. All of the following statements pertaining to this are true except:

a. Chemical or mechanical stimulation of the oropharynx leads to apnea and bradycardia.

b. Stimulation of laryngeal receptors produces cough and wheezing in experimental animals.

c. Excess interstitial fluid results in bradycardia, hypotension, and even apnea via stimulation of juxtacapillary receptors.

d. Laryngeal and bronchial receptors respond to CO_2 in an exponential fashion.

62. The resting $PaCO_2$ in the neonate is 33–34 torr as opposed to 40 torr in the older child or adult. Which one of the following statements least accurately explains the reason for this phenomenon?

a. The O_2 demand for the young infant is double of that for the adult based on a kilogram per kilogram of body weight basis.

b. Lower CO_2 is the result of higher minute ventilation required to meet the increased O_2 demand.

c. The CO_2 response curve is shifted to the left.

d. The CO_2 response curve is shifted to the right.

63. Chemical and neural control of respirations in the preterm infant differ from that of the full-term infant. All of the following statements are true except:

a. In preterm infants with periodic breathing, the CO_2 response curve is shifted to the right.

b. The $PaCO_2$ is closer to 40 torr as in adults.

c. The CO_2 response is flatter than in the term infant.

d. Premature infants do not have carotid bodies.

64. In children, the reason for the progressive reduction in total respiratory system compliance from birth until middle childhood is:

a. Individual variations of the operator performing the test.

b. A progressive reduction in lung compliance with age.

c. A progressive increase in airway resistance with age.

d. A progressive reduction in chest wall compliance with age.

e. None of the above.

65. The majority of tidal breathing in the infant takes place in the range of closing capacity. Which of the following statements pertaining to this phenomenon is true?

a. This increases the risk of atelectasis.

b. This is because of the very low elastic recoil pressure of the newborn chest wall.

c. Closing capacity refers to the volume of the lung below the functional residual capacity at which the alveoli and airways in the dependent regions of the lung close.

d. All of the above.

66. The highly compliant chest wall of the infant:

a. Means that the infant must generate more pressure and perform more work to move the same tidal volume.

b Is clinically manifested as retractions.

c. Is responsible for respiratory muscle fatigue and ultimate apnea, with any respiratory distress.

d. All of the above.

67. When infants are confronted with the need to increase work of breathing because of underlying pulmonary disease, a certain percentage of them will fatigue and ultimately develop apnea. Which of the following is a contributing factor?
    a. Functional residual capacity is much greater than closing capacity in infants.
    b. The small tidal volume in infants.
    c. The highly compliant chest wall.
    d. The CO_2 response curve of infants is shifted to the right.

68. Infants and newborns are more susceptible to diaphragmatic muscle fatigue because:
    a. Closing volume is lower than in adults.
    b. Of smaller residual volume.
    c. Of abundant sarcoplasmic reticulum in the muscle fibers of the diaphragm.
    d. Of the long contraction–relaxation time of diaphragmatic muscle fibers.

69. In the face of prolonged respiratory distress, some infants develop fatigue and apnea. The reasons for this phenomenon include all of the following except:
    a. These infants are unable to recruit intercostal muscle activity.
    b. Rapid chest wall distortion with respiratory distress prematurely terminates inspiration.
    c. The young infant cannot compensate for this respiratory load during active sleep.
    d. The short contraction–relaxation time of the respiratory muscles.

70. Which of the following statements inaccurately describes apnea in infants and children?
    a. Premature infants less than 60 weeks conception are at risk of life-threatening apnea following general anesthesia.
    b. Aminophylline helps apnea by significantly altering the pH and $PaCO_2$ around the respiratory center.
    c. The association between apnea and gastroesophageal reflux is well accepted.
    d. Children with obstructive sleep apnea because of adenotonsillar hypertrophy, may have deranged central control of respiration postoperatively as a result of increased opioid activity in the cerebrospinal fluid.

71. Cervical spine injury below C5 in an infant will not result in:
    a. Ineffective cough.
    b. Chest wall retraction with each contraction of the diaphragm.
    c. Mucus plugging.
    d. Respiratory failure.
    e. Decreased work of breathing.

72. Unilateral phrenic nerve paralysis is clinically more significant in infants and young children compared with adults because of all of the following except:
    a. Hemidiaphragmatic paralysis in this age group is equivalent to massive flail chest in an adult
    b. The excessively compliant chest wall of the young child.
    c. The poor ability of intercostal muscles to stabilize the chest wall in the young infant.
    d. Less compliant chest wall of the young child.
    e. With inspiration, the ipsilateral intercostal muscles and the paralyzed diaphragm are sucked in.

73. Airway resistance would appear to be the most direct measurement of airway obstruction. It is not used as frequently as tests of forced expiration in children because:
    a. It requires use of plethysmography.
    b. It is not as accurate as forced expiratory volume in 1 second.
    c. Physiologically important changes in pulmonary airways can be obscured by less important changes in the upper airway which may be responsible for 50% of airway resistance.
    d. None of the above.

74. Match the statements to the curves in the figure below.

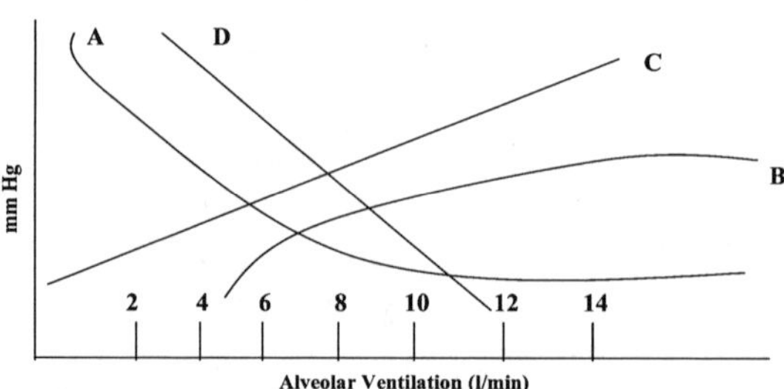

_____ Alveolar PO_2.
_____ Arterial PCO_2.

75. Which of the following does not increase the likelihood of having West "Zone 1" in the lungs?
    a. Mechanical positive pressure ventilation with hyperinflation.
    b. A pulmonary artery occlusion pressure of 22 mmHg.
    c. Pulmonary embolism.
    d. A capillary refill of 6 seconds in the lower extremity.

76. Regarding West "Zone 4" of the lung, which of the following is true?
    a. Blood flow in this zone is regulated by the gradient between pulmonary artery pressure and pulmonary venous pressure.
    b. Blood flow in this zone is regulated by the gradient between pulmonary artery pressure and alveolar pressure.
    c. Transduction of fluid across the capillary barrier exceeds the rate of lymphatic drainage from the lungs.
    d. Zone 4 blood flow exceeds Zone 3 blood flow.

77. In the pulmonary circulation, active vasoconstriction occurs when:
    a. Cardiac output decreases and pulmonary artery pressure increases or remains constant.
    b. Cardiac output increases and pulmonary artery pressure is constant.
    c. Cardiac output decreases and pulmonary artery pressure decreases.
    d. All of the above.

78. Match the statements with their correct associated outcome.

    | a. Generalized hypoxic pulmonary vasoconstriction. |
    | b. Regional hypoxic pulmonary vasoconstriction. |
    | c. Both. |
    | d. Neither. |

    _____ Result(s) in elevation of pulmonary artery pressure.
    _____ Protective mechanism(s) for the host.

79. Compliance is the relationship between changes in volume (ΔV) for a given change in the distending pressure (ΔP). Regarding this relationship, all of the following statements are true except:
    a. Compliance of the lungs is determined by DV and the difference between alveolar pressure and pleural pressure.
    b. Compliance of the chest wall is determined by ΔV and the difference between alveolar pressure and ambient pressure.
    c. Compliance of the total respiratory system is determined by ΔV and the difference between alveolar pressure and the ambient pressure.
    d. Chest wall compliance is the ΔV divided by the difference between pleural pressure and the ambient pressure.

80. Conditions associated with decreased total respiratory system compliance as a result of increased elastic recoil of the lungs include all of the following except:
    a. Adult respiratory distress syndrome (ARDS).
    b Pneumocystis carinii pneumonia.
    c. Pulmonary edema caused by severe mitral stenosis with circulatory failure.
    d. Near-drowning.
    e. Bronchiolitis.

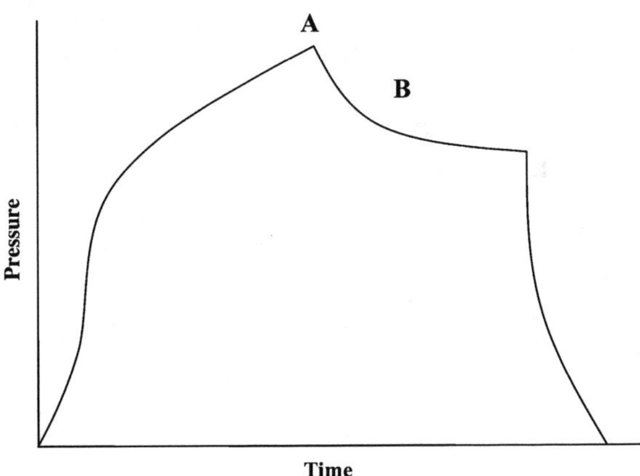

81. The above diagram relates the transthoracic pressure to time during a positive pressure inspiration. Which one of the following statements pertaining to Fig. 3 is least accurate?
    a. The decrease in pressure from A to B is because of the redistribution of gas into more compliant alveoli.
    b. This diagram indicates that dynamic compliance is greater than static compliance.
    c. The diagram indicates that static compliance is greater than dynamic compliance.
    d. A and C are true statements.

82. Conditions associated with decreased total respiratory system compliance include all of the following except:
    a. Thermal injury of the lower respiratory tract.
    b. Erect posture.
    c. Atelectasis.
    d. Abdominal distention.
    e. High peak end-expiratory pressure (PEEP).

83. All of the following statements about airway resistance in children are true except:
    a. Airway resistance accounts for less than 50% of total nonelastic resistance.
    b. With laminar flow, the pressure drop down the airway is proportional to the flow rate.
    c. With turbulent flow, the pressure drop down the airway is proportional to the square of the flow rate.
    d. Peripheral airways account for 50% of total airway resistance in children younger than 5 years.
    e. Airway resistance increases with increased flow and decreased functional residual capacity.

84. The time constant (t) describes the time required for the lung compartments to achieve a change in volume following the application or withdrawal of a constant distending pressure and is the product of compliance and resistance. Regarding this concept, which of the following statements is most accurate?
    a. t is expressed in terms of flow in liters per second.
    b. When a constant pressure is applied to the mouth, the component overcoming air flow resistance is maximal at first and declines exponentially.
    c. When a constant pressure is applied to the mouth the pressure required to overcome compliance is maximal initially and decreases exponentially.
    d. Mathematically, 63% of lung inflation or deflation occurs within 3 t.

85. An 8-year-old male with posttraumatic ARDS is being ventilated with a pressure limited "mode" of ventilation with an inspiratory time of 1 second, synchronized intermittent mandatory ventilation of 20 bpm, peak inspiratory pressure (PIP) of 30 cm H_2O, and PEEP of 8 cm H_2O. The chest radiograph has shown significant improvement over the past 24 hours, and FiO_2 has been decreased from 0.7 to 0.55. Failure to decrease the inspiratory time may result in all of the following except:
    a. Decreased venous return.
    b. Decreased physiological dead space.
    c. Auto PEEP.
    d. Pneumomediastinum.

86. Closing capacity is the sum of residual volume and closing volume. An increase in closing capacity leads to a situation where lung volume is reduced so far below functional residual capacity that small alveoli and airways in the dependent regions of the lungs are closed. Which of the following conditions is least likely to lead to elevation of closing capacity?
    a. Infancy.
    b. Bronchiolitis.
    c. Cystic fibrosis.
    d. Asthma.
    e. Pulmonary edema

87. In conditions associated with increased closing capacity, the most appropriate therapeutic intervention includes:
    a. Increase residual volume.
    b. Control pulmonary secretions and use of bronchodilators.
    c. Use of continuous positive airway pressure (CPAP).
    d. Use of PEEP when on mechanical ventilation.

88. The V/Q ratio remains stable as one moves from the base of the lung up to the third rib, but then as one moves toward the apex, the V/Q ratio changes exponentially because:
    a. Blood flow falls more rapidly than ventilation with distance up the lung.
    b. Ventilation increases more rapidly down the lungs than perfusion.
    c. Both ventilation and perfusion increase exponentially down the lungs.
    d. Ventilation decreases linearly but perfusion exponentially down the lungs.

89. Which of the following statements is most accurate regarding the compliance and resistance of the ventilatory circuits and their interaction with the patient?
    a. If the compliance of the ventilator circuit and the patient are equal, adequate delivery of tidal volume to the patient is assured.
    b. Large circuit compliance leads to delay in the delivery of an assisted breath.
    c. Use of rigid short tubing aggravates loss of tidal volume.

d. Distribution of volume delivered by a positive pressure ventilator between the ventilator circuit and the patient is determined entirely by the patient's respiratory compliance and resistance.

90. Modifications of ventilator circuiting for pediatric mechanical ventilators, in order to substantially reduce the ventilator system compliance, include all of the following except:
    a. Small diameter circuit tubing.
    b. Rigid tubing with inspiratory circuit as short as possible.
    c. Decreasing humidifier size.
    d. Positioning of exhalation valve away from the airway opening.
    e. Maintaining humidifier fluid level.

91. The most common clinical application of hyperbaric oxygen therapy is:
    a. Carbon monoxide poisoning.
    b. Decompression sickness.
    c. Gas embolism.
    d. Radiation necrosis.
    e. Crush injury.

92. Use of hyperbaric O_2 therapy for CO poisoning is probably the most common application of this technology. All of the following statements regarding this application are true except:
    a. The beneficial effect of hyperbaric O_2 therapy is directly related to the associated increase in PaO_2.
    b. The half-life of CO as measured by carboxyhemoglobin (HbCO) is decreased to 53 minutes at 3 atmospheric pressure (atm).
    c. Hyperbaric O_2 therapy helps reverse binding of carbon monoxide to cytochrome α_3.
    d. Hyperbaric O_2 therapy is indicated in patients who suffer unconsciousness or display signs of central nervous system depression.

93. The least likely complication of hyperbaric oxygen therapy is:
    a. Tympanic membrane perforation.
    b. Pneumomediastinum.
    c. Fire and ignition accidents.
    d. Significant central nervous system toxicity at 2.5 atm pressure.

94. Helium is a low-density gas that, when used in combination with oxygen, has proven particularly useful. All of the following statements are true except:
    a. The use of HeliOx is less dense than air.
    b. HeliOx may improve gas exchange and decrease peak inspiratory pressure in asthmatics requiring ventilatory support.
    c. In children with large airway obstruction HeliOx improves alveolar oxygen component.
    d. HeliOx decreases work of breathing.
    e. HeliOx can not be used in patients whose airway has been instrumented.

95. A 6-kg infant with pneumonia is being ventilated with conventional mechanical ventilation at a rate of 35 bpm on an FiO_2 of 0.6. The PIP is 32 cm H_2O and PEEP is 6 cm H_2O. The inspiratory time is set at 0.5 seconds and the flow of gas through the ventilator circuit is set at 8 L/minute. The approximate tidal volume is:
    a. 11 mL/kg.
    b. 5 mL/kg.
    c. 7 mL/kg.
    d. 9 mL/kg.
    e. None of the above.

96. Most of gas exchange during mechanical ventilation with a normal inspiration:exhalation ratio occurs during:
    a. Inspiration.
    b. The inspiratory plateau.
    c. Exhalation.
    d. Gas exchange is uniform throughout the respiratory cycle.

97. Time-limited, constant-flow ventilators are one category of ventilators that are sometimes used in the pediatric ICU. True statements pertaining to this category of ventilators include all of the following except:
    a. Use is restricted to the asynchronous mode.
    b. Tidal volume can only be estimated.
    c. Inspiratory flow limits of these ventilators do not provide adequate flow for patients weighing in excess of 15 kg.
    d. The peak inspiratory pressure relief valve is housed in the inspiratory circuit in these ventilators.

98. In the assist–control mode of mechanical ventilation:
    a. A preset tidal volume is delivered in response to every patient-initiated effort.
    b. The patient must perform inspiratory work to open the inspiratory valve and initiate each tidal volume.

   c. Ventilator trigger sensitivity and peak inspiratory flow are controlled by the operator.
   d. Ventilator peak inspiratory flow and trigger sensitivity affect work of breathing.
   e. All of the above.

99. Intermittent mandatory ventilation allows spontaneous breathing between positive pressure breaths with a preset tidal volume and frequency. Which one of the following statements least accurately describes intermittent mandatory ventilation?
   a. To minimize work of breathing, the inspiratory gas flow in continuous flow circuit should not exceed the patient's own peak inspiratory flow rate.
   b. A flow-by system avoids problems associated with continuous flow and demand flow systems in terms of work of breathing.
   c. Intermittent mandatory ventilation is likely to be associated with more stable hemodynamics compared with continuous mandatory ventilation.
   d. Intermittent mandatory ventilation is more likely to be associated with improved V/Q matching compared with continuous mandatory ventilation.
   e. The need for frequent administration of sedatives and/or muscle relaxants seems to be decreased by using intermittent mandatory ventilation compared with continuous mandatory ventilation.

100. In describing pressure support ventilation, which one of the following options is least accurate?
   a. The ventilator retains control of the cycle length, as well as the depth and flow characteristics.
   b. It has been shown to abolish diaphragmatic muscle fatigue in patients who fail conventional weaning attempts.
   c. Pressure support ventilation helps compensate for work of breathing owing to the inspiratory demand valve and endotracheal tube impedance
   d. Patient effort, length of pressure support, and the respiratory system impedance determine the tidal volume.

101. Inverse-ratio ventilation is performed using:
   a. Pressure-limited breaths with decelerating inspiratory flow rates and adjustment of inspiratory time to the desired level.
   b. Volume-limited breaths with low inspiratory flow rates to achieve the desired inspiratory time.
   c. Volume-limited breaths with normal inspiratory flow rate and prolonged inspiratory pause to maintain a prolonged inspiratory phase.
   d. All of the above.

102. During pressure-control, inverse-ratio ventilation, tidal volume is a function of:
   a. Respiratory system compliance and resistance.
   b. The preset pressure limit.
   c. The ratio of inspiratory time to total duty cycle.
   d. Frequency.
   e. All of the above.

103. Positive pressure ventilatory support in the setting of respiratory failure is aimed at elevating the functional residual capacity or mean lung volume through the application of CPAP or PEEP. Appropriate statements pertaining to this application include all of the following except:
   a. Application of appropriate levels of PEEP/CPAP can decrease work of breathing.
   b. High levels of PEEP have the potential to increase work of breathing.
   c. The decrease in DO_2 associated with high levels of PEEP is often resistant to fluid resuscitation and inotropic support.
   d. In the absence of pulmonary artery catheter, PEEP should be gradually increased to maintain an A-a gradient less than 250 torr with adequate perfusion.
   e. As a general rule, a pulmonary artery catheter is recommended to monitor cardiac output when PEEP of greater than 15 cm is used.

104. When deciding to discharge a patient who is ventilator-dependent, the least important factor to consider is:
   a. Presence of an established tracheostomy with healed stoma.
   b. PaO_2 greater than 60 torr with FiO_2 less than 0.3 and $PaCO_2$ less than 50 torr using home ventilatory settings.
   c. No need for PEEP.
   d. The underlying disease.
   e. Stable ventilatory settings for 1 month.

105. Adverse hemodynamic effects of PEEP are related to:
   a. Decreased venous return.
   b. Ventricular interdependence.
   c. Increased residual volume.

    d. Reflex neurohormonal factors leading to ventricular dysfunction.
    e. All of the above.

106. Barotrauma is a recognized complication of mechanical ventilatory support and has a number of clinical manifestations. Which of the following is always considered clinically significant?
    a. Pulmonary interstitial emphysema.
    b. Pneumomediastinum.
    c. Subcutaneous emphysema.
    d. Pneumoperitoneum.
    e. None of the above.

107. Tension pneumothorax is a life-threatening complication of trauma or positive pressure ventilation that requires immediate intervention. All of the following statements are true except:
    a. Tension pneumothorax occurs when a communication exists between the pleural space and either the alveoli or the atmosphere, so that air enters the pleural space during inspiration, but is unable to exit during exhalation.
    b. Tension pneumothorax occurs when intrapleural pressure continues to remain subatmospheric.
    c. Obstruction of venous return occurs.
    d. Treatment is by closed chest thoracotomy tube.

108. Features of veno-venous extracorporeal life support include all of the following except:
    a. It depends on patient's native heart for DO_2 to tissue.
    b. Usually requires lower extracorporeal flow.
    c. It reduces the risk of embolization with an intact heart.
    d. It maintains well-oxygenated pulmonary blood flow.
    e. It requires the right ventricle to work unremittingly in the face of pulmonary hypertension.

109. Match the statements with their correct associated descriptions.

> a. Veno-arterial extracorporeal life support.
> b. Veno-venous extracorporeal life support.
> c. Both.
> d. Neither.

    _____ Maintain(s) pulmonary blood flow with oxygenated blood.
    _____ Assist(s) systemic circulation.
    _____ Decrease(s) pulmonary artery pressure.

110. Which of the following equations best describes the O_2 saturation that is obtained using the pulse oximetry?
    a. $= HbO_2 / HbO_2 + Hb + HbCO + Hb$ met.
    b. $= HbO_2 / Hb$.
    c. $= HbO_2 / HbO_2 + Hb$.
    d. $= HbO_2 + Hb / HbO_2$.

111. You have made a diagnosis of nitrite poisoning and decide to administer methylene blue intravenously at a dose of 1 mg/kg over few minutes. As the nurse is injecting the methylene blue, you notice that the saturation on pulse oximetry decreases precipitously from 99 to 85%. The most likely explanation and the appropriate course of action is:
    a. Shock with hypotension; stop the medication.
    b. Formation of HbCO.
    c. Methylene blue is misinterpreted by the pulse oximeter as reduced Hb resulting in a low saturation; this should resolve in 2 minutes without any intervention.
    d. None of the above.

112. Match the correct hemoglobin to the statement below.

> a. HbCO.
> b. Hb.
> c. Oxyhemoglobin.

    _____ A high level of this compound leads to a low fractional saturation but relatively high functional saturation.

113. Which of the following is least likely to interfere with an accurate reading of saturation on pulse oximetry?
    a. High levels of HbCO.
    b. High levels of met Hb.
    c. An external light source such as a surgical lamp, bilirubin lamps, or fluorescent lights.
    d. Hyperbilirubinemia.
    e. Shock with low perfusion states.

114. Which of the following clinical conditions is not associated with a low mixed venous oxygen saturation?
    a. Low Hb.
    b. Low arterial oxygen saturation.
    c. Low cardiac output.
    d. Increased DO_2.
    e. Increased VO_2.

115. Which of the following clinical conditions is not associated with a high mixed venous oxygen saturation?
    a. Increased DO_2.
    b. Decreased O_2 extraction by the tissue.
    c. Severe mitral regurgitation.
    d. A wedged pulmonary artery catheter.
    e. Increased VO_2.

116. The figure below represents the capnogram obtained from a patient on SIMV mode of mechanical ventilation and a ventilator with a demand valve mechanism. The best course of action would be:

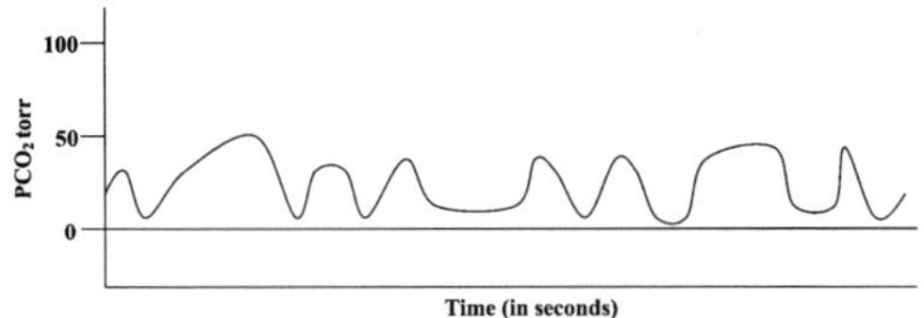

    a. Substitute the neuromuscular blockade agent used with a nondepolarizing agent.
    b. Calm the patient and reassure him.
    c. Add a bronchodilator and intravenous corticosteroid.
    d. Add 20 cm water of pressure support.
    e. None of the above, as this represents a normal variation of capnography.

117. Which one of the clinical conditions listed below is not expected to be associated with a sudden decline in end tidal carbon dioxide?
    a. Cardiac standstill.
    b. Air embolism.
    c. Obstruction of the endotracheal tube.
    d. Leakage in the circuit or discontinuation of the ventilator suddenly.
    e. Hypoventilation.

118. You are preparing to draw an arterial blood gas sample from a patient in the pediatric ICU. In discussing with your medical students, the technical errors associated with this process, which one of the following statements would you not make?
    a. A gas bubble in the syringe will falsely elevate $PaCO_2$.
    b. The major blood gas error associated with excess heparin in the sample is a drop in $PaCO_2$.
    c. When a sample that is obtained from a patient breathing room air is interfaced with a bubble, the PaO_2 obtained will be close to 150 torr.

    d. In a patient on high FiO_2 with normal lungs, the presence of an air bubble in the syringe may spuriously lower PaO_2.

119. Alterations in blood gas values occur if the sample is not immediately analyzed leading to spurious results; generally, this effect is most noticeable in patients with:
    a. Hyponatremia and hypercalcemia.
    b. Leukopenia.
    c. Neutropenia.
    d. Leukocytosis and reticulocytopenia.
    e. Reticulocytosis with high band forms.

120. Which one of the following drugs leads to a high anion gap metabolic acidosis?
    a. Acetazolamide.
    b. Aldactone.
    c. Arginine HCl.
    d. Aspirin.
    e. Cholestyramine and sulfamylon.

121. Which of the following is not a characteristic feature of posterior choanal atresia?
    a. Clinical symptoms have been noted to persist after surgical correction in some infants.
    b. Most cases are unilateral.
    c. Has a familiar occurrence.
    d. Other associated anomalies are extremely uncommon.

122. Nasal encephalocele is a recognized cause of nasal obstruction in children. Which one of the following statements does not accurately describe this condition?
    a. Usually communicates with the subarachnoid space.
    b. May be seen as a nasofrontal or a nasoethmoidal mass.
    c. The mass is soft, compressible and may be pulsatile, but biopsy is contraindicated.
    d. Nasal obstruction does not occur when the mass is located at the base of skull.

123. Nasopharyngeal angiofibromas
    a. May extend to the nasal passages and cause obstruction.
    b. Tend to cause symptoms typically at puberty.
    c. Rhinorrhea and epistaxis are common symptoms.
    d. Treatment is radiation therapy or surgery.
    e. All of the above.

124. Match the correct associations.

> | a. Infant | c. Both |
> |---|---|
> | b. Adult | d. Neither |

   _____ Vocal cords are concave and at an angle to the trachea.
   _____ The main bronchi branch from the trachea at equal angles.
   _____ The glottis is located at C6.
   _____ The tracheal length from glottis to bifurcation is 11 cm.

125. Which of the following statements regarding the pediatric airway is true?
   a. The lateral diameter of the newborn glottis is 10 mm.
   b. At birth, the trachea is approx 10–12 cm in length.
   c. At 4–6 months, the epiglottis loses contact with the soft palate and becomes more erect.
   d. The glottis assumes the adult location at the level of the sixth cervical vertebra by 6 years of age.

126. During spontaneous respirations, the major contribution to total respiratory resistance is by:
   a. Nasal airway and mouth.
   b. Glottis.
   c. Trachea.
   d. Bronchi.

127. A child with an airway that has a diameter of 8 mm develops a respiratory infection with airway inflammation and circumferential edema, which leads to a 1-mm uniform reduction in the size of the airway; this will decrease the cross-sectional area of the airway by:
   a. 34%.
   b. 44%.
   c. 56%.
   d. 64%.
   e. 74%.

128. Laryngospasm is induced by reflexes in the nose, oropharynx, epiglottis, and vocal cords and may be seen in response to mucous, saliva, emesis, or blood. It necessitates immediate interventions, which may include:
   a. Positive pressure ventilation by a mask.
   b. Removal of the offending agent.
   c. Elevation of the mandible.
   d. Use of a muscle relaxant.
   e. All of the above.

129. In children younger than two and a half years with chronic stridor, the most common etiology is:
   a. Infection of the larynx and surrounding structures.
   b. Congenital anomalies of the larynx.
   c. Foreign body aspiration.
   d. Trauma.

130. Laryngomalacia is characterized by all of the following except:
   a. It is the most common congenital laryngeal anomaly.
   b. Aryepiglottic folds fall into the glottis on inspiration.
   c. Voice is hoarse leading to abnormal cry.
   d. Resolves by 18–24 months.
   e. Tracheostomy may be required if the problem interferes with feeding and growth.

131. All of the following congenital abnormalities lead to abnormal cry and hoarseness of voice except:
   a. Laryngocele.
   b. Laryngeal web.
   c. Laryngomalacia.
   d. Laryngeal cyst.
   e. Laryngotracheoesophageal cleft.

132. Match the correct associations.

> | a. Laryngomalacia | c. Both |
> |---|---|
> | b. Airway hemangioma | d. Neither |

   _____ Symptoms usually occur before six months of age.
   _____ Treatment is conservative, since most cases resolve by two years of age.

133. Syndromes associated with difficult airway management due to micrognathia is/are:
   a. Hallermann-Streiff Syndrome (Oculomandibulodyscephaly).
   b. Mobius Syndrome.
   c. Noonan's Syndrome.
   d. DiGeorge Syndrome.
   e. All of the above.

134. Postoperative complications associated with cleft lip/palate repair include:
   a. Edema leading to nasopharyngeal obstruction.
   b. Nasopharyngeal blockage from secretions.
   c. Laryngospasm from excessive secretion and bloody drainage.
   d. All of the above.

135. Macroglossia with a short neck combines to produce a difficult airway in which of the following clinical disorders?
    a. Hurler's Syndrome.
    b. Scheie's Syndrome.
    c. Both.
    d. Neither.

136. A difficult airway owing to a short and rigid neck is seen in:
    a. Hurler's and Marqio's mucopolysaccharidoses.
    b. Klippel-Feil Syndrome.
    c. Myositis ossificans.
    d. Ankylosing spondylitis.
    e. All of the above.

137. A two and a half-year-old white male who has a 2-day history of an upper respiratory tract infection and fever is now having mild stridor and dysphagia. His immunizations are up to date. You suspect retropharyngeal abscess. Which one of the following statements is incorrect regarding this patient?
    a. Age of the patient is somewhat atypical.
    b. Inspiratory radiograph films are more informative than expiratory films.
    c. A chest radiograph should be obtained to evaluate mediastinal extension.
    d. The retropharyngeal space extends from the base of the skull to the level of the second thoracic vertebra
    e. The usual organisms are staphylococci, group A streptococci, and anerobes.

138. A 3-year-old is admitted to the pediatric ICU with a diagnosis of bacterial tracheitis. All of the following statements are true except:
    a. Diagnosis is confirmed by thick purulent secretions suctioned from the trachea or the presence of a pseudomembrane, or ulcerations intratracheally.
    b. Intermittent tracheal suctioning should be avoided.
    c. Intubation may be required in cases of severe airway obstruction.
    d. Repeated bronchoscopy aids secretion removal and assessment of disease progression.
    e. Extubation criteria include lack of fever, presence of air leak around the tube, signs of healing at bronchoscopy, and a decreased need for suctioning.

139. A two and a half-year-old with viral croup required intubation for increasing CO_2 and acidemia 3 days ago. Extubation is recommended when:
    a. An air leak around the tube can be heard with coughing.
    b. An air leak around the tube can be heard with a positive pressure insufflation of less than 40 cm H_2O.
    c. The amount of endotracheal secretions has diminished.
    d. All of the above.

140. With regard to orofacial trauma caused by external forces, all of the following statements are true except:
    a. Nasotracheal intubation should be avoided with midfacial fractures.
    b. Provided the cervical spine is stable, hemorrhage at the base of the tongue should be managed by having the patient in the prone, or lateral position with the head down to allow drainage of blood.
    c. A skateboard-associated injury to the neck usually involves an area of soft tissue and an underlying skeletal injury.
    d. The amount of subcutaneous emphysema of the neck correlates with the severity of airway injury.

141. In children with acquired subglottic stenosis, the most common etiology is:
    a. Endotracheal intubation.
    b. External neck trauma.
    c. Burns.
    d. High tracheostomy sites.
    e. Tumors.

142. Among the risk factors for the development of subglottic stenosis is the duration of mechanical ventilation. The acceptable time for the duration of intubation is:
    a. 2 days.
    b. 4 days.
    c. 7 days.
    d. 10 days.
    e. None of the above.

143. With regard to thermal and chemical injuries to the head and neck region, all of the following statements are true except:
    a. If there are flame burns of the face or singed facial hairs, the temperature is high enough to result in a respiratory burn.
    b. Thermal injury usually affects the nasopharynx and larynx.

   c. A child with a history of caustic ingestion requires examination of the larynx.

   d. HeliOx has not been shown to be effective in the management of postextubation stridor in burn victims.

144. Papillomas are the most common airway tumors in children with symptoms usually appearing before 7 years of age. True statements about papillomas include all of the following except:
   a. Most commonly located on vocal cords.
   b. Initial symptoms involve a change in voice such as stridor.
   c. Often these children have personality changes.
   d. The natural history is life-long recurrence.
   e. The goal of therapy is to remove most of the lesions to prevent spreading while preserving airway anatomy.

145. The predominant pathophysiological abnormality leading to hypoxemia in bronchiolitis caused by respiratory syncytial virus infection is:
   a. V/Q mismatch.
   b. Right-to-left intrapulmonary shunting.
   c. Hypoventilation with relative alveolar hypoxemia.
   d. Diffusion barrier.
   e. All of the above.

146. A 5-month-old with severe respiratory syncytial virus bronchiolitis is noted to be slightly edematous with puffiness of the periorbital area and low urine output. Past medical history is unremarkable for prematurity or other perinatal disorders. It is also negative for any liver or kidney diseases. Physical examination does not reveal evidence of hepatomegaly or pronounced component of the second heart sound. Laboratory data shows that serum electrolytes are within normal limits. The most likely explanation for this finding is:
   a. Hypoalbuminemia.
   b. Hyponatremia with low urine Na^+.
   c. Congestive heart failure owing to cor pulmonale.
   d. High antidiuretic hormone levels with hyperaldosteronism.
   e. None of the above.

147. Evaluation of urine for the patient in the previous question will most likely show:
   a. Low urine Na^+.
   b. High urine Na^+.
   c. Normal urine Na^+.
   d. Any of the above.

148. In acute asthma, which one of the following demonstrates the most severe decrease?
   a. Maximum mid-expiratory flow rate.
   b. Mean expiratory forced reserve.
   c. Functional vital capacity.
   d. Forced expiratory volume 1.0 ($FEV_{1.0}$).

149. After treatment of an acute attack of asthma, which of the following is least likely to improve?
   a. Maximum mid-expiratory flow rate.
   b. Mean expiratory forced reserve.
   c. Functional vital capacity.
   d. $FEV_{1.0}$.

150. Which one of the following parameters is least likely to decrease during an acute attack of asthma?
   a. Inspiratory capacity.
   b. Vital capacity.
   c. Expiratory reserve volume.
   d. Maximum expiratory flow rate.
   e. Residual volume.

151. Pathophysiological changes that occur in an acute episode of asthma include all of the following except:
   a. Hypocapnia is caused by alveolar hyperventilation secondary to activation of pulmonary reflexes.
   b. Hypocapnia correlates with the degree of airway obstruction.
   c. The degree of hyperoxia correlates well with the degree of airway obstruction as measured by $FEV_{1.0}$.
   d. Elevated $PaCO_2$ occurs when $FEV_{1.0}$ falls below 20% predicted.
   e. Elevated $PaCO_2$ is not seen if peak expiratory flow rate is greater than 25% predicted.

152. True statements regarding an acute asthmatic attack include:
   a. Left ventricular afterload is advantageously lowered by the significantly negative intrathoracic pressure with inspiration.
   b. A decrease in pulsus paradoxus always indicates an improvement in the patient's clinical condition.
   c. Hypocapnia seen in the early stages of an attack correlates with the degree of airway obstruction.
   d. Pulsus paradoxus is because of a combination of increased left ventricular afterload and ventricular interdependence during inspiration.
   e. None of the above.

153. Hypoxemia during status asthmaticus results from:
   a. V/Q mismatch.
   b. Increased O_2 requirement.
   c. Increased interstitial lung fluid.
   d. All of the above.

154. $FEV_{1.0}$ is an important parameter in the evaluation of a patient in status asthmaticus because of all of the following, except:
   a. $FEV_{1.0}$ correlates with PaO_2.
   b. $FEV_{1.0}$ inversely correlates with $PaCO_2$.
   c. $PaCO_2$ elevation occurs when $FEV_{1.0}$ falls below 20% predicted.
   d. Pulsus paradoxus is present in all patients with an $FEV_{1.0}$ less than 20% predicted.

155. At an $FEV_{1.0}$ less than 20% predicted:
   a. $PaCO_2$ rises.
   b. Hypoxemia occurs.
   c. Pulsus paradoxus is present in all patients.
   d. All of the above.

156. A 3-year-old boy developed acute airway obstruction possibly secondary to pneumococcal epiglottitis at home. An emergency cricothyrotomy was performed using a 16-gage angiocath, which was connected to a size 3.0 endotracheal tube adapter. Oxygen is delivered at a rate of 4 L/minute from an E-cylinder. The pressure gauge reading on the E-cylinder is at 1100 PSI. The transport team leader asks you, "How much time do we have before we run out of O_2?" (The cylinder factor for the E-cylinder is 0.3 L/PSI) Your answer should be:
   a. 8.2 minutes.
   b. 82 minutes.
   c. 820 minutes.
   d. 8 hours.
   e. Cannot be determined with the information provided.

157. Which one of the combinations of values below best describes ventilation/perfusion ratio in the normal lung in the upright posture?

	Apices	Bases
a.	>1	>1
b.	>1	<1
c.	<1	>1
d.	<1	<1
e.	1	1

158. Which of the following would be the most compelling indication for tracheostomy in a fire victim?
   a. Full thickness facial burns.
   b. Apnea.
   c. Proximal laryngeal damage.
   d. Severe pulmonary edema.
   e. Circumferential full-thickness burns of the neck.

159. Which of the following statements is true regarding the growth and development of lung units in infants?
   a. The lungs of newborn infants lack true alveoli
   b. Terminal bronchioles grow and bifurcate to give rise to respiratory bronchioles during infancy.
   c. Interalveolar Pores of Kohn are well developed in the neonate.
   d. Alveoli form via septation of saccules.
   e. The number of secondary acini increases during the first year of life.

160. A patient with pneumonia is breathing an FiO_2 of 0.4. The $PaCO_2$ on arterial blood gases is 40 torr, and the PaO_2 is 100. The patient's temperature is 37°C and the barometric pressure is 747. Assuming that the respiratory quotient is 0.8, what is the alveolar–arterial O_2 gradient in this patient?
   a. 30.
   b. 130.
   c. 180.
   d. 430.
   e. 140.

161. Which of the following is primarily responsible for the production of tumor necrosis factor?
   a. Platelets.
   b. Macrophages.
   c. B-lymphocytes.
   d. T-lymphocytes.
   e. Neutrophils.

162. A 10-year-old girl was involved in a motor vehicle collision, and is noted to have moderate respiratory distress. A chest radiograph shows a large left-sided pneumothorax. BP is normal. After a chest tube is inserted and is functioning properly, a persistent large air leak is noted. A repeat chest radiograph shows that there is still persistent pneumothorax. The patient's condition remains stable. The most appropriate next step in the management of this patient is:

    a. Insert a second chest tube.
    b. Perform an immediate thoracotomy.
    c. Repeat a chest radiograph in 8 hours.
    d. Initiate jet ventilation.
    e. Perform a bronchoscopy.

163. When ketamine is administered by the intramuscular route, a larger dose is necessary to induce general anesthesia, compared with the intravenous route. The most likely explanation for this is:
    a. Upregulation of drug receptors.
    b. Tachyphylaxis.
    c. Slower absorption.
    d. Incomplete absorption.
    e. Tissue metabolism.

164. Recovery after alveolar injury is characterized by which of the following processes:
    a. Serum factors enter the alveoli and delay the healing process.
    b. Polymorphonuclear leukocytes clear the alveolar debris.
    c. Alveolar type I cells divide and multiply to reconstitute the alveolar surface.
    d. The surface is first reconstituted by alveolar type II cells that, in turn, evolve into alveolar type I cells.
    e. The pericytes multiply and evolve into alveolar type I cells.

165. Which of the following is the earliest evidence of inspiratory muscle fatigue after discontinuation of mechanical ventilation?
    a. An increase in respiratory rate.
    b. An increase in $PaCO_2$.
    c. Alternation of abdominal and thoracic breathing every few breaths.
    d. Primary thoracic inspirator effort when supine.
    e. Abdomen moving inward during inspiration.

166. Which of the following statements is correct regarding the physiology of hemeproteins within the Hb or myoglobin?
    a. CO_2 increases the affinity of Hb for O_2.
    b. O_2 has a stronger affinity for Hb than myoglobin.
    c. CO_2 combines with nonoxygenated Hb to form carbaminohemoglobin.
    d. 2,3-DPG increases Hb affinity for O_2 by competing with hydrogen ion for binding sites.
    e. O_2 and hydrogen ions bind to the same sites on Hb.

167. An 18-day-old infant male underwent insertion of an aorticopulmonary shunt estimated to be 5 mm in diameter for pulmonary atresia. Postoperatively it is noted that he has a large left-to-right shunt and continues to receive conventional mechanical ventilation. Which of the following interventions is most likely to reduce the left-to-right shunt flow?
    a. Intravenous hydralazine.
    b. Intravenous nitroprussid.
    c. Increase arterial pH.
    d. Increase FiO_2.
    e. Increase PEEP.

168. Which of the following is the major precursor of arachidonic acid?
    a. Glutamic acid.
    b. Leucine.
    c. Isoleucine.
    d. Linoleic acid.
    e. Valine.

169. A child with pneumonia and respiratory failure is receiving conventional mechanical ventilation. Minute ventilation (MV) is 2 L/min and the PEEP is set at 5 cmH_2O. Hb is 9 gm% and arterial blood gases show that arterial O_2 saturation is 85%. Cardiac output is estimated to be 2 L/min. O_2 Transport from lungs to tissues will be most improved by which of the following:
    a. Increasing MV to 3 L/min.
    b. Increasing PEEP to 10 cmH_2O.
    c. Increasing Hb to 14 gm%.
    d. Increasing O_2 saturation to 95%.
    e. Increasing cardiac output to 2.4 L/min.

170. Stimulation of juxtacapillary receptors (J receptors) produces:
    a. Rapid shallow breathing.
    b. Bronchodilation.
    c. Hypotension.
    d. Cough.
    e. Tachycardia.

171. Which of the following types of cells is most likely to manifest injury at the onset of ARDS?:
    a Clara cells.
    b. Pulmonary macrophages.
    c. Pulmonary endothelial cells.
    d. Type I epithelial pneumocytes.
    e. Type II epithelial pneumocytes.

172. Rebreathing during the use of Mapleson D breathing circuit while under anesthesia can be minimized by:
    a. Increasing fresh gas flow.
    b. Decreasing fresh gas flow.
    c. A short expiratory flow.
    d. Fast respiratory rate.
    e. None of the above.

173. Barotrauma is a recognized complication of positive pressure ventilation. Which of the following ventilatory strategies is expected to be associated with the least risk of barotrauma:
    a. A tidal volume (TV) of 5 mL/kg and a PEEP of 10 cmH$_2$O.
    b. A TV of 7 mL/kg and a PEEP of 15 cmH$_2$O.
    c. A plateau pressure less than 35 cmH$_2$O with a decelerating waveform.
    d. Peak airway pressure of 50 cmH$_2$O with a square waveform inspiratory flow.
    e. A TV of 10 mL/kg and a mean inspiratory flow of 60 L/minute.

174. Regional lung overdistention at end-inspiration rarely occurs during mechanical ventilation in which of the following settings:
    a. Diffuse idiopathic pulmonary fibrosis.
    b. ARDS.
    c. Acute exacerbation of chronic obstructive pulmonary disease (COPD).
    d. Auto-PEEP of 15 cmH$_2$O without bronchospasm (emphysema).
    e. Acute bronchospasm with hyperinflation.

175. When a patient is receiving conventional positive pressure ventilation at a specific fixed TV, which of the following fixed end points will result as conditions change?
    a. A uniform expansion of all lung units based on the plateau pressure.
    b. A constant plateau pressure in spite of changing respiratory rate.
    c. A constant end-inspiratory lung volume in spite of varying airway resistance.
    d. A constant increase in intrathoracic pressure in spite of changes in lung compliance.
    e. None of the above.

176. A 1-year-old boy with ARDS is on pressure-limited ventilation with an inspiratory time of 1 second, SIMV of 20 bpm, PIP of 30 cmH$_2$O, and PEEP of 8 cmH$_2$O. The chest radiograph has shown signifi-cant improvement over the past 24 hours, and the FiO$_2$ has been weaned from 0.7 to 0.45. Failure to decrease the inspiratory time may result in all of the following except:
    a. Decreased venous return.
    b. Decreased physiological dead space.
    c. Auto-PEEP.
    d. Pneumomediastinum.

177. Nitric oxide is synthesized from which of the following?
    a. Arginine.
    b. Glutamic acid.
    c. Leucine.
    d. Isoleucine.
    e. Linoleic acid.

178. A 1-day-old infant underwent insertion of an aorticopulmonary shunt measuring 5 mm in diameter for an underlying cyanotic congenital heart disease. He has been admitted to the ICU for postoperative care and is on conventional positive pressure ventilation. A large left-to-right shunt is noted while he is on the ventilator. Which of the following is most likely to reduce the left-to-right shunt blood flow?
    a. Hydralazine.
    b. Increasing FiO$_2$.
    c. Administration of inhaled nitric oxide.
    d. Increasing PEEP on the ventilator.
    e. Increasing arterial pH.

179. A 9-month-old infant who was on mechanical ventilation for pneumonia and respiratory failure was extubated. Which of the following is the earliest evidence of inspiratory muscle fatigue after discontinuation of mechanical ventilation?
    a. Alternation of abdominal and thoracic breathing every few breaths.
    b. Primary thoracic inspiratory efforts when supine.
    c. An increase in respiratory rate.
    d. An increase in arterial CO$_2$.
    e. Abdomen moving inward during inspiration.

180. What is the toxic byproduct of the combination of nitric oxide with oxygen?
    a. Nitric oxide.
    b. Nitric dioxide.
    c. Nitrous oxide.
    d. Hb.
    e. All of the above.

181. A HeliOx has been shown to be of benefit in which of the following clinical situations?
    a. Croup.
    b. COPD.
    c. Asthma.
    d. Fixed upper airway narrowing.
    e. All of the above.

182. Marked hypertrophy of smooth muscles in the bronchial arteries and bronchial tree is present in a lung biopsy specimen from a 19-month-old infant. Which of the following is the most likely underlying lung disease in this patient?
    a. Primary pulmonary hypertension.
    b. Chronic asthma.
    c. BPD.
    d. Dysmotile cilia syndrome.
    e. Tracheobronchomegaly.

183. Respiratory failure characterized by hypercapnia, but a normal P_AO_2–P_aO_2 difference would most likely occur in which of the following conditions?
    a. Pneumonia with a lobar pattern.
    b. ARDS.
    c. Upper airway obstruction.
    d. Pulmonary edema is association with severe head injury.
    e. Severe status asthmaticus.

184. Which of the following is equivalent to intrapleural pressure at rest?
    a. Airway pressure and the surface tension of the pleura.
    b. Pressure exerted by the weight of the lung at vertical levels.
    c. Airway pressure minus alveolar pressure.
    d. The surface tension of the alveoli.
    e. The net pressure resulting from the elastic recoil of the lung and chest wall.

185. Bronchogenic cyst is most likely to occur in which of the following locations?
    a. Subpleural region.
    b. Middle mediastinum.
    c. Upper lobe.
    d. Anterior mediastinum.
    e. Lingula.

186. Which of the following is the most important factor responsible for the hysteresis of the pressure–volume curve of the normal lung in vivo?

    a. Elastin and collagen properties.
    b. The Laplace relationship.
    c. Airway compliance.
    d. Frequency dependence of compliance.
    e. Air–surface interface.

187. Which of the following results in increased mechanical efficiency of the diaphragm?
    a. Increasing the curvature of the dome of the diaphragm.
    b. Shortening of the muscle fibers.
    c. Increasing end-expiratory lung volume above the relaxed volume of the rib cage and the abdomen.
    d. Completely relaxing the abdomen.
    e. Inspiration against a resistive load.

188. Which of the following distributions of cell types in bronchoalveolar lavage fluid is more consistent with ARDS?

	Alveolar macrophages	*Lymphocytes*	*PMNs*
a.	25%	4%	70%
b.	25%	2%	4%
c.	85%	2%	12%
d.	85%	12%	2%
e.	92%	5%	2%

189. A 16-year-old adolescent female with cystic fibrosis is admitted to the pediatric ICU with hemoptysis of sufficient severity to require several blood transfusion therapies. Of the following, which procedure would be most appropriate at this time?
    a. Perfusion lung scan.
    b. Bronchial arteriography.
    c. Pulmonary arteriography.
    d. MRI of the chest.
    e. CT scan of the chest.

190. From birth until 6 years of age, functional residual capacity (FRC) increases as a function of total lung capacity because:
    a. Airway resistance increases.
    b. Chest wall compliance decreases.
    c. The t for expiratory flow increases.
    d. A child spends progressively more time in the erect posture.
    e. Laryngeal adductors become active during expiration.

191. Therapy with a helium–oxygen mixture (HeliOx) can be used in children with severe subglottic stenosis because:
    a. HeliOx is a bronchodilator.
    b. HeliOx is less dense than air.
    c. HeliOx is less viscous than air.
    d. Flow through large airways is dependent on gas viscosity.
    e. Flow through large airways is always transitional.

192. Which of the following is the most prominent histological feature of BPD?
    a. Disrupted airway branching pattern.
    b. Decreased number of alveoli.
    c. Deficient bronchial cartilage.
    d. Eosinophilic infiltration of alveolar septa.
    e. Capillary hyperplasia.

193. An infant with BPD is on oxygen. The current fraction of inspired oxygen that maintains a PaO_2 of 55 mmHg and a barometric pressure of 760 mmHg is 0.27. The infant is being transferred to another hospital via a plane flying at a high altitude, which results in a reduction in the barometric pressure to 623 mmHg. What FiO_2 will be required to maintain the same PaO_2 assuming a constant respiratory quotient of 0.8, a constant $PaCO_2$ of 40 mmHg, and a body temperature of 37°C:
    a. 0.24.   d. 0.33.
    b. 0.27.   e. 0.37.
    c. 0.30.

194. The function of surfactant associated with protein C is:
    a. To stimulate surfactant synthesis.
    b. To facilitate formation of surfactant films at air–liquid interface.
    c. To regulate surfactant release.
    d. To inhibit enzymes that inactivate surfactant.
    e. Not related to normal surfactant function.

195. Type I pulmonary pneumocytes are best described as:
    a. Cells involved in surfactant synthesis.
    b. Cells involved in neurohumoral release and synthesis.
    c. Cells involved in glycoprotein synthesis.
    d. Cells that function as stem cells for type II alveolar cells.
    e. Cells that minimize the barrier to gas exchange.

196. Forced vital capacity is useful as an index of pulmonary impairment because:
    a. It shows the least decline in the supine position.
    b. It is affected only in obstructive lung diseases.
    c. It has a high intrasubject reproducibility.
    d. It has a large standard deviation.
    e. It remains stable with increasing height.

197. Which of the following is used to calculate work of breathing?
    a. Pressure–volume curve.
    b. Flow–volume curve.
    c. Pressure–flow curve.
    d. Volume–time curve.
    e. Flow–time curve.

198. A 14-year-old male is admitted to the pediatric ICU for heroin overdose. Alveolar carbon dioxide is 85 mmHg at a barometric pressure of 760 mmHg and water vapor pressure of 47 mmHg. Upon arrival and while breathing room air, his alveolar–arterial oxygen tension difference was 10 mmHg. Assuming that the fraction of inspired oxygen of room air is 0.21 and the respiratory quotient is 0.8, the patient's arterial oxygen tension would be:
    a. 23 mmHg.
    b. 33 mmHg.
    c. 43 mmHg.
    d. 53 mmHg.
    e. 63 mmHg.

199. A medication is being administered to a patient at intervals equivalent to its half-life. How many half-lives will it take for the plasma concentration of the medication to reach 97% of the final steady-state levels?
    a. One half-life.   d. Four half-lives.
    b. Two half-lives.   e. Five half-lives.
    c. Three half-lives.

200. If the patient in Question 199 requires extracorporeal life support, what would be the effect of this modality of therapy on the half-life of the medication?
    a. Increase.
    b. Decrease.
    c. Remain the same.
    d. Volume of distribution decreases dramatically.

2 Cardiovascular System

The following chapter will focus on the cardiovascular system. Pertinent questions, answers, and rationale will be reviewed. Answers for this chapter can be found beginning on page 115.

Key Words: Heart; cardiovascular; rhythm; ventricles; atrial.

1. All of the following are true regarding the interaction between respirations and circulation except:
   a. The Mueller maneuver decreases afterload.
   b. The hemodynamic effects of changing intrathoracic pressure dominates over changing intrathoracic volume.
   c. Hypoxic pulmonary vasoconstriction is noted when alveolar oxygen pressure (PaO_2) drops to less than 60 torr.
   d. The single most important cardiopulmonary interaction is the effect that ventilator induced changes in intrathoracic pressure have on right ventricular preload.
   e. Venous return parallels transmural pressure of the right atrium.

2. Ventricular afterload is best approximated by which of the following?
   a. Ventricular end-diastolic pressure.
   b. Ventricular end-diastolic volume.
   c. Systolic blood pressure.
   d. Mean blood pressure.
   e. Ventricular wall stress.

3. The mechanism operative in ventricular interdependence is:
   a. Right-to-left shift of the interventricular septum.
   b. Constraint of left ventricular expansion by stretch of common ventricular myofibrils.
   c. Restriction of left ventricular filling by the stretched pericardium.
   d. All of the above.

4. Which of the following statements is true pertaining to cardiopulmonary interaction?
   a. The cardiopulmonary interaction is of greatest clinical importance for the failing left ventricle.
   b. In the failing heart, the effect of changes in intrathoracic pressure on preload will dominate over the effects on afterload.
   c. In young infants with less compliant ventricles with a limited contractile reserve, positive pressure ventilation with increased intrathoracic pressure may be detrimental.
   d. Afterload is best approximated by left ventricle preload.

5. All of the following statements are true regarding the fetal circulation except:
   a. The foramen ovale allows equalization of preload of the right and left ventricles.
   b. The right ventricle ejects more highly oxygenated blood than the left ventricle, because it receives the umbilical vein blood.
   c. The right and left ventricular pressures are nearly equal *in utero*.
   d. The right ventricle ejects more blood than the left ventricle owing to the difference in afterload.

From: *Pediatric Critical Care Review*
Edited by: R. A. Hasan and M. D. Pappas © Humana Press Inc., Totowa, NJ

6. Which of the following is true regarding the fetal and newborn myocardium?
   a. A low contractile element concentration is present in the newborn myocardium.
   b. Because fetal heart functions at the peak of the ventricular function curve, combined ventricular output is maximum at a resting atrial pressure of 3–5 mmHg.
   c. Compared with the adult, the newborn heart has higher indices of myocardial performance at rest, but is unable to significantly improve ventricular performance.
   d. Small increases in afterload decrease cardiac output more significantly in the fetus and the infant compared with the adult, and nitroglycerin increases cardiac output more in the adult compared with the infant.
   e. All of the above.

7. Hemodynamic changes at birth include:
   a. Right ventricular afterload decreases, and left ventricular afterload decreases.
   b. Right ventricular afterload decreases, and left ventricular afterload increases.
   c. Both right ventricular and left ventricular afterload increase.
   d. Right ventricular afterload increases, and left ventricular afterload decreases.
   e. None of the above.

8. Which of the following contributes the most to the total peripheral resistance?
   a. Aorta and large arteries.
   b. Small arteries.
   c. Arterioles.
   d. Capillaries.

9. The major portion of cardiac O_2 consumption is used to support which of the following?
   a. Myocardial wall tension.
   b. The product of stroke volume and mean arterial pressure.
   c. Electrical activation of the myocardium.
   d. None of the above.

10. Which of the following situations is considered to be least efficient with regard to myocardial O_2 consumption and myocardial wall tension?
    a. Poor myocardial compliance.
    b. A heart with left ventricular hypertrophy.
    c. A dilated heart with a small preload.
    d. A dilated heart with a large preload and a thin left ventricular wall.

11. Ischemia of the myocardium with associated symptoms and signs is rarely seen with aortic regurgitation, but is commonly seen with aortic stenosis. Which of the following underlying pathophysiological phenomena related to these clinical entities is true?
    a. Maintaining blood pressure by increasing stroke volume rather than vasoconstriction is more O_2 efficient.
    b. The O_2 cost of isometric contraction (pressure work) is much greater than isotonic contraction (volume work).
    c. Increasing cardiac output by afterload reduction, which increases stroke volume, but decreases pressure, greatly improves the efficiency of the heart.
    d. All of the above statements are true.

12. Regarding the figure below, match the following statement(s) with their correct answer below:

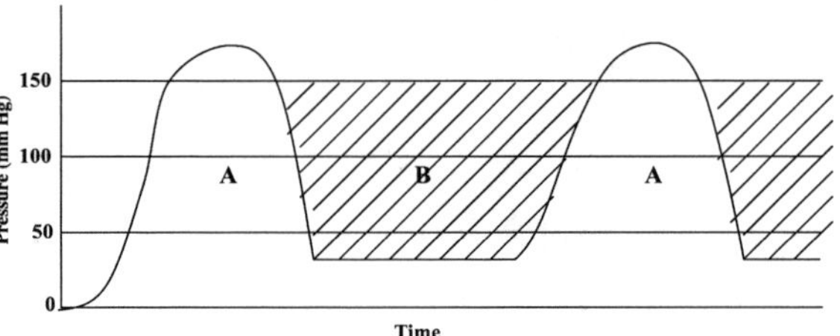

    a. Area A.
    b. Area B.
    c. Both.
    d. Neither.
    _____ Represent(s) myocardial O_2 supply.

13. Ischemic heart disease (IHD) should be sought as a diagnosis in neonates who are critically ill. Risk factors for IHD in neonates include:
    a. Increased intracavity pressure.
    b. Variable aortic pressure.
    c. Ductal run-off.
    d. Global hypoxia and episodes of arterial desaturation.
    e. All of the above.

14. Which of the following statements is true regarding IHD in critically ill neonates?
    a. IHD is almost unheard of.
    b. IHD is treated with O_2, positive pressure ventilation, and inotropes.
    c. Symptoms resolve in 48 hours with supportive care, whereas the electrocardiogram and radiographic changes resolve in 2 weeks.

d. The clinical picture is that of hypoxemia, cardiomegaly, cardiogenic shock, and tricuspid insufficiency.
e. All except A are true.

15. Clinical situations in which myocardial ischemia and infarction are recognized in children with congenital heart disease include:
a. Right ventricular infarction in total anomalous pulmonary venous drainage.
b. Left ventricular infarction in aortic stenosis.
c. Biventricular infarction in transposition of the great arteries.
d. All of the above.
e. None of the above.

16. Which of the following is a true statement concerning anomalous left coronary artery?
a. By 4 months of age, the majority of infants will have developed a coronary fistula.
b. Without treatment, 80% of infants will survive to adulthood.
c. There is frequently a history of cyanosis at birth.
d. The clinical condition may mimic gastroschisis.
e. All of the above.

17. The leading cause of IHD in children is:
a. Kawasaki syndrome.
b. Left anomalous coronary artery.
c. Severe aortic stenosis.
d. Atherosclerotic disease.
e. None of the above.

18. Coronary artery involvement and cardiac abnormalities are more common in children with Kawasaki syndrome who exhibit which of the following characteristics?
a. Are female older than 8 years of age.
b. Have associated torus fracture.
c. Have had a fever less than 2 days.
d. Have an erythrocyte sedimentation rate of less than 20 mm/hour.
e. None of the above.

19. A 13-year-old male victim of a motor vehicle accident with multiple trauma and closed head injury is in the pediatric intensive care unit (PICU) with elevated intracranial pressure. Poor peripheral perfusion and low urine output is noted with a central venous pressure of 18 mmHg. True statements pertaining to this patient include:
a. Impaired left and right ventricular function has been reported in patients with closed head injury.

b. Head injury causes an enhanced autonomic response with direct sympathetic cardiac stimulation and an enhanced level of circulating catecholamines.
c. ST-T changes on the electrocardiogram are seen in head injury patients.
d. Myocardial injury is seen frequently in the setting of thoracic trauma.
e. All of the above.

20. During high permeability pulmonary edema:
a. The ratio of extravascular lung water to dry lung weight is decreased.
b. The blood-free dry weight of the lung is increased.
c. The dry weight of the lung is decreased.
d. None of the above is true.

21. Which of the following statements pertaining to this equation is true?

$$Q = K_f (Pc\text{-}Pi) - \sigma (\Pi_c - \Pi_i)$$

a. K_f is the reflection coefficient.
b. σ is the filtration coefficient.
c. When $\sigma = 1$, there is no restriction to passage of protein across the capillary membrane.
d. When $\sigma = 0$ there is absolute restriction to the passage of protein across the capillary membrane.
e. None of the above.

22. Of the various causes of heart failure that produce pulmonary edema not related to congenital heart disease, anthracycline cardiotoxicity is an important type. A factor that potentiates the incidence of heart failure because of anthracycline is:
a. Administration of bleomycin.
b. Administration of cyclophosphamide.
c. Mediastinal radiotherapy.
d. All of the above.
e. None of the above.

23. A 13-year-old boy with a previous history of acute lymphoblastic leukemia treated with chemotherapy including doxorubicin presents to the PICU in florid pulmonary edema. The chest radiograph shows an enlarged heart with evidence of alveolar edema. All of the following statements are true of this clinical scenario except:
a. Symptoms of congestive cardiac failure caused by doxorubicin toxicity may appear years after the last dose of doxorubicin.

b. The mortality rate for this patient is at least 50–60%.
c. Cardiotoxicity as a result of doxorubicin is dose independent.
d. Cardiac enzyme assay and serial chest radiographs have not been useful in the prediction of cardiomyopathy.
e. Because anthracyclin cardiomyopathy may be reversible in children, intensive cardiac support with tracheal intubation and positive pressure ventilation may be warranted to treat an acute episode of pulmonary edema.

24. Which of the following is not a cause of high permeability pulmonary edema?
a. Salicylate intoxication.
b. Prolonged exposure to high fraction of inspired oxygen (FiO_2).
c. Anaphylaxis associated with pulmonary edema.
d. A combination of doxorubicin and cyclophosphamide.
e. Heroin overdose.

25. Which of the following organ systems is most frequently affected by heroin overdose?
a. Kidney.
b. Heart.
c. Brain.
d. Lung.
e. Skeletal muscle.

26. Which of the following statements describing pulmonary vascular tree physiology is true?
a. Normal matching of ventilation to perfusion is achieved by local hypoxic pulmonary vasoconstriction.
b. Hypoxic pulmonary vasoconstriction is usually localized and reversible.
c. In neonates, hypoxic pulmonary vasoconstriction may persist even after the hypoxia has been corrected.
d. Potential anatomic shunts that are present inside the lungs can open up and may account for the cyanosis noted during conditions of elevated pulmonary pressure.
e. All of the above.

27. Which of the following physiological changes in response to hypoxia is not likely?
a. Impairment of short term memory occurs at approximately PaO_2 of 60 torr.
b. When the PaO_2 falls to less than 60 torr, carotid and aortic bodies are activated leading to tachycardia and hyperventilation.
c. Levels of 2,3 diphosphoglycerate increase in 20 minutes.
d. Tubular reabsorption of Na^+ is impaired at a low PaO_2.
e. PaO_2 of less than 40 torr produces twitching and seizures.

28. A two and a half-month-old baby with Tetralogy of Fallot is brought to the emergency department and subsequently to the PICU for progressively turning blue soon after waking when his mother began to feed him. He became fussy, began to cry, and since then, has been getting progressively more cyanotic and limp. All of the following are true statements except:
a. The onset of these symptoms in early morning and with feeding is characteristic.
b. The peak incidence is seen at this age.
c. There is a strong negative correlation between PaO_2 and the incidence of attacks.
d. Squatting or knee–chest position redistributes systemic blood flow to the upper body to improve pulmonary blood flow, but does not affect arterial oxygen saturation.
e. Propranolol can abort the attack and may decrease the frequency of these episodes when used chronically.

29. Cyanosis at a normal PaO_2 occurs in:
a. A victim of smoke inhalation.
b. A child overdosed on shoe dye.
c. A patient with a hematocrit of 75%.
d. All of the above.

30. In the postoperative period, a right-to-left shunt helps preserve cardiac output and decreases postoperative complications in children with which of the following conditions?
a. Repair of Tetralogy of Fallot.
b. Repair of truncus arteriosis.
c. Fenestrated modified Fontan procedure.
d. All of the above.
e. None of the above.

31. A 6-month-old child with Down's syndrome who underwent repair of an atrioventricular canal defect was admitted to the PICU 6 hours ago. High pulmonary artery pressure is noted along with a decreased O_2 saturation to the 80s and evidence of low cardiac output. The first priority after stabilization of the patient is:
a. Adjust the vent settings.
b. Increase FiO_2.

c. Obtain a chest radiograph.
d. Obtain an echocardiogram to rule out any residual abnormality.
e. None of the above.

32. All of the following statements are true regarding pulmonary circulation in this patient except:
    a. O_2 is a very strong pulmonary vasodilator after cardiopulmonary bypass.
    b. The effect of hyperventilation on pulmonary vascular resistance is mediated by changes in pH rather than PCO_2.
    c. Pulmonary vascular resistance increases with increasing postoperative hematocrit.
    d. Pulmonary vascular resistance increases in the postoperative night as pulmonary artery pressure is maintained or increases, thus cardiac output decreases.
    e. Pulmonary vascular endothelial dysfunction after cardiopulmonary bypass is common.

33. A 5-day-old who presented with rapid onset of shock a few hours ago is found to have hypoplastic left heart syndrome and is on a prostaglandin-E_2 infusion. The patient is being mechanically ventilated. You notice that the O_2 saturation on pulse oximetry is 92%. You anticipate all of the following except:
    a. Pulmonary congestion.
    b. Right ventricle may suffer from diastolic overload.
    c. Use of hyperventilation and tolazoline will improve saturation and the patient's overall condition.
    d. Pulmonary blood flow is increased.

34. All of the following are true regarding chylothorax except:
    a. Malnutrition is a recognized complication.
    b. Most frequently seen with intrapericardial procedures.
    c. May occur without damage to the thoracic duct.
    d. Pleural fluid may appear serosanguinous and will not clot.
    e. Pleural effusion may develop as late as 1 month after surgery.

35. Regarding treatment of chylothorax:
    a. Pleural drainage is required to improve ventilation and prevent atelectasis.
    b. To decrease lymph flow, a high-carbohydrate, high-protein, medium-chain triglyceride diet with reduced fat is recommended.

c. Malnutrition is an important complication.
d. All of the above.

36. Which of the following is an indication for surgical ligation of the thoracic duct for chylothorax?
    a. Average daily chyle loss of greater than 100 mL/year of the patient's age, after 5 days of medical therapy.
    b. A flow of chyle that does not diminish after 2 weeks.
    c. Nutritional complications that are severe.
    d. All of the above.

37. Match the selections listed below with their appropriate descriptions.

> a. The modified Fontan procedure.
> b. Stage I Norwood procedure.
> c. Both.
> d. Neither.

_____ Increased pulmonary vascular resistance results in hypoxemia.

_____ Increased pulmonary vascular resistance results in cardiogenic shock.

_____ Improve(s) systemic oxygenation and reduces the obligatory diastolic overload.

38. Which of the following statements is not true regarding fenestrated Fontan procedure?
    a. Maintains the systemic perfusion when pulmonary vascular resistance is elevated.
    b. Decreases the incidence of pleural effusion.
    c. Increases the mortality rate in patients undergoing the procedure.
    d. Can be closed in the cardiac catheterization laboratory later during hospitalization.

39. When an infant with transposition of the great arteries and an intact ventricular septum presents for repair at 3 months of age, the best approach is:
    a. Senning procedure.
    b. Mustard procedure.
    c. Immediate correction by arterial switch.
    d. Pulmonary artery banding and a Blalock-Taussig shunt.
    e. None of the above.

40. The two issues of paramount importance after arterial switch are:
    a. Mustard vs Senning's procedures.
    b. Presence of atrial septal defect and patent ductus arteriosus.

    c. Global performance of left ventricle and focal myocardial ischemia.
    e. None of the above.

41. Chylothorax is least likely to occur with repair of:
    a. Aortic or pulmonary valve surgery or ventricular septal defect.
    b. Patent ductus arteriosus ligation.
    c. Repair of coarctation.
    d. Glenn anastomosis.
    e. Shunt procedure (Blalock-Taussig, Waterston, Pott).

42. Postoperatively, patients with transposition of the great arteries undergoing arterial switch are characterized by all of the following except:
    a. Unrecognized left-to-right shunts or overzealous volume administration that can precipitate sudden hemodynamic compromise.
    b. Focal ischemia is a recognized complication.
    c. Compromised cardiac output responds favorably to afterload reduction.
    d. Global left ventricular systolic dysfunction is not seen.
    e. The left ventricle is typically dilated and tolerates any further load poorly.

43. Following a Blalock-Taussig shunt, true statements include all of the following except:
    a. The ipsilateral arm may be cold and pulseless for 48–72 hours.
    b. Blalock-Taussig shunt is generally performed on the side opposite the aortic arch.
    c. Ipsilateral pulmonary edema is a recognized complication.
    d. Flow is determined by the size of the subclavian artery; size of the graft itself is not critical.
    e. Diuretics should be avoided if possible.

44. Which of the following statements is inaccurate regarding cardiac transplantation?
    a. A major cause of early postoperative failure is right ventricular failure from increased pulmonary vascular resistance.
    b. Matching is based on ABO compatibility.
    c. Systemic hypertension is frequently seen postoperatively caused by cyclosporin-A.
    d. Endomyocardial biopsy is the best way to diagnose rejection when done weekly postoperatively.
    e. Ketamine will enhance myocardial function.

45. A 5-month-old underwent repair of Tetralogy of Fallot through a ventriculotomy with a transannular patch. Central venous pressure is 10 mmHg. Poor perfusion of the extremities is noted with low urine output. A bolus of colloid 15 mL/kg is given over 20 minutes. It is noted that the central venous pressure has decreased to 7 mmHg. This suggests that:
    a. Ventricular compliance has improved.
    b. Afterload has decreased following volume expansion.
    c. Myocardial perfusion has improved.
    d. This clinical scenario is not possible.
    e. A, B, and C.

46. A 12-year-old is admitted to the PICU with septic shock. A pulmonary artery catheter is inserted for hemodynamic monitoring. Left ventricular stroke work index was 30 g/minute/m^2 4 hours ago. Now left ventricular stroke work index is 55 g/minute/m^2. This indicates that:
    a. Afterload has increased.
    b. Afterload has decreased.
    c. Contractility has improved.
    d. None of the above.

47. The compensatory state of shock is least likely with:
    a. Cardiogenic shock.
    b. Septic shock.
    c. Hypovolemic shock.
    d. Obstructive shock.

48. Match the selections listed below with their appropriate descriptions.

a. An adolescent with extensive orthopedic injury receiving positive mechanical ventilation.
b. An infant with critical aortic stenosis receiving positive pressure ventilation.
c. Both.
d. Neither.

_____ With inspiration, there is a decrease in pulse pressure without a phase lag and diastolic pressure falls.

_____ With inspiration, there is an increase in pulse pressure without a phase lag and diastolic pressure increases.

49. A mechanism responsible for pulmonary edema associated with upper airway obstruction does not include which of the following?
    a. Increased right ventricular afterload.
    b. Ventricular interdependence.
    c. Increased left ventricular afterload.
    d. Decreased left ventricular afterload.

50. An infant with congestive cardiac failure is admitted to the PICU. Intermittent "grunting" is noted. All of the following are true statements regarding this clinical scenario except:
    a. Grunting is a form of the Valsalva maneuver.
    b. Grunting decreases left ventricular afterload.
    c. Grunting is a form of the Mueller maneuver.
    d. A decrease in left ventricular preload may shift the Starling curve to a more favorable position, thus decreasing myocardial O_2 consumption.
    e. This patient is likely to benefit from inotropic drugs.

51. Nitroprusside would be least effective for:
    a. Congestive heart failure as a result of cardiomyopathy.
    b. Mitral regurgitation.
    c. Ventricular septal defect with congestive cardiac failure because of significant left-to-right shunt.
    d. Myocardial dysfunction following cardiopulmonary bypass.
    e. Hypotensive anesthesia.

52. Which of the following statements is least accurate regarding the toxicity of nitroprusside?
    a. Neuroexcitatory symptoms of delirium, confusion, and convulsions are a result of thiocyanate accumulation.
    b. Thiocyanate tends to accumulate in patients with renal dysfunction.
    c. Thiocyanate is not removed by either hemo or peritoneal dialysis.
    d. Measurement of thiocyanate concentration does not have relevance to detecting cyanide toxicity.
    e. Methemoglobin levels should be determined during prolonged infusion of nitroprusside.

53. Match the selections listed below with their appropriate descriptions.

a. Nitroprusside.	c. Both.
b. Nitroglycerin.	d. Neither.

_____ The preferred drug when treating a child with congestive cardiac failure, pulmonary edema, and marginal blood pressure.

_____ The preferred drug for the treatment of congestive cardiac failure induced by mitral or aortic regurgitation.

_____ The preferred drug for congestive cardiac failure with preserved blood pressure, because it produces a greater increase in cardiac output in this setting.

54. Which of the following is true regarding volume resuscitation in shock state?
    a. Isotonic solutions may be administered safely up to an amount equivalent to 200% of the patient's circulating blood volume.
    b. Hetastarch and Dextran administration should not exceed 200 mL/kg/dose because of concerns about hemostasis.
    c. Rapid fluid resuscitation in excess of 40 mL/kg in the first hour of evaluation is associated with improved survival and no increased risk of pulmonary edema in patients with septic shock.
    d. Plasma catecholamines increase only marginally in shock states.
    e. None of the above.

55. In the United States, trauma is the leading cause of death in children older than 1 year. The major contributor to mortality is:
    a. Hypovolemic shock.   d. Head injury.
    b. Cardiogenic shock.   e. Infection.
    c. Septic shock.

56. In the PICU, the major cause of cardiogenic shock is:
    a. Myocarditis.
    b. Kawasaki syndrome.
    c. Anomalous left coronary artery.
    d. Postoperative repair of congenital cardiac lesions.
    e. Isoproterenol treated asthmatics.

57. Impaired cellular metabolism occurs earliest during the clinical course of which type of shock?
    a. Cardiogenic shock.
    b. Septic shock.
    c. Hypovolemic shock.
    d. Obstructive shock.
    e. Anaphylactic shock.

58. In a child who presents with a temperature of 42°C, poor peripheral circulatory status, altered mental status, and acidosis:
    a. Heat shock protein is released in excessive amounts.
    b. Anhydrosis results from cellular sweat gland damage.
    c. Disseminated intravascular coagulation is a recognized complication.
    d. Riley-Day syndrome is a possibility.
    e. All of the above.

59. A 14-year-old who sustained a fractured femur suddenly develops chest pain and dyspnea. Pathophysiological changes likely leading to this clinical picture include:
    a. Sudden right ventricular failure leading to shock.
    b. Pulmonary vasoconstriction and pulmonary capillary endothelial damage.
    c. Massive release of vasoactive mediators from pulmonary circulation leading to circulatory failure.
    d. All of the above.

60. Useful diagnostic work-ups include:
    a. Microscopic urinalysis.
    b. Ventilation–perfusion scan.
    c. Pulmonary angiography.
    d. All of the above.

61. Therapy for the patient referenced in Question 60 would include all except:
    a. Optimizing hemodynamics.
    b. Optimizing oxygenation.
    c. Prevention of further episodes.
    d. Removal of emboli.

62. Air embolism with fatal cerebral complications occurs with:
    a. Laceration of a large vessel following trauma.
    b. Spinal surgery.
    c. Cranial surgery.
    A. All of the above.

Questions 63–65: A 12-year-old child who has had renal transplantation presents with sudden onset of acute, severe abdominal pain with prostration. He has been receiving azathioprine and prednisone for the last 4 months. He is hypotensive, poorly perfused, and pale with marked abdominal rigidity. No hematemesis or melena are noted. Urinalysis is unremarkable. Amylase and lipase are 850 and 500 IU/dL, respectively.

63. The most likely diagnosis is:
    a. Pyelonephritis.
    b. Chronic rejection.
    c. Pancreatic shock.
    d. Perforated duodenal ulcer preceded by hemorrhage.
    e. None of the above.

64. Anticipated complications in this patient include:
    a. Hypercalcemia.
    b. Hyperuricemia.
    c. Acute respiratory distress syndrome.
    d. Hypervolemia.
    e. Appendicitis.

65. Appropriate interventions in the patient would include which of the following?
    a. Volume restriction.
    b. Appropriate management of hypercalcemia.
    c. Surgical exploration.
    d. Appropriate management of respiratory dysfunction.

66. When managing children at risk of developing shock states, all of the following are true except:
    a. Urine output in children is normally 2–3 mL/kg/hour.
    b. It is usual for oliguria to occur before the alterations in blood pressure or the development of significant tachycardia.
    c. Central filling pressure always reflects intravascular volume accurately.
    d. Intravascular volume expansion by as much as 30% may not significantly alter right atrial pressure .
    e. The major determinants of cardiac filling pressure are ventricular function and compliance.

67. A 3-year-old with a 2-day history of frequent episodes of diarrhea is admitted to the PICU with a diagnosis of hypovolemic shock. There is no evidence of systemic infection and chest radiograph shows a normal size heart and normal lung fields. Which of the following statements regarding management of this patient is least accurate?
    a. It is unlikely that monitoring of central venous pressure adds significantly to careful, repeated physical exams and monitoring of urine output.
    b. Every attempt should be made to elevate the central venous pressure to greater than 14 mmHg.
    c. The concept that central filling pressure always reflects intravascular volume accurately is misleading.

d. If this patient develops oliguria or anuria, central venous pressure monitoring becomes essential to avoid fluid overload.

68. Regarding metabolic acidosis in the shock state, all of the following are true except:
    a. Base deficits greater than 10 mEq/L in cardiogenic and septic shock are associated with a worse outcome than a similar situation in hypovolemic shock.
    b. Hepatic conversion of lactate or acetate to correct acidosis is impaired in most shock states.
    c. Severe metabolic acidosis associated with organic acidemia can be treated with peritoneal dialysis.
    d. With correction of acidosis, serious hypercalcemia and hyperkalemia may occur.

69. Which of the following is true of hemodynamic management of shock states?
    a. When volume resuscitation greater than 50–70 mL/kg is administered in the first 4–6 hours, invasive monitoring should be considered.
    b. In patients with acute respiratory distress syndrome, central filling pressures should be maintained at a lower level (≤10 mmHg).
    c. In patients with increased intracranial pressure, inotropic support may be warranted before preload is fully augmented.
    d. Application of pneumatic antishock garments in the field does not alter survival.
    e. All of the above.

70. The functional reserve of the cardiovascular system in the infant is limited owing to:
    a. Abundance of contractile elements in the neonatal myocardium.
    b. Sarcoplasmic reticulum is more abundant.
    c. Less compliant myocardium leading to increased myocardial wall stress.
    d. Pulmonary vascular bed is minimally recruited under basal conditions.

71. The Bezold-Jarisch Reflex refers to:
    a. Under basal conditions, sympathetic tone to the heart is relatively low, whereas parasympathetic tone is dominant.
    b. Stretching of the carotid sinus triggers a parasympathetic-efferent activity resulting in bradycardia and vasodilation.
    c. Hypovolemia with a decreased stretching of aortic arch baroreceptors causes a sympathetic output with tachycardia and vasoconstriction.

d. Activation of cardiopulmonary baroreceptors localized in the atrial and ventricular wall result in vagal stimulation with bradycardia and vasodilation.
    e. None of the above.

72. Risk factors for infection following radial artery cannulation include:
    a. Insertion by surgical cut down.
    b. Inflammation at the insertion site.
    c. Cannulation for more than 4 days.
    d. All of the above.

73. The most serious complication of axillary artery cannulation is:
    a. Thrombosis.
    b. Distal ischemia.
    c. Embolism.
    d. Brachial plexus injury.
    e. Infection.

74. Precautions to be taken during pulmonary artery catheter insertion include all of the following except:
    a. When withdrawing the catheter, always deflate the balloon by disconnecting the syringe and opening the valve to the atmosphere.
    b. Dysrhythmias occur most commonly during insertion into the right atrium, probably because of irritation of the arterioventricular mode.
    c. The catheter should not be advanced more than 10 cm without seeing a change in waveform after entering the right atrium.
    d. Balloon rupture is more commonly seen in pediatric patients.
    e. Risk of infection is reduced if the catheter is left in place for less than 3 days.

75. The figure below shows various curves that represent cardiac output as measured by the thermodilution technique. Which of the following statements is most accurate?

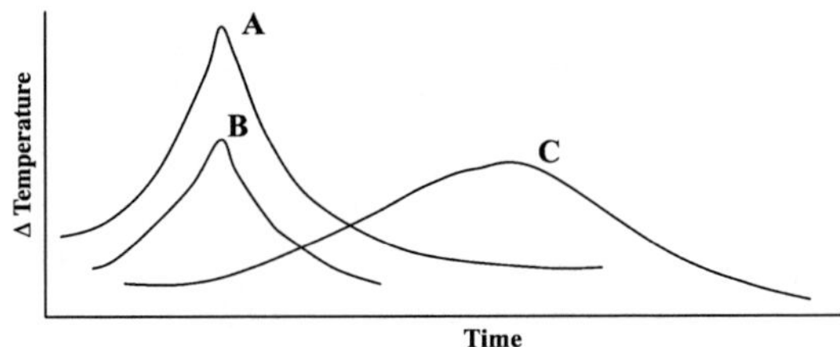

a. Curve "A" represents a patient with a ventricular septal defect.
    b. Curve "C" is likely to give a falsely high cardiac output.

   c. Cardiac output obtained by Curve "B" will be higher than Curve "A".

   d. Curve "A" will correspond to a higher cardiac output than Curve "B".

   e. All of the above.

Questions 76–79: Please reference the figure below. Loop A–B–C–D is the normal pressure volume loop of the cardiac cycle.

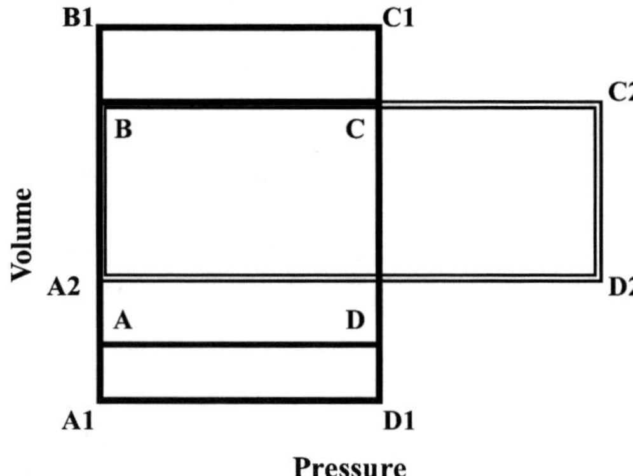

76. In the normal loop (A–B–C–D), the point at which the aortic valve opens is:

   a. Point B.

   b. Point C.

   c. Point A.

   d. Point E.

   e. Point D.

77. An intervention is performed which results in loop $A–B_1–C_1–D$. The most likely explanation for this change is:

   a. A bolus of intravenous fluid.

   b. An increase in afterload.

   c. An increase in contractility.

   d. All of the above.

78. Provided there is no change in pressure, loop $A_1–B–C–D_1$ is most likely a result of:

   a. Increased preload.

   b. Increased contractility.

   c. Decreased contractility.

   d. None of the above.

79. Provided the contractility is unchanged, loop $A_2–B–C_2–D_2$ is most likely a result of:

   a. Increased end-diastolic pressure.

   b. Increased afterload.

   c. Increased contractility.

   d. Decreased afterload.

   e. None of the above.

3   Central Nervous System

The following chapter will focus on the central nervous system. Pertinent questions, answers, and rationale will be reviewed. Answers for this chapter can be found beginning on page 119.

Key Words: Brain; trauma; parenchyma; hydrocephalus; hemorrhage.

---

1. Central hypoventilation syndrome is characterized by dysfunction of the respiratory center responsible for autonomic control of breathing. True statements pertaining to this syndrome include all of the following except:
   a. Apnea typically occurs during rapid eye movement sleep.
   b. Central hypoventilation syndrome usually presents with cyanosis at birth that requires positive pressure ventilation.
   c. Diminished school performance, hypersomnolence, or morning headache may be the clinical presentation.
   d. Cor pulmonale is a recognized complication.
   d. Acquired causes are well recognized.

2. Acquired central hypoventilation syndrome may be a result of:
   a. Posterior fossa tumors.
   b. Brain stem encephalitis.
   c. Severe asphyxia following near-drowning.
   d. Medullary infarction.
   e. All of the above.

3. Central hypoventilation syndrome is seen in which of the following conditions?
   a. Neoplasms of the cerebellum.
   b. Encephalitis.
   c. Idiopathic hypothalamic syndrome.
   d. Pyruvate dehydrogenase deficiency.
   e. All of the above.

4. Match the selections listed below with their appropriate descriptions.

   > a. Achondroplasia.
   > b. Arnold-Chiari malformation.
   > c. Both.
   > d. Neither.

   ____ When apnea is seen, it is usually mixed apnea.
   ____ Typically causes central apnea.

5. The case illustrated in Question 4 (*see* figure below) is most compatible with:

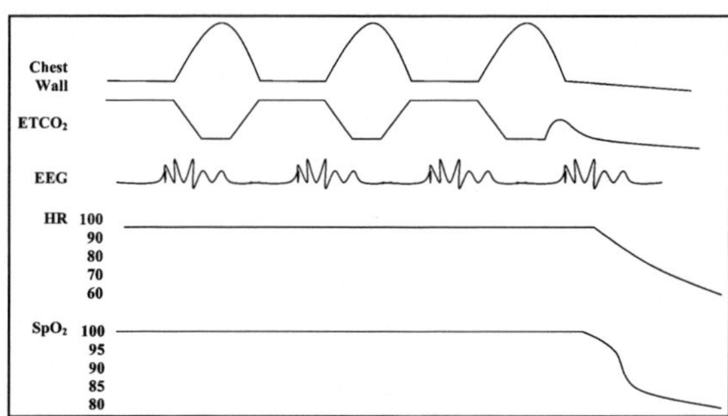

   a. Obstructive apnea.
   b. Central hypoventilation syndrome with central apnea.
   c. Mixed apnea.
   d. None of the above.

From: *Pediatric Critical Care Review*
Edited by: R. A. Hasan and M. D. Pappas © Humana Press Inc., Totowa, NJ

6. Fortunately, spinal cord injuries are uncommon in children. True statements pertaining to this disorder include all of the following except:
   a. Lower thoracic and lumbar spine injuries do not produce any abnormalities in respiratory function because of the preservation of diaphragm and intercostal muscles.
   b. Ventilation/perfusion mismatch is a recognized phenomenon with C3–C5 injury.
   c. Hypoventilation is a recognized phenomenon in infants with lesions below C5.
   d. High cervical spine lesions (C1–C2) result in apnea and early death.
   d. Pulmonary edema is a recognized associated complication.

7. Traumatic spinal cord injury should be suspected in a child with:
   a. Hypotension.
   b. Flaccidity.
   c. Hypoventilation.
   d. Coma.
   e. All of the above.

8. A 5-year-old involved in a motor vehicle accident is intubated for hypoventilation. His increased intracranial pressure is controlled with moderate hyperventilation and intravenous mannitol. No seizure activity has been noted. The most appropriate neurodiagnostic test for evaluation of possible spinal cord injury is:
   a. Magnetic resonance imaging (MRI).
   b. Portable cervical spine radiographs.
   c. Somatosensory evoked potential.
   d. Auditory evoked potential.
   e. None of the above.

9. Following spinal cord injury in children, important facts to remember when caring for the patient include all of the following except:
   a. Radiographic bony abnormality is evident in the vast majority of cases.
   b. Gastric and intestinal motility are depressed.
   c. Suctioning of the trachea may induce bradycardia owing to an exaggerated vagal response.
   d. Upper airway occlusion may occur because of asynchronous stimulation of the diaphragm and upper airway.
   e. Pulmonary edema may occur.

10. Mortality from tetanus is most commonly secondary to abnormalities in the:
    a. Respiratory system.
    b. Cardiovascular system.
    c. Neurological system.
    d. Immunological system.

11. Tetanus can develop following entry of the organism into the body in which of the following conditions?
    a. Otitis media.
    b. Intravenous drug abuse.
    c. Contaminated umbilical cord.
    d. Septic abortion.
    e. All of the above.

12. Which of the following characteristics of tetanus is least likely in a newborn?
    a. Clinical presentation usually occurs at the end of the first week.
    b. Poor feeding is an early sign of the disease.
    c. Reflex spasm and rigidity.
    d. Generalized seizures.
    e. Extremely painful muscle spasms are provoked by stimulation.

13. Which of the following is true regarding clinical and laboratory features of tetanus?
    a. Wound cultures reliably and consistently yield the causative organism.
    b. Cerebrospinal fluid (CSF) abnormalities are fairly typical.
    c. Leukocytosis is a consistent finding.
    d. Absence of a portal of entry is rarely seen.
    e. None of the above.

14. In a patient with tetanus, "respiratory convulsions" can be described by which of the following conditions?
    a. Respiratory convulsions often arise unexpectedly.
    b. Respiratory convulsions may lead to severe hypoxia.
    c. Treatment involves rapid administration of a fast-acting muscle relaxant followed by endotracheal intubation.
    d. Continued muscle relaxation following intubation is advised.
    e. All of the above.

15. Characteristics of neonatal tetany include:
    a. A high predisposition to aspiration pneumonia.
    b. Prolonged nasotracheal intubation compares favorably to tracheostomy.
    c. Infants are particularly prone to laryngeal spasm following extubation.

d. The need for mechanical ventilatory support for 3–5 weeks.

e. All of the above.

16. Match the selections listed below with their appropriate descriptions.

> a. Poliomyelitis.
> b. Guillain-Barre Syndrome.
> c. Both.
> d. Neither.

_____ Autonomic nervous system dysfunction is a recognized complication.

_____ Mortality is largely attributed to the respiratory dysfunction.

_____ Distal symmetrical weakness in lower extremities is an early sign of the disease.

_____ Weakness usually progresses over a period of several days.

17. A 5-year-old Vietnamese child presents to the emergency department with cyanosis, increased respiratory secretions, and excessive salivation. He is intubated and transferred to the pediatric intensive care unit (PICU). History reveals that his family moved to the United States about 5 weeks ago and that he has not received any immunizations. The father indicates that a 7-year-old neighbor died of some unknown respiratory disease in Vietnam about 3 weeks prior to their departure. The patient has had upper respiratory infection symptoms for 3–4 days, but today he was complaining of shortness of breath and became progressively cyanotic with the inability to move his left arm. Physical examination reveals absent deep tendon reflexes in the right knee and left elbow. An appropriate statement pertaining to this case is:

a. The alarming rapidity of progression of the muscle weakness is typical of this condition.

b. CSF pleocytosis with elevated protein may be noted, and the causative agent may be isolated from fecal or oropharyngeal specimens.

c. A clinical picture similar to this may be seen in an immunocompromised patient in the United States.

d. Survival from this disease is the rule.

e. All of the above.

18. The syndrome of inappropriate antidiuretic hormone secretion is a recognized complication in which of the following?

a. Respiratory syncytial virus infection.

b. Guillain-Barré syndrome.

c. Both.

d. Neither.

19. Indications for endotracheal intubation for a child with Guillain-Barré syndrome include all of the following except:

a. Forced vital capacity of less than 15 mL/kg.

b. Maximum inspiratory pressure below −20 cm H_2O.

c. Decreased residual volume.

d. $PaCO_2$ greater than 50 torr with acidemia.

e. A weak cough or gag, or the presence of atelectasis.

20. When preparing to intubate a patient with Guillain-Barré syndrome:

a. Depolarizing muscle relaxants should be avoided.

b. Absence of protective airway reflexes is an indication for tracheal intubation.

c. Circulatory response to intravenous sedatives is exaggerated.

d. All of the above.

21. All of the following are true regarding mechanical ventilatory support of patients with Guillain-Barré syndrome except:

a. Pneumonia is an uncommon complication in these patients.

b. Timely tracheal suctioning and provision of chest physiotherapy is of utmost importance in these patients.

c. Recovery from the respiratory insufficiency is the rule, despite the presence of residual weakness in 20% of patients.

d. Initially, total ventilatory support should be provided followed by partial withdrawal slowly.

22. The most common form of cardiac rate/rhythm abnormality in Guillain-Barré syndrome is:

a. Sinus tachycardia.

b. Sinus bradycardia.

c. Sinus node dysfunction.

d. Ventricular fibrillation.

e. Ventricular tachycardia.

23. Adults with unilateral diaphragmatic paralysis maintain normal oxygenation in the upright posture despite loss of 25% of vital capacity. Infants, on the other hand, develop significant gas exchange abnormalities related to:
    a. The very compliant chest wall of the infant.
    b. Horizontal orientation of the rib cage.
    c. The fact that infants are usually cared for in the supine position.
    d. All of the above.

24. The most common cause of a unilateral diaphragmatic paralysis in infants is:
    a. Trauma from a motor vehicle accident.
    b. Trauma from cardiothoracic surgery.
    c. Birth trauma.
    d. None of the above.

25. Regarding juvenile myasthenia gravis, all of the following are true except:
    a. Early symptoms frequently follow an acute viral illness.
    b. Early symptoms predominantly involve cranial nerves.
    c. Hyperthyroidism is a recognized association.
    d. Other autoimmune diseases, such as systemic lupus erythematosus, are not associated with myasthenia gravis.

26. Congenital myasthenia gravis is not characterized by which of the following?
    a. Onset a few days after birth.
    b. History of myasthenia in the mother during pregnancy.
    c. History of myasthenia in a sibling.
    d. Poor feeding.
    e. Respiratory failure is unusual.

27. Neonatal myasthenia gravis is characterized by all of the following except:
    a. Dysphagia and dysphasia within 24 hours after delivery.
    b. Uniformly born to mothers with myasthenia gravis.
    c. Symptoms respond poorly to anticholinesterase therapy.
    d. Symptoms subside by 5 weeks after birth.

28. Familial infantile myasthenia gravis is characterized by:
    a. Not being born to a mother with myasthenia gravis.
    b. History of myasthenia gravis in a sibling.

    c. Marked respiratory depression to the point of apnea at birth.
    d. Episodes of weakness and apnea in the first 2 years of life which respond to anticholinesterase therapy.
    e. All of the above.

29. A 14-year-old with myasthenia gravis is noted to have stridor following extubation after surgical removal of a lump in the breast. The stridor in this patient could be a result of:
    a. Vocal cord paralysis.
    b. Laryngeal muscle weakness.
    c. Postextubation stridor caused by glottic/subglottic edema.
    d. All of the above.

30. In a patient with myasthenia gravis, which of the following statements is most accurate regarding the need for and necessary precautions for endotracheal intubation?
    a. Vocal cord paralysis and laryngeal muscle weakness are recognized causes of airway obstruction following general anesthesia.
    b. Succinylcholine is the agent of choice to facilitate intubation.
    c. Peripheral muscle weakness correlates well with respiratory muscle weakness.
    d. Extubation can be done within a few days in those requiring ventilatory support.
    e. Plasmapheresis has not been shown to decrease the duration of endotracheal intubation and mechanical ventilation postoperatively.

31. Which of the following statements is incorrect regarding pathophysiology of botulism?
    a. The toxin binds to presynaptic, pre- and postganglionic parasympathetic neurons, and at the neuromuscular junction.
    b. The vast majority of cases are associated with ingestion of home-canned food.
    c. Binding of the toxin to the neurons is irreversible.
    d. Level of consciousness is often disturbed.
    e. The need for prolonged ventilatory support is typical.

32. All of the following are true regarding infantile botulism except:
    a. Endotracheal intubation is recommended whenever significant depression of the gag reflex is noted.

   b. Signs of severe occulomotor nerve dysfunction has been linked to the eventual development of respiratory failure.

   c. Recovery of peripheral muscles is noted before recovery of the diaphragm.

   d. Return of head control can be used in timing attempts at aggressive weaning and extubation.

   e. Autonomic disturbances, such as alteration in heart rate and blood pressure, do occur but do not require any intervention.

33. Evoked potentials are tools that are available to neurointensive care. Which of the following statements regarding evoked potentials is true?

   a. Evoked potentials are employed primarily as diagnostic and prognostic aids.

   b. With somatosensory evoked potentials, absence of the cortical wave bilaterally in comatose patients is predictive of a vegetative state.

   c. Absence of brainstem auditory evoked potentials in the presence of wave I are highly predictive of brain death.

   d. All of the above.

34. Which one of the following statements about traumatic brain injury is least correct?

   a. The integrity of CO_2 vasoresponsivity has prognostic value in that outcome is better in those patients with intact vasoresponsivity.

   b. In severe head injury, vasoresponsivity to CO_2 is lost much more than vasoresponsivity to changes in blood pressure.

   c. Low cerebral blood flow in the frontoparietal cortex suggests a poor neurological outcome.

   d. After head injury, cerebral blood flow may become pressure-dependent.

35. All of the following are true regarding the pathophysiology of meningitis except:

   a. Markedly reduced cerebral blood flow is recognized, and this is associated with a poor prognosis.

   b. In those patients with normal cerebral blood flow, regional hypoperfusion is common.

   c. Reduced cerebral perfusion pressure, primarily caused by increased intracranial pressure which occurs early in the course of meningitis, is associated with a poor prognosis.

   d. Autoregulation is lost.

   e. The reactivity of cerebral blood flow in response to changes in PCO_2 is well preserved and raises the possibility that severe hyperventilation may cause further ischemic damage.

36. Which of the following would be the most useful technique for prognostication in a setting of head injury?

   a. Somatosensory evoked potentials.

   b. Visual evoked potentials.

   c. Brainstem audio evoked potentials.

   d. Compressed spectral array.

   e. Cerebral function monitor.

37. The severity of cerebral edema can inherently impact prognosis of brain injury patients. Which one of the following statements regarding cerebral edema is false?

   a. Vasogenic edema has a better prognosis than cytotoxic edema because neurons are not primarily injured.

   b. Cytotoxic edema involves failure of adenosine triphosphatase-dependent sodium exchange.

   c. Cerebral blood volume is the important determinant of intracranial pressure.

   d. Cerebral blood flow is the primary determinant of intracranial pressure.

38. Which of the following is a true statement regarding treatment of intracranial pressure?

   a. Ketamine may cause cerebral vasodilation secondary to a cholinergic mechanism.

   b. High positive end-expiratory pressure when used at high levels may increase intracranial pressure.

   c. Mannitol may decrease cerebral blood flow via vasoconstriction.

   d. All of the above.

39. Select the most accurate events following global cerebral ischemia.

   a. Ischemia, hyperemia, hypoperfusion.

   b. Ischemia, hypoperfusion, hyperemia.

   c. Ischemia with persistent hyperemia.

   d. Ischemia with persistent hypoperfusion.

40. All of the following are true regarding histological changes in the brain following ischemia except:

   a. Intracellular organic disruption indicates irreversible injury.

   b. Reperfusion may liberate toxic metabolites.

   c. Cellular swelling is seen in the early stages and is reversible.

   d. The most vulnerable area of the cortex are layers three, five and six.

   e. CA_1 and CA_3 sectors of the hippocampus are spared from injury.

41. Which one of the following statements is incorrect regarding clinical and imaging evaluation of the central nervous system?
    a. The computed tomography (CT) scan is more sensitive for the detection of acute subarachnoid hemorrhage than the MRI.
    b. The posterior fossa is more clearly visualized by the MRI than CT scan.
    c. The oculomotor nerve can be assessed by the corneal reflex.
    d. Decerebrate posture correlates with high pontine and mid brain lesions.

42. Match the pupillary change with the corresponding location of that lesion in the brain.

> a. Small reactive bilateral.
> b. Unilateral-dilated and fixed.
> c. Large fixed-hippus bilateral.
> d. Pinpoint bilateral.
> e. Midposition-fixed bilateral.

_____ Pons.   _____ Midbrain.

43. All of the following statements regarding status epilepticus are true except:
    a. It is defined as epileptic activity lasting longer than 30 minutes without recovery of a level of consciousness.
    b. In experimental models, phase I is characterized by hypertension, lactic acidosis, and hyperglycemia.
    c. Phase I lasts approximately 30 minutes.
    d. Phase II is characterized by hypothermia, hypokalemia, and hyperglycemia.
    e. Cerebral blood flow, glucose, and O_2 consumption diminish during phase II.

44. Which of the following statements is inaccurate regarding the pharmacology of lipid soluble anticonvulsants?
    a. A lipid soluble drug possesses a "distribution" phase and an "elimination" phase.
    b. The volume of distribution of a lipid soluble drug is directly proportionatal to the degree of its solubility.

   c. With highly lipid soluble drugs, free brain concentration does not correspond to free serum concentration.

   d. Without a loading dose, a time equivalent to five or more elimination half-lives is required to attain a steady-state serum concentration.

45. Diazepam and lorazepam are commonly used to abort seizures. Which of the following statements most accurately describes these two medications?
    a. Diazepam is the least lipid soluble of the anticonvulsants.
    b. Lorazepam has more associated side effects of respiratory depression and apnea than diazepam.
    c. Diazepam has a very small volume of distribution owing to its poor lipid solubility.
    d. Lorazepam does not have any significant metabolites.
    e. The volume distribution of lorazepam is at least five times that of diazepam.

46. Which of the following statements inaccurately describes the pharmacology of anticonvulsants?
    a. Phenobarbital has a very slow onset of action because of its very low lipid solubility.
    b. Elimination kinetics of phenytoin is linear.
    c. When used repeatedly for status epilepticus, lorazepam may become progressively less effective.
    d. Thiopental and paraldehyde can be used as alternative choices in the treatment of status epilepticus.
    e. Infants have a higher elimination capacity for anticonvulsants than older children.

47. Of all trauma admissions involving children, the vast majority are attributable to:
    a. Head injury.
    b. Chest injury.
    c. Abdominal injury.
    d. Pelvic injury.
    e. Genitourinary injury.

48. Which of the following statements is incorrect with regard to mechanisms of brain injury?
    a. Primary brain injury can occur from direct impact, causing neuronal injury, or oblique acceleration forces to long white matter tracts, resulting in axonal shear injury.
    b. Most gray matter contusions are seen on the inferior aspect of the temporal and frontal lobes.

c. Diffuse white matter injury is often seen in the areas of the corpus callosum and brainstem.
d. Cytotoxic edema is more likely to be seen in the white matter, and vasogenic edema in the gray matter.
e. Most head injuries in children do not involve a skull fracture.

49. Which of the following statements is most accurate regarding glutamic acid in the brain?
  a. It is released normally in high concentrations from glial cells.
  b. When released from glial cells, it is a source of nutrition for astrocytes.
  c. Its concentration in the brain interstitium is inversely related to intracranial pressure.
  d. It is usually found in negligible concentrations in the brain extracellular fluid.

50. A 2-year-old toddler receives 200 mg of phenobarbital intravenously. The patient's weight is 10 kg and the volume distribution for phenobarbital is 1 L/kg of body weight. The initial blood concentration is expected to be:
  a. 10 mg/L.
  b. 20 mg/L.
  c. 30 mg/L.
  d. 40 mg/L.

51. Which of the following statements below most accurately describes the anatomy and physiology of the brain?
  a. The majority of the blood flow to the brain is committed to the white matter.
  b. Arterial oxygen tension has no influence on cerebral blood flow.
  c. A change of 1 mmHg in $PaCO_2$ results in a 4% change in cerebral blood flow.
  d. Water constitutes only 30% of the total white matter and gray matter contents.

52. Match the following sign/symptom with the expected location of the lesion in the brain:

a. Hypothalamus.	e. Midbrain tectum.
b. Deafferented pupil.	f. Pons.
c. Cerebellum.	g. Cribriform plate
d. Ipsilateral cortex.	of ethmoid.

_____ Nystagmus.
_____ Tonic deviation of the eye(s).
_____ Marcus Gunn pupil.
_____ Horner's syndrome.

_____ Midposition pupils with hippus.
_____ Pinpoint pupils (reactive).
_____ Leakage of CSF from nose.

53. Which of the following cardiorespiratory abnormalities is recognized to be associated with head injury?
  a. Ventricular and supraventricular tachycardia.
  b. Sinus arrest.
  c. Pulmonary edema.
  d. All of the above.
  e. None of the above.

54. The figure below represents the relationship between intracranial volume and the intracranial pressure. Most of the initial compensation that leads to a shift from position A to B on the curve is a result of:

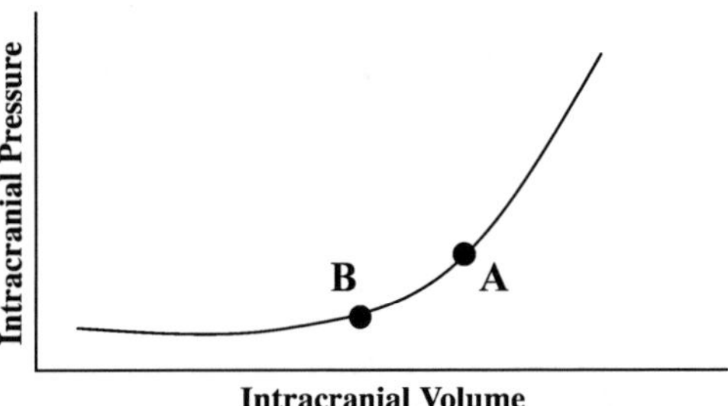

  a. Compression of lateral ventricles.
  b. Decreased CSF production.
  c. Egress of CSF from intracranial to intraspinal space.
  d. Decreased O_2 delivery to the brain.

55. Match the following central nervous system lesions with the corresponding descriptions below:

a. Contusion.
b. Penetrating injury.
c. Epidural hematoma.
d. Subdural hematoma.
e. Intracerebral hematoma.

_____ In most cases, treatment is nonoperative and outcome is poor.
_____ Dense crescentic lesion on brain CT scan.
_____ Localized lenticular lesion on brain CT scan.
_____ Clostridium perfringes abscess.
_____ An area of bruising or microscopic hemorrhage caused by trauma.
_____ May occur secondary to birth trauma.

56. A 6-year-old boy has developed a cerebrovascular accident (stroke) involving the distribution of the middle cerebral artery. Which one of the following metabolic disorders is most likely to be the underlying predisposing factor?
    a. Homocystinuria.
    b. Congenital adrenal hyperplasia.
    c. Phenylketonuria.
    d. Vitamin D deficiency.
    e. Wilson's Disease.

57. A 10-year-old girl presents with a sudden onset of excruciating headache followed by progression to a coma over a very short period of time. CT scan was suggestive of a ruptured arteriovenous malformation with extensive subarachnoid hemorrhage. She was admitted to the PICU where she slowly recovered over a period of several days. Now 3 weeks after discharge, she presents with somnolence and papilledema which is detected on physical examination. The most likely explanation for this neurological deterioration is:
    a. Arterial spasm.
    b. Astrocytoma.
    c. Communicating hydrocephalus.
    d. Obstructive hydrocephalus.
    e. Pseudotumor cerebri.

58. A 5-year-old who has been struck by an automobile has been admitted to the PICU. In evaluating this patient, which of the following clinical descriptions is most accurate?
    a. CSF rhinorrhea develops in 70% of cases of basilar skull fracture and is permanent in the vast majority of cases.
    b. Ecchymosis with bluish discoloration in the periorbital area in this patient is referred to as Battle's sign.
    c. Use of corticosteroids will definitely be beneficial in this patient if significant head injury is suspected.
    d. If a basilar skull fracture is suspected in this patient, radiographic studies will positively identify the fracture site in greater than 90% of cases.
    e. Because of the underdevelopment of sinuses at this age, CSF rhinorrhea would be rare in this patient.

59. Select which of the following requires definitive debridement and elevation within 48 hours.
    a. Depressed skull fracture.

    b. Linear skull fracture.
    c. Both.
    d. Neither.

60. A 3-year-old white male suffers a 2-hour seizure after abruptly losing consciousness while at play. An initial CT scan of his brain reveals a 3-cm aneurysm involving the circle of Willis. Which of the following statements is true regarding cerebral vasculature?
    a. The posterior circulation (paired vertebral arteries and basilar artery) supplies brainstem and cranial nerves.
    b. The circle of Willis is formed by the internal carotid artery, the middle cerebral arteries, and the anterior and posterior communicating arteries.
    c. Wallenberg's Syndrome is caused by the compromise of the posterior–inferior cerebellar artery.
    d. Ischemia in the vascular distribution of the superior cerebellar artery will cause dizziness, tremor, and contralateral weakness.
    e. All of the above.

61. Match the disease process with its most closely associated finding:

    > a. Rete mirabile of Moyamoya.
    > b. Right-to-left cardiac shunt.
    > c. Arteriovenous malformations.

    _____ Thrombotic stroke.
    _____ Embolic stroke.
    _____ Intracerebral hemorrhage.

62. Which of the following regarding strokes in children is true?
    a. Basilar artery migraine is a differential diagnosis.
    b. Exchange transfusion does not help treat a child with stroke and polycythemia.
    c. Hyperventilation improves clinical outcome of ischemic strokes.
    d. Steroid administration improves clinical outcome in stroke patients.
    e. Anticoagulation is indicated in evolving strokes.

63. State whether the following statements are true or false regarding arteriovenous malformations in children:
    _____ a. Single most common causes of cerebral hemorrhage in children.

_____ b. Vascular resistance is high causing high blood flow.

_____ c. Most patients remain asymptomatic throughout the adolescent period.

_____ d. Most common presentation is headache.

_____ e. The "gold standard" test for diagnosis is four-vessel angiography.

_____ f. Resection is the procedure of choice.

64. All of the following statements are true regarding intracranial aneurysms except:
    a. Relatively rare in children.
    b. Saccular or "berry" type is the most common.
    c. Mycotic aneurysms are associated with congenital heart disease.
    d. Fusiform aneurysms occur following trauma.
    e. A large majority occur at the posterior and anterior communicating arteries.

65. State whether the following statements regarding aneurysms in children are true or false.
    _____ a. Aneurysms rarely cause seizures.
    _____ b. Vein of Galen aneurysm presents in the neonate with congestive heart failure.
    _____ c. Polycystic kidney disease, aortic coarctation, Marfan syndrome, and Moyamoya are associated with an increased risk of intracranial aneurysm.

The following chapter will focus on infectious diseases. Pertinent questions, answers, and rationale will be reviewed. Answers for this chapter can be found beginning on page 123.

Key Words: Infection; antibiotics; sepsis; cascade; fever.

1. Nosocomial infections are an unfortunate complication of hospitalization. All of the following statements regarding nosocomial infections in children are true except:
   a. Hospital acquired infections are generally highest in teaching hospitals.
   b. Surgical services have the highest rate of nosocomial infections.
   c. In the pediatric services, respiratory infection is the most common nosocomial infection.
   c. *Eschericha coli* is the most common cause of pediatric urinary tract infection (UTI).
   d. *Klebsiella* is the most common cause of lower respiratory infections in newborns.

2. Which of the following is least accurate regarding nosocomial upper respiratory infection?
   a. When patients with nasotracheal tubes in place develop maxillary sinusitis, *Pneumococcus* is the most common organism.
   b. It has been shown that in acute sinusitis, culture of the nose or throat does not yield the organisms responsible for the sinusitis.
   c. Corneal ulcers, if discovered, must be treated aggressively to prevent progression to hypopyon.
   d. Data suggest that there is little overall effect of a different physical plant of the hospital, whether new or old, on the resultant nosocomial infection.

3. Respiratory-born nosocomial infections are associated with increased morbidity and mortality, which is likely to increase hospital costs. Regarding this topic, which of the following statements is not true?
   a. Patients treated with H_2-blockers are at higher risk of tracheal colonization with Gram-negative bacilli.
   b. Ventilators with humidifying cascades, rather than nebulizers, have little role in contaminating patients if the tubing is changed every 48 hours.
   c. Aspiration occurs more often in children with an uncuffed endotracheal tube compared with those having a cuffed tube.
   d. Initial colonization begins in the stomach or hypopharynx with subsequent spread to the trachea.
   e. Anerobes are the dominant organisms that colonize the trachea in intubatedpatients.

4. All of the following statements regarding infections associated with arterial catheterization are true except:
   a. Insertion by a surgical cutdown is associated with a significantly higher risk of localized and systemic infection compared with percutaneous insertion.
   b. Catheters in place for more than 4 days have a twofold higher risk of being infected.
   c. Local inflammation correlates well with duration of catheter insertion.
   d. Single patient disposable transducers can be used up to 4 days without bacteremia prevalence.
   e. *Candida albicans* and *Enterococcus* are the most common organisms involved in infection.

5. All of the following statements regarding central venous catheterization are true except:
   a. Catheters placed during an active infection may become colonized with the same organism causing the bacteremia.
   b. The proximity of a tracheostomy tube may be a relative contraindication for a subclavian catheter placement.

    c. Pulmonary artery catheters have a significantly higher incidence of positive catheter tip cultures after 72 hours of insertion.

    d. *Staphylococcus epidermidis* and *Staphylococcus aureus* are the most common causes of parenteral nutrition-associated infections.

    e. Fifty percent of parenteral nutrition-associated infections are fungal.

6. Select whether the following statements regarding nosocomial infections in children are true or false.

    _____ a. Skin site erythema greater than 4 mm in diameter, fever, and positive skin cultures are predictive of catheter-associated infection.

    _____ b. Asymptomatic pseudomonas bacteremia in dialysis patients has been reported.

    _____ c. External shunts for hemodialysis are most commonly infected by *S. aureus*.

    _____ d. Approximately 10% of cannulas placed for extracorporeal life support become infected.

    _____ e. Coagulase-negative staphylococci are the most common cause of catheter-related sepsis.

7. All of the following statements regarding UTI in children are true except:

    a. During infancy, males outnumber females 3:1.

    b. In the pediatric intensive care unit, the cumulative risk of UTI in catheterized patients approaches 30%.

    c. In a midstream "clean catch" specimen, greater than 10^5 organisms/mL indicates infection.

    d. Meatal cleansing with providone-iodine and use of impregnated catheters significantly decrease incidence of UTI.

    e. Urinary catheters are more likely to be colonized with Gram-positive, rather than Gram-negative bacteria.

8. All of the following statements regarding intracranial pressure devices are true except:

    a. Increasing frequency of breaks in the system increases the risk of infection.

    b. Prophylactic antibiotic coverage significantly decreases the incidence of infection.

    c. Duration of placement is directly related to infection rate.

    d. Placement either in the intensive care unit or in the operating room appears to have no relationship to the rate of infection.

    e. Intraventricular hemorrhage in the presence of an intracranial pressure greater than 20 cm H_2O increases the rate of infection.

9. All of the following statements regarding childhood infections are true except:

    a. Common offending organisms during the first 7 days of life are Group B streptococci, *E. coli*, and *Listeria monocytogenes*.

    b. Ampicillin and a third generation cephalosporin will effectively cover the organisms in Answer A.

    c. *Haemophilus influenzae, Streptococcus pneumoniae* and *Neisseria meningitidis* are the three most common causes of bacterial meningitis and pneumonia in children.

    d. In the septic child with an abdominal focus, ampicillin, gentamicin and tobramycin are adequate.

    e. Avoiding monotherapy with cephalosporin in the treatment of catheter sepsis decreases the risks of emerging resistant organisms.

10. Match the clinical features with the corresponding type of Group B streptococcal infection.

> a. Early-onset neonatal Group B streptococcal infection.
> b. Late-onset Group B streptococcal infection.

    _____ Higher association with pneumonia.
    _____ Higher association with meningitis.
    _____ Type III isolated 95% of the time.
    _____ Poor correlation with maternal colonization.

11. Both the choice of antibiotics and the population at risk being treated, affect bacterial complications of a disease. Select whether the following statements are true or false.

    _____ a. Ampicillin/gentamicin combination is synergistic against Group B streptococcal infection.

    _____ b. Ampicillin/chloramphenicol combination is synergistic against Group B streptococcal infection.

    _____ c. Low complement levels, poor opsonization capacity, and decreased immunoglobulin levels account for an infant's susceptibility to Group B streptococcal infection.

    _____ d. Simple and exchange transfusions improve short-term outcome in Group B streptococcal infection.

    _____ e. Most babies with Group B streptococcal infection are born to mothers who possess antibodies against the infecting strain.

____ f. *L. monocytogenes* becomes more coccoid in morphology the longer it stays in culture.

____ g. High-risk groups for *L. monocytogenes* include neonates, pregnant women, and the elderly.

____ h. *L. monocytogenes* has a bimodal presentation similar to Group B streptococcal infection.

12. Match the following associated findings with the most accurate diagnosis, either A or B, regarding sepsis.

> a. Early-onset *L. monocytogenes* sepsis.
> b. Late-onset *L. monocytogenes* sepsis.

____ Mother has a "flu-like" illness.
____ Meningitis.
____ Type IV_b.
____ Mothers are asymptomatic.

13. A full-term infant is born by spontaneous vaginal delivery to a mother with active herpetic lesions. All of the following statements regarding herpes simplex virus infection are true except:
    a. Contraction during delivery is the most common.
    b. Approximately 6% of babies delivered by cesarean section within 4 hours of membrane rupture become infected.
    c. A total of 10–20% of adult genital diseases may be caused by type I herpes simplex virus
    d. Incubation period is approximately 2 days.
    e. Premature babies are more likely to be affected.

14. Select whether the following statements regarding herpes simplex virus are true or false.
    ____ a. Mucosal or skin lesions are present 20–30% of the time in neonatal diagnoses.
    ____ b. Meningoencephalitis occurs in 75% of neonatal diagnoses.
    ____ c. Disseminated diagnosis has a mortality rate of 40%.
    ____ d. Type 2 has an increased rate of pneumonitis and disseminated intravascular coagulopathy than type 1.
    ____ e. Mothers with genital lesions need to be isolated from their babies.
    ____ f. It may be wise to isolate the mother from the infant when the mother has oral lesions.

15. A 2-year-old male presents to the emergency department with tachycardia, hypotension, fever, and ecchymotic lesions on his trunk and lower extremities. You suspect meningococcemia. All of the following statements regarding *N. meningitis* are true except:
    a. The disease caused by *N. meningitidis* is usually endemic.
    b. Ninety percent of infections occur in children younger than 2 years of age.
    c. Prior infection with influenza A or B has been associated with increased susceptibility to infection with *N. meningitidis*.
    d. The disease is more common in males.
    e. Carriage of the organism in the nasopharynx is very rare.

16. Unfavorable prognostic features in meningococcal infection include all of the following except:
    a. Cerebrospinal fluid (CSF) white blood cell (WBC) count of three mononuclear cells/mm^3.
    b. Presence of petechiae for less than 12 hours prior to admission.
    c. Presence of shock.
    d. An erythrocyte sedimentation rate of 100 mm/hour.
    e. A peripheral WBC count of 3000/mm^3.

17. Which of the following is true regarding fulminant meningococcemia?
    a. Rarely fatal.
    b. Petechiae are universally absent.
    c. Large doses of exogenous corticosteroids always reverse the shock state.
    d. Cardiovascular collapse is secondary to endotoxemia.
    e. Mortality is approximately 35% in patients with unfavorable prognostic factors.

18. Which of the following statements is true regarding meningococcal infection?
    a. High-dose methylprednisolone always reverses the associated shock state.
    b. Myocarditis develops 24–48 hours after presentation in 3–5% of all patients.
    c. Pneumonia is always mild.
    d. Rifampin prophylaxis of household and day care center contacts is recommended.

19. Which of the following infections is associated with petechiae?
    a. *H. influenza*.
    b. *Neisseria gonorrhea*.

    c. *N. meningitidis.*
    d. *S. pneumoniae.*
    e. All of the above.

20. Which of the following statements regarding *H. influenzae* type B infection is least accurate?
    a. Acute sepsis may mimic meningococcemia.
    b. Adrenal hemorrhage is recognized in fatal cases.
    c. Death related to overwhelming sepsis is caused by intractable hypotension and cardiac dysfunction.
    d. Chemoprophylaxis with Rifampin is recommended for all household contacts.
    e. Rifampin prophylaxis should be administered 1 month after completion of the therapeutic antibiotic course.

21. Which of the following statements regarding meningitis in children is true?
    a. Otitis media has not been associated with *H. influenzae* meningitis.
    b. Contaminated lake water is a recognized source of *Naegleria* meningitis.
    c. Meningitis usually involves the parenchyma of the brain.
    d. Virchow-Robin spaces are continuous extensions of the subarachnoid space, which prevent bacteria from infecting the surface of the brain.
    e. The process of meningitis rarely includes cerebral edema.

22. Which of the following statements is the most appropriate responseregarding the pathophysiology of meningitis?
    a. Convulsions in the first 72 hours of the illness carry a grave prognosis.
    b. Children less than 5 years of age who attend a day care center are at a lower risk of meningitis than the average child.
    c. Limitation of ocular movement always indicates increased intracranial pressure.
    d. Papilledema that develops within the first day of presentation is more likely to be a result of a ruptured brain abscess, than meningitis itself.
    e. All of the above.

23. Which one of the following statements is incorrect regarding the clinical manifestations of bacterial meningitis?
    a. Convulsions occur in 30% of cases during the course of the illness.
    b. Convulsions that are limited to the first 48–72 hours of illness carry a better prognosis.
    c. Kernig's sign is positive when pain is elicited after extension of the leg.
    d. Limitations of extraocular movements are secondary to paresis of cranial nerve VII.
    e. Tuberculosis and cryptococcal meningitis are more likely to present with focal signs and papilledema.

24. All of the following statements regarding laboratory diagnosis of meningitis are true except:
    a. Definitive diagnosis is made by CSF culture.
    b. The normal opening pressure by spinal manometer in the neonate is 90–110 cmH_2O.
    c. The normal opening pressure of older children and adults is up to 180 cmH_2O.
    d. An acceptable upper limit for WBC numbers of CSF in the full-term baby is 32 WBCs/mm^3.
    e. In infants, neutrophils may comprise 90% of the WBCs in the CSF and still be considered normal.

25. CSF abnormalities can help to determine the etiology of meningitis. Select whether the following statements are true or false.
    _____ a. Spinal fluid remains clear with up to 500 WBCs/mm^3.
    _____ b. Red blood cells in the CSF may raise the protein by 5 mg/100 mL for every 1000 red blood cells/mm^3.
    _____ c. Abnormal CSF lactate is greater than 2 mg/100 mL.

26. Which of the following is true regarding partially treated meningitis?
    a. Clinical course and outcome are improved when prior treatment (oral antibiotics) has been administered prior to hospitalization.
    b. CSF becomes "sterile" within 1 hour of parenteral antibiotic administration.
    c. Specific antigens of the bacterial capsule are detectable for up to 2 weeks after antibiotic therapy.
    d. Approximately 50% of children receive antibiotics in some form prior to diagnosis.

27. Which of the following statements is least accurate regarding evaluation and therapy of a child with meningitis?
    a. Tuberculous meningitis is less likely to present with focal signs and papilledema than other causes of bacterial meningitis.
    b. Cryptococcal meningitis is more likely to present with focal signs and papilledema than bacterial meningitis.
    c. The presence of retinal hemorrhages suggests cortical vein thrombosis.
    d. The normal CSF opening pressure in the neonate is 100 mm H_2O.

28. The following statements regarding complications of meningitis are all true except:
    a. Syndrome of inappropriate antidiuretic hormone secretion has been noted in more than 50% of patients.
    b. Subdural effusions mostly occur beyond the first week of the illness and eventually resolve spontaneously.
    c. Cerebral vasculitis leading to capillary leakage is the likely pathogenesis of subdural effusions
    d. The most common cause of recurrent fever after initial treatment of meningitis is a nosocomial infection.
    e. By day 5 of treatment, only 30% of children with *H. influenzae* meningitis will be afebrile.

29. Select whether the following statements regarding childhood meningitis are true or false.
    _____ a. Fever which persists beyond the tenth hospital day is most likely because of subdural effusions, drug fever, arthritis, brain abscess, and nosocomial infection (in descending order).
    _____ b. 30–50% of persistent fevers have an unknown etiology despite adequate treatment for meningitis with negative blood cultures.
    _____ c. The outcome of children is directly proportional to the persistence of positive CSF cultures.
    _____ d. Gram-negative endotoxin may be related to the formation of intracranial abscesses, hydrocephalus, and parencephalic cysts in children with Gram-negative meningitis.

30. All of the following statements regarding therapy of meningitis are true except:
    a. Respiratory isolation is required for 24–48 hours after initiation of antibiotic treatment.
    b. Hyperglycemia may worsen the outcome for children with cerebral ischemia.
    c. The American Academy of Pediatrics recommends dexamethasone as a treatment option for children with suspected bacterial meningitis.
    d. Aztreonam, a synthetic monocyclic β-lactam antibiotic, has been shown to be effective in therapy of Gram-negative infections.
    e. The child with a ventriculoperitoneal shunt and suspected meningitis should receive a combination of ampicillin and clindamycin for adequate antimicrobial coverage.

31. Select whether the following statements regarding childhood meningitis are true or false.
    _____ a. Most neonatal meningitis cases require greater than or equal to 21 days of intravenous antibiotics.
    _____ b. With tuberculous meningitis, a lymphocytic reaction in the CSF may mimic a viral etiology.
    _____ c. In the first several weeks of tuberculous meningitis, cerebral fluid glucose and protein may remain normal.
    _____ d. Acid-fast smear in tuberculous meningitis is positive in more than 90% of patients.
    _____ e. Long-term sequelae for bacterial meningitis occur in 30–50% of affected patients.

32. Singer criteria for hospital admission of patients with probable aseptic meningitis include all of the following except:
    a. Deteriorating clinical condition.
    b. Patients younger than 1 year of age.
    c. All children who have received antibiotics in the week prior to presentation.
    d. CSF: increased protein, decreased glucose, less than 1000 WBC/mm³.
    e. An older sibling with upper respiratory infection symptomatology.

33. The following statements are all true regarding ECHO and Coxsackie viruses except:
    a. Typical incubation period is 3–5 days.
    b. Group B is most common in Coxsackie virus, and type 9 among ECHO virus.

c. Peak incidence occurs in late summer.
d. Meningitis is usually benign.
e. Incidence rates increase with higher socioeconomic groups.

34. Select whether the following statements regarding meningitis are true or false.
    _____ a. Lymphocytic choriomeningitis develops after contact with infected rodents.
    _____ b. Corticosteroids greatly enhance recovery time of aseptic meningitis.

35. All of the following statements regarding viral encephalitis are true except:
    a. Arbor viruses are the most common etiological agents.
    b. In 75% of cases, no specific etiology can be established.
    c. The hallmark of the disease is disturbed higher cerebral function.
    d. The majority of cases are secondary to hematogenous spread.
    e. With herpes simplex virus, the electroencephalogram displays abnormalities in the occipital cortical region.

36. Which of the following statements is true regarding arboviruses?
    a. Highest mortality occurs with California equine encephalitis.
    b. Transmitted by rodents.
    c. Occurs in late autumn and early winter.
    d. St. Louis encephalitis is the most common arbovirus infection in the United States.

37. Match each of the following arboviruses with its most likely clinical presentation.

> A. Eastern equine encephalitis.
> B. Californian equine encephalitis.
> C. Western equine encephalitis.
> D. Venezuelan equine encephalitis.

    _____ Midwest, "LaCrosse strain," school-age children, most recover without sequelae.
    _____ Abrupt onset, children less than 1 year of age, and extensive neuronal death with devastating sequelae.
    _____ California and Texas, hyperplasia and occlusion of small blood vessels, and elevation of intracranial pressure.
    _____ Affects adults more than children, rare neurological involvement.

38. All of the following statements regarding Rocky Mountain spotted fever are true except:
    a. It is a tick-born disease.
    b. Occurs primarily in the Rocky Mountain area.
    c. Complicated by meningoencephalitis in 30% of cases.
    d. 10% of cases progress to coma.

39. A 6-year-old female presents with a high temperature for 3 days despite negative blood and CSF cultures. A computed tomography scan of the brain reveals a 2-cm ring-enhanced lesion consistent with a brain abscess. The most likely predisposing condition is:
    a. Suppurative otitis media.
    b. Suppurative mastoiditis.
    c. Suppurative frontal sinusitis.
    d. An uncorrected Tetralogy.

40. Which of the following statements about brain abscess is most accurate?
    a. Abscess formation occurs in areas of the brain with generous blood supply, and is therefore most commonly seen in gray matter.
    b. Brain abscess formation very commonly complicates bacterial meningitis beyond the neonatal period.
    c. When seizures develop, they are always focal in type.
    d. Brain abscess formed by hematogenous seeding is usually in the distribution of the middle cerebral artery.
    e. All of the above.

41. Which of the following is most accurate regarding the microbiology and chemotherapeutic treatment strategies for brain abscess?
    a. The overwhelming majority of brain abscesses is caused by a single organism; polymicrobial etiology is very rare.
    b. Suppurative otitis media caused by *H. influenzae* type B is the most common predisposing factor.
    c. Aminoglycosides are drugs of first choice.
    d. In the neonatal period, *Citrobacter diversus* and *Proteus mirabilis* are the most common etiological agents.
    e. All of the above.

42. Which of the following statements regarding sub-
    dural empyema is true?
    a. The subdural space at the base of the brain is
       most frequently involved.
    b. It is usually restricted from spreading by the
       suture lines where the dura is firmly adherent.
    c. *H. influenzae* is the most common etiological
       agent in infants.
    d. Magnetic resonance imaging is the diagnostic
       imaging procedure of choice.
    e. All of the above.

43. Match the most likely organism with its disease
    process.

    > a. Brain abscess in a child with a
    >   cyanotic congenital heart disease.
    > b. Subdural empyema.
    > c. Spinal epidural abscess.

    _____ *S. aureus*.
    _____ Aerobic streptococci.
    _____ Hemolytic streptococci.

44. Which of the following is not a proposed diagnos-
    tic criterion for toxic shock syndrome in children?
    a. Fever greater than 39°C.
    b. Diffuse or palmar erythema.
    c. Hypotension.
    d. Lymphocytosis.
    e. Diarrhea or vomiting.

45. Which of the following is true regarding toxic
    shock syndrome?
    a. It is caused by coagulase-negative staphylococci.
    b. Neutralizing antibodies are formed immediately
       by the body against the toxin.
    c. Menstrual cases are seen exclusively in African
       Americans.
    d. A serum creatinine greater than 3 mg% at pres-
       entation predicts a prolonged hospital course.
    e. All of the above.

46. Which of the following statements regarding Rocky
    Mountain spotted fever is true?
    a. Most victims are adults.
    b. *Dermacentor variabilis* is the most common tick
       involved in the eastern regions of the United
       States, and *Dermacentor andersoni* is the most
       common tick in the West.
    c. Peaks in winter.
    d. Incubation period is 24 hours.
    e. Man is the primary host of *Rickettsia rickettsii*.

47. All of the following statements are true regarding
    Rocky Mountain spotted fever except:
    a. Initial presentation consists of fever, headache,
       and malaise.
    b. Rash appears 10 days after the onset of fever,
       and begins on the trunk.
    c. Erythematous macules become petechial over
       the course of several days.
    d. Complement fixation or indirect fluorescent anti-
       body titers are used to confirm the diagnosis.
    e. Diffuse vasculitis affects many organ systems.

48. All of the following statements regarding Legion-
    naire's disease are true except:
    a. The disease mostly affects adult males.
    b. It may present with cerebellar ataxia.
    c. Lung disease is lobar.
    d. Fever, nonproductive cough, hematuria, and
       encephalopathy are presenting signs.
    e. It accounts for 50% of pneumonias in adults.

49. Superantigens are potentially involved in which of
    the following disorders?
    a. Toxic shock syndrome.
    b. HIV infection.
    c. Kawasaki syndrome.
    d. All of the above.
    e. None of the above.

50. Match the clinical sign of toxic shock syndrome in:

    > a. An adult.   b. A child.

    _____ Prodromal symptoms of fever, mucosal ery-
          thema, vomiting, and dizziness are almost
          always seen.
    _____ Hypotension is prominent at admission.

51. Match the clinical presentation with the correct
    infectious agent.

    > a. Brain abscess in an infant with meningitis.
    > b. Brain abscess in a child with uncorrected
    >   Tetralogy of Fallot.
    > c. Brain abscess is secondary to a penetrating
    >   brain injury.
    > d. Brain abscess in a patient with a compro-
    >   mised immune system.

    _____ *Nocardia* spp.
    _____ *C. diversus*.
    _____ α-Hemolytic streptococci.
    _____ *S. aureus*.

5 Hematology and Oncology

The following chapter will focus on hematology and oncology. Pertinent questions, answers, and rational will be reviewed. Answers for this chapter can be found beginning on page 129.

Key Words: White blood cells; malignancy; chemotherapy; bleeding.

1. Despite great advances in the treatment of childhood diseases, malignancy remains an ominous threat. All of the following statements regarding malignant diseases in children are true except:
   a. Neoplastic disease is the leading cause of death in the 1–15-year-old population.
   b. The leukemias are the most common malignancies of childhood.
   c. Brain tumor is the most common solid tumor in childhood.
   d. Ectodermal and endodermal carcinomas are rarely seen in children.

2. With regard to the association of infection with long-term catheter insertion in the pediatric population, which one of the following is most accurate?
   a. Infus-a-port carries a lower rate of infection than Broviac single lumen catheter.
   b. Infus-a-port has a lower rate of infection than both single lumen Broviac and double lumen Hickman catheters.
   c. Double lumen catheters have a higher rate of infection compared with single lumen catheters.
   d. There is no significant difference in infection rate between the externalized and the subcutaneously implanted catheters.

3. A 4-year-old boy with leukemia is being evaluated for fevers. Physical examination does not reveal any focus of infection. The complete blood count shows a total white blood cell count of 1235 cells/mm^3 with 12% neutrophils and 2% band form. The rest of the differential count is lymphocytes. The platelet count is 32,000/mm^3. Which of the following statements is most accurate regarding this clinical scenario?
   a. Fifty to seventy percent of febrile episodes in oncology patients are noninfectious.
   b. Blood culture is positive in more than 75% of disseminated fungal infections.
   c. The degree of neutropenia does not correlate with the morbidity and mortality caused by bacterial infections.
   d. Bronchoscopy should be done at this point in this patient to evaluate for pneumocystis.
   e. *Candida* and *Aspergillus* species are the two most common fungal agents causing fungal infections in pediatric oncology patients.

4. All of the following statements regarding the child with malignant disease are true except:
   a. *Pneumocystis carinii* will be identified in 15% of patients despite previous treatment with trimethoprim-sulfamethoxazole.
   b. Granulocyte transfusions may be beneficial in the setting of neutropenia and culture proven sepsis.
   c. Pneumonitis, as a result of granulocyte transfusion can usually be avoided with appropriate premedication.
   d. The half-life of transfused platelets is longer than 4 weeks.
   e. Spontaneous bleeding may occur when the platelet count is less than 20,000/mm^3.

From: *Pediatric Critical Care Review*
Edited by: R. A. Hasan and M. D. Pappas © Humana Press Inc., Totowa, NJ

5. Match the following chemotherapeutic drug with its most likely hematological effect:

a.	Actinomycin D.	d.	Methotrexate.
b.	Anthracycline.	e.	Vincristine.
c.	L-Asparaginase.	f.	Glucocorticoids.

_____ Antithrombin III deficiency.
_____ Chronic hepatic dysfunction.
_____ Hypofibrinogenemia.
_____ Increases fibrinolysis.
_____ Increases factors II, VII, VIII, X.
_____ Decreases vitamin K-dependent factors.

6. All of the following statements are true regarding pulmonary parenchymal disease in children with malignancies except:
   a. The pulmonary parenchyma is commonly involved in leukemia.
   b. The initial lesion from radiation exposure occurs within 6 hours of radiation therapy and involves capillary endothelial damage.
   c. Bleomycin- and Busulfan-associated pulmonary fibrosis is dose-dependent.
   d. Cyclophosphamide and methotrexate have been associated with pulmonary fibrosis.

7. Select whether the following statements regarding malignancies and chemotherapy in children are true or false.
   _____ a. Cyclophosphamide is associated with hemorrhagic cardiac necrosis.
   _____ b. Anthracycline induced cardiomyopathy manifests as myofibrillar loss and cytoplasmic vacuolization.
   _____ c. Cardiomyopathy is unrelated to radiotherapy.
   _____ d. Vincristine may induce syndrome of inappropriate antidiuretic hormone secretion.
   _____ e. Intrathecal chemotherapy may cause seizures.
   _____ f. When *P. carinii* infection occurs after bone marrow transplant, it is most commonly seen at 2–4 weeks.

8. Match the following chemotherapeutic drug with its most closely associated adverse neurological effect.

a.	Methotrexate.	c.	Vincristine.
b.	Cisplatin.	d.	5-Fluorouracil.

_____ Ototoxicity.

_____ Acute cerebellar ataxia.
_____ Aseptic meningitis.
_____ Syndrome of inappropriate antidiuretic hormone secretion.

9. Match the following chemotherapeutic drug with its most commonly associated complication.

a.	Methotrexate (high dose).
b.	Cisplatin.
c.	L-Asparaginase.
d.	Cyclophosphamide.

_____ Tubular necrosis.
_____ Hemorrhagic cystitis.
_____ Tubular precipitation.

10. All of the following statements regarding bone marrow transplantation are true except:
    a. The most common indications are acute myelogenous leukemia and acute lymphoblastic leukemia in remission.
    b. In patients who receive allogeneic bone marrow transplantation, the mortality rate is 20–35%.
    c. The risk periods for pneumonitis and pulmonary insufficiency are 2 weeks, 6–12 weeks, and 3–6 months after bone marrow transplantation.
    d. Cytomegalovirus infection is most common 6 months after a bone marrow transplant.
    e. Cyclosporin may prevent acute rejection.

11. Match the chemotherapy drug with its mechanism of action:

a.	Methotrexate.	d.	Cyclophosphamide.
b.	Vincristine.	e.	Glucocorticoids.
c.	Doxorubicin.		

_____ Antimetabolite.
_____ Breaks DNA strands.
_____ Inhibits microtubule function.
_____ Antibiotic.
_____ Lymphocytotoxic.

12. A 5-year-old girl has prolonged bleeding after a tooth is pulled by her dentist. Additionally, her 16-year-old sister has protracted monthly menses of 7–9 days. You suspect von Willebrand's disease. Which of the following statements regarding the coagulation system is true?
    a. The prothrombin time measures the extrinsic and common pathways.

b. The activated partial thromboplastin time measures the intrinsic and common pathways.

c. The thrombin time measures the coagulation cascade from prothrombin to stable fibrin.

d. Factors XII, XI, IX, and X comprise the intrinsic system.

e. All of the above.

13. Select whether the following statements regarding the clotting system and blood products are true or false.

_____ a. The only source for Factors V and XI is fresh frozen plasma.

_____ b. The preferred source for Factors II, VII, X, and antithrombin III is cryoprecipitate.

_____ c. Cryoprecipitate contains fibrinogen, Factor VIII, and von Willebrand's factor.

_____ d. The main components of the antithrombotic system include antithrombin III, protein C, and protein S.

_____ e. Protein C induces proteolysis of Factors V and VIII, and neutralizes plasminogen activator inhibitor.

_____ f. Vitamin K-dependent factors include II, VII, IX, and X.

_____ g. Vitamin K is a vitamin that is stored in the body, and therefore no exogenous supplementation is necessary.

14. All of the following are the main components of the antithrombotic system except:
a. Antithrombin III.
b. Protein C.
c. Protein S.
d. Protein B.

15. An 11-month-old male with a history of biliary atresia has developed fulminant hepatic failure with gastrointestinal bleeding and bleeding from his central line site. You suspect a hepatic coagulopathy. Which of the following statements regarding this situation is true?

a. Dietary inadequacy and total parenteral nutrition are causes of vitamin K deficiency.

b. Fibrinogen, Factors V, VIII, and proteins C and S are depleted during disseminated intravascular coagulopathy.

c. In hepatic coagulopathy, a prolonged PT indicates decreased synthesis of vitamin K-dependent factors.

d. Factor V synthesis is independent of vitamin K availability.

e. All of the above.

16. Which of the following is a true statement regarding coagulopathy associated with cardiopulmonary bypass?

a. Protamine is used to potentiate heparinization.

b. Hyperfibrinogenolysis causing significant bleeding can be treated with epsilon aminocaproic acid intravenously.

c. Vitamin K deficiency is rarely a noted effect.

d. D-dimers are frequently elevated.

17. Which of the following is a true statement regarding coagulopathy associated with massive transfusion?

a. Hemolysis always occurs.

b. Platelet destruction occurs, necessitating platelet transfusion to maintain a platelet count of 80,000–100,000/mm^3.

c. Changing the transfusion circuit may temporarily reduce the activity of the coagulation cascade.

d. A, B and C.

e. B and C.

18. Which of the following biochemical changes is least likely to be associated with massive transfusion?

a. Disseminated intravascular coagulopathy.

b. Abnormal platelet function.

c. An increase in 2,3-diphosphoglycerate.

d. Hyperkalemia.

e. Hypothermia and metabolic acidosis.

19. Which of the following regarding antithrombin III and heparin is true?

a. Antithrombin III is synthesized in the liver and inhibits thrombin and factor Xa.

b. Acquired antithrombin III deficiency is more common than the autosomal-dominant inherited congenital type.

c. Antithrombin III concentrations less than 70% are associated with thromboses.

d. Heparin-induced antiplatelet antibodies occur in approximately 5% of patients receiving heparin.

e. All of the above.

20. Which of the following statements is true regarding heparin-induced antiplatelet antibodies?

a. Typically occur 4–15 days after first exposure to heparin.

b. Typically occur 1–9 days following the second exposure to heparin.

c. Are associated with thromboses.

d. All of the above.

21. Which of the following statements is true regarding protein C and protein S anticoagulant systems?
    a. Protein C is a vitamin K dependent protease which is produced by the liver.
    b. Protein C is deactivated by thrombin.
    c. Protein C is catalyzed by thrombomodulin.
    d. Protein C deficiency is most commonly an acquired abnormality, rather than a congenital one.
    e. A, C, and D.

22. Which of the following statements regarding fibrinolytic therapy is true?
    a. Streptokinase is produced by β-streptococci; it attaches to plasminogen and is subsequently rapidly inactivated by naturally occurring antibodies with a half life of 30 minutes.
    b. Urokinase can be produced from human urine; it hydrolyzes plasminogen to plasmin with a half-life of 30 minutes.
    c. Tissue plasminogen activator is produced in vascular endothelium; it converts plasminogen to plasmin.
    d. Absolute contraindications to fibrinolytic therapy include acute hemorrhage, recent cerebral vascular accident, and aneurysm.
    e. All of the above.

23. A 1-week-old infant undergoes a cardiac catheterization for a diagnosis of a cardiac defect. His right femoral artery is cannulated. After the procedure, his right leg is cold and his femoral pulse is barely palpable. You suspect a thrombus. Which of the following statements are true regarding thrombolytic therapy?
    a. Heparinization is standard management until recannulization or vascular integrity improves.
    b. Partial thromboplastin time should be 2.5–3.0 times normal during heparin therapy.
    c. Streptokinase and tissue plasminogen activator are contraindicated for femoral artery spasm after catheterization.

    d. Indications for surgical intervention of pulmonary emboli include pulmonary artery cross-sectional obstruction greater than 50%, right ventricular failure, or shock.
    e. A and D.

24. Which of the following is/are true statements regarding chronic anticoagulation therapy?
    a. Warfarin inhibits synthesis of Factors II, VII, IX, X, protein C, and protein S.
    b. Platelet aggregation is decreased by blocking the synthesis of thromboxane A_2 with cyclooxygenase inhibitors.
    c. Sulfinpyrazone or aspirin may be used.
    d. Platelet aggregation is decreased by administration of a phosphodiesterase inhibitor.
    e. All of the above.

25. Match the following drug with its site of action.

    | a. Aspirin. | c. Both. |
    | b. Sulfinpyrazone. | d. Neither. |

    _____ Cyclo-oxygenase inhibition.
    _____ Phosphodiesterase inhibition.
    _____ Irreversibly bound to thromboxane A_2.

26. All of the following regarding thrombosis of prosthetic valves are true except:
    a. Biological valves are less thromboembolic than mechanical valves.
    b. Mitral valves are more thromboembolic than aortic valves.
    c. Recommendations by the National Heart, Lung, and Blood Institute for mechanical valves include long-term anticoagulation.
    d. Thromboprophylaxis for prosthetic valves in pediatric patients does not decrease the occurrence of acute thromboembolic effects.

6   Renal System

The following chapter will focus on the renal system. Pertinent questions, answers, and rationale will be reviewed. Answers for this chapter can be found beginning on page 132.

Key Words: Diuretics; kidney failure; bypass; hypovolemia; filtration.

1. The risk of development of acute renal failure after cardiac surgery is highest in:
   a. Neonates.
   b. Infants.
   c. Children.
   d. Adults.

2. Which of the following causes vasodilation of the cortical vasculature?
   a. Mannitol.
   b. Furosemide.
   c. Both.
   d. Neither.

3. Clinical settings in which mannitol has definitely been shown to be effective in preventing the deterioration of renal function is:
   a. During and after cardiopulmonary bypass.
   b. During and after aortic cross-clamping.
   c. During and after hypovolemic shock.
   d. Before the administration of cisplatin.
   e. None of the above.

4. A neonate with gastroschisis underwent surgical repair and was subsequently admitted to the neonatal intensive care unit for postoperative care. Anuria has persisted for 8 hours in spite of aggressive fluid resuscitation to a central venous pressure of 12 mmHg. The echocardiogram shows normal myocardial function, and abdominal ultrasound does not show any evidence of urinary outflow obstruction. The complete blood count is within normal limits, and urinalysis does not show any hematuria or sediments. The most likely explanation for the anuria is:
   a. Acute tubular degeneration.
   b. Acute cortical necrosis.
   c. Increased intra-abdominal pressure.
   d. Dysplastic kidneys.
   e. None of the above.

5. Which of the following statements is least accurate regarding acute renal failure?
   a. Adults with no underlying renal disease who develop acute renal failure have a worse prognosis compared with children.
   b. Following cardiac surgery, the incidence of acute renal failure is higher in children than in adults.
   c. Children over the age of 2 years with acute renal failure have a much better outlook with meticulous medical care.
   d. Spontaneous recovery from acute renal failure is likely to begin 1–3 weeks after onset.
   e. The mortality rate for children with acute renal failure is much higher than in adults.

6. The earliest electrocardiogram changes of an elevated serum K^+ is:
   a. First-degree atrioventricular block and peaked T-wave.
   b. Widened QRS complex and peaked T-wave.
   c. Absent P-waves, wide QRS, and peaked T-wave.
   d. Shortened QT interval.
   e. None of the above.

7. Which of the following statements is true regarding management of suspected acute renal failure?
   a. In euvolemic patients, the rapid intravenous administration of mannitol should result in a urine output greater than 0.5 mL/kg within 1 hour if a prerenal etiology dominates.
   b. The vasodilatory and natriuretic properties of furosemide are beneficial when administered early in the course of acute renal failure.
   c. In euvolemic patients, furosemide in an incremental dose of up to 10 mg/kg may be used.
   d. If there is no response to a fluid challenge, low-dose dopamine could be added.
   e. All of the above.

From: *Pediatric Critical Care Review*
Edited by: R. A. Hasan and M. D. Pappas © Humana Press Inc., Totowa, NJ

8. In a patient who has just been admitted to the pediatric intensive care unit with new onset of acute renal failure, which of the following pathophysiological changes is least likely to occur?
   a. Blood urea nitrogen (BUN) and creatinine will rise at 10 and 0.5 mg/dL/day, respectively.
   b. Serum HCO_3 decreases by 2 mEq/L/day because of release of tissue phosphate.
   c. Serum K^+ increases by 0.3–0.5 mEq/L/day.
   d. Hypernatremia is commonly observed.
   e. Hypophosphatemia and associated hypocalcemia may develop rapidly after the onset of acute renal failure.

9. Which of the following is least appropriate in the treatment of acute renal failure?
   a. Treatment of hyperkalemia.
   b. Aggressive treatment of hypocalcemia in the absence of tetany.
   c. Treatment of hyperphosphatemia with calcium carbonate or lactate.
   d. Early institution of dialysis in patients with hemolytic-uremic syndrome.
   e. Aggressive correction of respiratory acidosis.

10. Which of the following statements least accurately describes the process of dialysis?
    a. When compared with HCO_3, acetate dialysis is characterized by greater hemodynamic stability.
    b. To prevent the dysequilibrium syndrome, mannitol may be administered in the first hour of an acute dialysis in patients with BUN greater than 150 mg/dL.
    c. Hemodialysis seems to be more efficient than peritoneal dialysis in decreasing blood uric acid when it is the etiological factor in acute renal failure.
    d. The efficacy of peritoneal dialysis is greatest in infants, compared with children and adults.
    e. The dysequilibrium syndrome results from a rapid decline in serum osmolality caused by the overly rapid removal of solutes from the circulation, and manifests itself as seizures.

11. Correct statements regarding the "dysequilibrium syndrome" include all of the following except:
    a. Can be prevented by limiting the rate of flow through the hemodialysis to approximately 4 mL/kg/minute.
    b. Can be prevented by limiting the total dialysis time to 2 hours at the initiation of hemodialysis.
    c. Can be prevented by using a dialysate with a higher Na^+ concentration.
    d. Is seen with the same frequency with peritoneal dialysis compared with hemodialysis.

12. Which of the following options is not true regarding nutritional support of patients with acute renal failure?

> a. Supplementation of calories from carbohydrate, protein, and fat spares the breakdown of endogenous protein and minimizes the need for dialysis.
> b. Higher amounts of B-complex vitamins are required.
> c. Vitamin C intake should be increased to 1000 mg/day.
> d. Providing a hypertonic glucose and amino acids solution is more beneficial than glucose alone.

    a. Renal failure caused by rapidly progressive glomerulonephritis.
    b. Postoperative renal failure.
    c. Both.
    d. Neither.

13. True or false?
    _____ Hypertension with hypertensive encephalopathy is common.

14. Calculation of the loading dose of gentamycin to be used in the treatment of gram negative urinary tract infection in a 6-year-old girl depends on:
    a. Desired plasma concentration and volume of distribution.
    b. Volume of distribution and clearance.
    c. Clearance and desired plasma concentration.
    d. Plasma half-life and volume of distribution.
    e. Plasma half-life and clearance.

15. The most appropriate therapeutic intervention for severe hypercalcemia is:
    a. Intravenous dimercaprol.
    b. Oral dimercaprol.
    c. Intravenous ethelene diamine tetraacetic acid.
    d. Intravenous furosemide.
    e. Hydrochlorothiazide.

16. Match the following drug with its most likely effect.

> a. Captopril.
> b. Enalapril.
> c. Both.
> d. Neither.

_____ Pruritus, rash, and eosinophilia.
_____ Temporary loss of taste.
_____ Initial severe hypotensive response.
_____ Inhibits the breakdown of bradykinin.
_____ Postural hypotension and reflex tachycardia.
_____ Neutropenia.

17. Which of the following is the most accurate statement regarding the perioperative management of a patient with end-stage renal disease who is undergoing cadaveric kidney transplantation?
    a. Acute preoperative dialysis should be performed since very high BUN is undesirable postoperatively.
    b. Postoperatively, high normal intravascular volume (central venous pressure 10–15 mmHg) should be avoided because of loss of autoregulation in the cadaveric kidney.
    c. Preoperative transfusion to a hematocrit of 40% is essential.
    d. After the clamps are released, a dose of furosemide (1–2 mg/kg) is useful in inducing renal vasodilatation and solute diuresis.
    e. Cadaveric transplant survival is reduced in patients who have received multiple blood transfusions.

18. Which of the following statements is true regarding the relationship between transfusion of blood products and graft survival in the recipients of cadaveric kidney transplantation?
    a. Graft survival improves with increasing number of blood transfusions received.
    b. The positive effect of transfusion on the graft is greatest with packed red blood cells and whole blood transfusion.
    c. Patients receiving intraoperative transfusions have some improvement in survival, compared with patients who do not receive transfusions.
    d. All of the above.
    e. None of the above.

19. Match the diagnosis(es) below with the most likely effect(s).

> a. Hemolytic uremic syndrome.
> b. Disseminated intravascular coagulopathy.
> c. Both.
> d. Neither.

_____ Increased platelet consumption.
_____ Deficiency of prostaglandin I_2 activity.

20. Degradation of atracurium is primarily via:
    a. Hepatic conjugation.
    b. Renal excretion unchanged.
    c. Ester hydrolysis.
    d. Hoffman degradation.

21. Which of the following statements is true regarding adjustment of drug dosage for renal failure?
    a. Adjustment of dosage is not indicated for drugs with a very wide therapeutic range, such as penicillins, unless renal failure is profound.
    b. Adjustment for drugs with a narrow therapeutic index is not indicated unless renal function is less than 70% of normal.
    c. Dosage adjustments of less than or equal to 25% are not worthwhile.
    d. When f (fraction filtered unchanged by kidneys) is less than 25%, the adjustment for renal failure is not necessary unless nonrenal routes of elimination are also decreased.
    e. All of the above.

22. The letters in the figure below represent the site of action for the medications listed below. Match the medications to their appropriate site(s) of action.

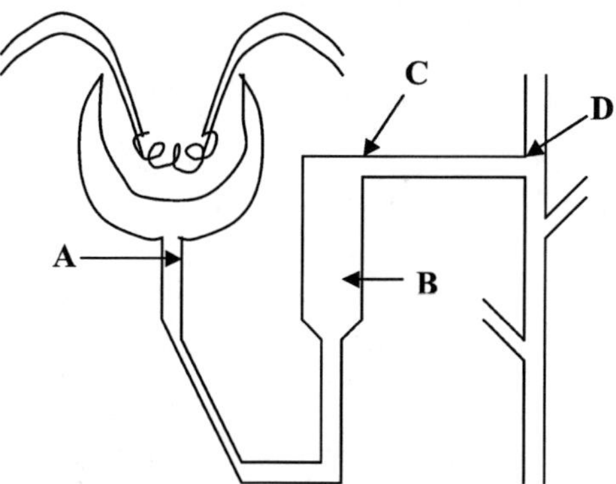

_____ 1. Furosemide.
_____ 2. Chlorothiazide.
_____ 3. Spironolactone.
_____ 4. Mannitol.

23. A 6-month-old infant presents with generalized tonic-clonic seizures and is poorly responsive to intravenous lorazepam and phenytoin. The trachea is intubated and he has been admitted to the pediatric intensive care uint on mechanical ventilation. Physical examination shows a heart rate of 95 beats per minute, blood pressue of 90/65 mmHg, and capillary refill is 3 seconds. Examination of genitalia is within normal limits. Laboratory analysis shows: Na 114, K 3.9, Cl 88, total CO_2 20 mEq/L. Urine specific gravity is 1.008, urine osmolality is 288 mOsmol/L and urine Na is 20 mEq/L. No urinary sediments are seen. BUN is 10 mg%, creatinine is 0.5 mg%, and blood glucose is 95 mg%.

24. The most likely diagnosis is:
    a. Syndrome of inappropriate antidiuretic hormone secretion.
    b. Severe dehydration.
    c. Acute cortical necrosis.
    d. Water intoxication.
    e. Congenital adrenal hyperplasia.

25. The most appropriate initial intervention is:
    a. 3% NaCl.
    b. Antidiuretic hormone.
    c. Cortisol.
    d. Dialysis.
    e. Massive fluid resuscitation.

7
Endocrine System

The following chapter will focus on the endocrine system. Pertinent questions, answers, and rationale will be reviewed. Answers for this chapter can be found beginning on page 134.

Key Words: Ketosis; cerebral edema; diabetes; coma; osmolality.

1. Diabetic ketoacidosis is a potentially life-threatening medical condition that complicates insulin-dependent diabetes. A true statement regarding diabetic ketoacidosis is:
   a. The metabolic acidosis is a ketoacidosis and, hence, is always a high anion gap metabolic acidosis.
   b. The degree of acidosis is closely related to the degree of hyperglycemia.
   c. The degree of anion gap bears no relationship to the degree of azotemia.
   d. Patients presenting with diabetic ketoacidosis and a normal anion gap recover from acidosis more rapidly if bicarbonate is used in place of chloride in the intravenous fluids.
   e. Because diabetic ketoacidosis is a catabolic state, it is accompanied by a shift of extracellular phosphate into the intracellular space.

2. In children with established insulin-dependent diabetes, the most common precipitating factor for diabetic ketoacidosis is:
   a. Inadvertent or deliberate omission of insulin.
   b. Severe emotional stress.
   c. Infection.
   d. Use of drugs.
   e. None of the above.

3. The degree of cerebral obtundation during diabetic ketoacidosis correlates most closely with the degree of:
   a. Hyperosmolality.
   b. Hyponatremia.
   c. Acidosis.
   d. Hypophosphatemia.
   e. Hyperapnea.

4. A 4-year-old with insulin-dependent diabetes presented to the emergency department with fever and Kussmaul respirations. Blood glucose is 600 mg/dL and arterial blood gases show a pH of 7.1, bicarbonate of 7 mEq/L, and serum sodium is 129 mEq/L. Therapy with intravenous saline (0.9 NaCl) and insulin is initiated. Within a few hours clouded sensorium is noted. Appropriate statements pertaining to this clinical scenario include:
   a. Deepening coma during diabetic ketoacidosis treatment is more likely in children.
   b. Antibiotics should be given during the initial resuscitation phase in this patient.
   c. If the patient's neurological status fails to improve, a cranial computed tomography scan of the head needs to be done.
   d. Intracranial pressure monitoring need not be instituted at this time.
   e. All of the above.

5. Which of the following has been shown to occur in proportion to the severity of brain injury?
   a. Hyperglycemia.
   b. Coagulopathy.
   c. Both.
   d. Neither.

6. Hypoglycemia is a life-threatening medical emergency that requires immediate attention. One measure used is the administration of glucagon. Glucagon is likely to be effective against hypoglycemia in which of the following clinical conditions?
   a. Starvation.
   b. Ketotic hypoglycemia.
   c. Glycogen storage disease.
   d. Cirrhosis with hepatocellular failure.
   e. None of the above.

From: *Pediatric Critical Care Review*
Edited by: R. A. Hasan and M. D. Pappas © Humana Press Inc., Totowa, NJ

7. Which of the following statements is true regarding hypoglycemia in newborns, infants, and children?
   a. A neonate may need up to 20 mg/kg/minute of glucose in the perioperative period to maintain normoglycemia.
   b. Hepatic glycogen stores fall by 90% in the first 3 postnatal hours.
   c. Hypoglycemia caused by documented high insulin levels that are resistant to medical therapy, warrants a consideration for laparotomy.
   d. Ketotic hypoglycemia is the most common form of childhood hypoglycemia.
   e. All of the above.

8. Which of the following statements is inaccurate regarding water homeostasis?
   a. The maximum effect of arginine–vasopressin is to produce a urine osmolality of 1400 mOsmol/L and a urine output of 0.5 mL/kg/hour.
   b. In the absence of arginine–vasopressin, urine flow will stabilize at 5 mL/kg/hour and an osmolality of 300 mOsmol/L.
   c. An infusion of DDAVP should be initiated as soon as the diagnosis of diabetes insipidus is made with the goal of establishing a urine osmolality double that of plasma, and a urine output of 2 mL/kg/hour.
   d. In the setting of global cerebral insult, the development of diabetes insipidus will most likely be followed by death in 1–5 days.
   e. In the absence of osmotic diuretics, urine osmolality of less than 300 mOsmol/L when the serum osmolality is greater than 295 mOsmol/L is highly suggestive of diabetes insipidus.

9. Match the diagnosis with its most likely description below:

a. Diabetes insipidus.
b. Osmotic diuresis.
c. Nonoliguric renal failure.
d. Fluid overload.

   _____ Urine osmolality is 268 mOsmol/L and plasma osmolality is 327 mOsmol/L.
   _____ Polyuria with a urine specific gravity of 1.008 and a plasma osmolality of 275 mOsmol/L.
   _____ Urine osmolality of 297 mOsmol/L and plasma osmolality of 299 mOsmol/L.
   _____ Fraction of excretion of sodium is equal to 3.

10. Match the most likely diagnosis with the following urine measurements.

	Urine $Na+$ (mEq/L)	FE_{NA+} (%)	Urine osmolality	Urine/Plasma osmolality
a.	<10	<1	>500	>1.59
b.	>60	>2.98	298	1.008
c.	>80	>1.98	695	2

    _____ Rotavirus gastroenteritis with profuse diarrhea.
    _____ Hemolytic uremic syndrome.
    _____ Syndrome of inappropriate anti-diuretic hormone secretion.

11. A newborn is admitted to the pediatric intenstive care unit (PICU) for hypoglycemia. Physical examination is significant for hepatomegaly. The urine does not reveal ketonuria and toxic screening is reported to be negative. The most likely etiology for this patient is:
    a. Endocrinopathies.
    b. Storage disease.
    c. Chemicals or toxins.
    d. Ketotic hypoglycemia.

12. Precautions that must be taken when measuring ionized calcium include all of the following except:
    a. Blood must be collected aerobically.
    b. Blood must be collected anaerobically.
    c. Red blood cells must be quickly removed.
    d. Anticoagulants that complex with calcium must be avoided.

13. With regard to hypercalcemia in the PICU, all of the following statements are true except:
    a. Lack of weight-bearing is the most important factor in the hypercalcemia associated with immobility, and is more severe in children.
    b. Total serum calcium of less than 15 mg% is regarded as not acutely life-threatening.
    c. Hypercalcemia is protective against digitalis toxicity.
    d. When hyperparathyroidism is suspected as the etiology of the hypercalcemia, mithromycin should be avoided if surgery is anticipated.
    e. When using phosphate for treatment of hypercalcemia, the product of the concentration of calcium and phosphorus should be kept below 60.

14. A 9-year-old boy is admitted to the PICU with hypocalcemia with an ionized calcium level of 0.7 mmol/L. The hypocalcemia has been resistant to administration of repeated doses of intravenous calcium chloride. Under these circumstances, which of the following management strategies would be considered least appropriate?
    a. Hypomagnesemia must be considered.
    b. Hypoparathyroidism must be considered.
    c. Vitamin D insufficiency must be considered.
    d. $MgSO_4$ is preferred to $MgCl$ in this setting.
    e. Rapid magnesium infusion leads to a poor clinical response because peak magnesium level is associated with a peak in renal excretion.

15. Appropriate statements regarding treatment of hypomagnesemia in the intensive care setting include all of the following except:
    a. The daily requirement is in the range of 0.3–0.4 mEq/kg/day intravenously.
    b. If the glomerular filtration rate is reduced, magnesium replacement may result in hypermagnesemia.
    c. Intravenous magnesium is best delivered as a rapid bolus to achieve a high peak serum level.
    d. Aminoglycosides are a recognized cause of hypomagnesemia.

16. Clearance of which of the following drugs is dependent on hepatic blood flow?
    a. Propranolol and labetalol.
    b. Lidocaine and nitroglycerine.
    c. Morphine and verapamil.
    d. All of the above.
    e. None of the above.

17. Which of the following is the most appropriate statement regarding intravenous steroid preparations?
    a. Dexamethasone has the largest sodium retaining property, and hydrocortisone the least.
    b. When anti-inflammatory properties and relative hypovolemia are desired, dexamethasone is the agent of choice.
    c. The anti-inflammatory properties of hydrocortisone do not increase when higher doses of hydrocortisone are used.

d. For the patient in shock and adrenal insufficiency, hydrocortisone is inappropriate.
    e. Synthetic steroids compared with hydrocortisone are more avidly protein-bound and undergo faster hepatic degradation.

18. Match the disease process with the correct association.

    > a. Congenital adrenal hypoplasia.
    > b. Pyloric stenosis.
    > c. Both.
    > d. Neither.

    _____ Hyponatremia.
    _____ Metabolic acidosis.
    _____ Emergency administration of "stress" doses of glucocorticoids is unlikely to be detrimental.

19. Drugs known to cause adrenal suppression include:
    a. Ketoconazole.
    b. Bactrim®
    c. Etomidate.
    d. All of the above.

20. A 12-year-old is admitted to the PICU with intractable shock and a poor response to volume administration. You suspect adrenal insufficiency. All of the following statements pertaining to this diagnosis are true except:
    a. With long-term steroid use, hypothalamic–pituitary–adrenal axis suppression can be minimized by steroid administration in the morning.
    b. Reliable evidence regarding adrenal suppression can be obtained by the 30-minute adrenocorticotropic hormone stimulation test.
    c. Clinically significant hypothalamic–pituitary–adrenal axis suppression does not occur with prolonged use of 12 mg/m^2/day of cortisol.
    d. Dexamethasone administration will interfere with subsequent measurement of cortisol.
    e. Methyl prednisolone interferes with the protein displacement method but not with the common radioimmune assay method of cortisol determination.

8 Nutrition and the Gastrointestinal System

The following chapter will focus on the gastrointestinal system and nutrition. Pertinent questions, answers, and rationale will be reviewed. Answers for this chapter can be found beginning on page 136.

Key Words: Calories; enteral; hyperalimentation; liver; stomach; intestine.

1. Which of the following statements regarding nutritional needs in infants and children is inaccurate?
   a. Storage of fat may constitute as much as 20% of gross body weight in normal infants.
   b. There are two essential fats: linoleic and linolenic acid.
   c. Daily normal nitrogen losses include 2 mg of nitrogen per basal kcal, 20% in feces, and 10 mg/kg body weight from skin.
   d. Protein requirement in infants and children is approximately 2 g/kg/day.
   e. Fat requirement in infants is approximately 1 g/kg/day.

2. All of the following statements regarding starvation are true except:
   a. Only glycogen, which is stored in the liver, is available for transport to the central nervous system.
   b. As glucose levels fall, insulin levels decrease.
   c. Ketonemia inhibits pyruvate dehydrogenase, and thus blocks glucose-derived substrate from entering the Krebs cycle.
   d. The ebb phase, followed by the flow phase, are characteristic features.

3. Which of the following statements are true regarding stressed starvation or hypermetabolism?
   a. Ebb phase is associated with an increase in metabolic rate.
   b. Flow phase corresponds to the period of hypermetabolism.
   c. Hypoglycemia is the hallmark of stressed metabolism.
   d. Peripheral oxidation of lipids is decreased.
   e. Enhanced and increased sensitivity to the effect of insulin on glucose uptake is noted.

4. After several days of starvation, the levels of which of the following continue to rise?
   a. Serum insulin.
   b. Serum ketones.
   c. Serum glucose.
   d. Urinary nitrogen excretion.

5. Match the following metabolic fuel with its respiratory quotient.

   | a. Carbohydrate. |
   | b. Fat. |
   | c. Protein. |

   ____ 0.7.
   ____ 0.8.
   ____ 1.0.

6. Preventive measures against stress ulceration in the intensive care unit (ICU) does not include which of the following?
   a. Enteral feeding of an elemental diet.
   b. H_2-blocker administration by continuous infusion.
   c. Hourly anti-acid administration enterally.
   d. Administration of sucralfate enterally.
   e. Administration of gastrin.

7. An elemental diet has been utilized in the prevention of stress ulceration in the ICU. Which one of the following statements is not a proposed mechanism by which enteral feeding protects against stress ulceration?
   a. Accelerating turnover of gastric mucosal cells.
   b. Releasing the hormone gastrin.
   c. Buffering gastric acid and maintaining a gastric pH greater than 4.0.
   d. Releasing cholecystokinin and catecholamines, such as norepinephrine.

From: *Pediatric Critical Care Review*
Edited by: R. A. Hasan and M. D. Pappas © Humana Press Inc., Totowa, NJ

8. A 9-year-old boy, a victim of a motor vehicle accident with a closed head injury, is in the pediatric ICU (PICU). Brisk fresh blood along with some coffee ground material is retrieved from the nasogastric tube. The procedure that is least helpful in the management of this patient is:
   a. Gastric lavage.
   b. Endoscopy.
   c. Arteriography.
   d. Upper gastrointestinal series.

9. Endoscopy in the patient from Question 8 revealed diffuse gastritis diagnosed as "stress gastritis." Which of the following statements most accurately describes the clinical course and management of this patient?
   a. A satisfactory clinical response to gastric lavage and hemodynamic support.
   b. H_2-blockers stop bleeding faster than lavage alone.
   c. Anti-acids stop bleeding faster than lavage alone.
   d. Prostaglandin analogs, such as Enprostil, have been shown to be superior to all other traditional measures combined.

10. Paralytic ileus is a common problem after laparotomy. Which of the following statements pertaining to this phenomenon is least accurate?
    a. Vasopressin is released during laparotomy and contributes to decreased small bowel contractility.
    b. Hypokalemia appears to exert its effects by interfering with the release of acetylcholine from the presynaptic area when serum K^+ is less than 2.5 mEq/L.
    c. The colon is the portion of the gut most sensitive to anesthesia-induced inhibition of motility, because it is most dependent on neural controls to achieve motility.
    d. The role that handling or direct manipulation of the gut plays in the development of ileus is very well established.

11. Ogilvies Syndrome (localized ileus or pseudo-obstruction) is associated with all of the following conditions except:
    a. Cholecystitis.
    b. Pancreatitis.
    c. Intra-abdominal abscess.
    d. Lower lobe pneumonia.
    e. Torus fracture.

12. Postoperative intussusception is a problem that is sometimes overlooked in the postoperative period in patients with evidence of gastrointestinal obstruction. True statements pertaining to this entity include all of the following except:
    a. A granulocytic leukocytosis of major proportions may be seen.
    b. Usually appears within the first postoperative week.
    c. Requires surgical correction.
    d. Usually ileocecal.
    e. Difficult to diagnose because symptoms are masked by nasogastric suctioning and the use of postoperative pain medications.

13. Which part of the gastrointestinal tract is most sensitive to inhibition of motility by anesthesia, with consequent development of ileus in the postoperative period?
    a. Stomach.   d. Ileum.
    b. Duodenum.   e. Colon.
    c. Jejunum.

14. Which of the following statements is least accurate regarding management of postoperative ileus?
    a. If the cecum is dilated to more than 12 cm in diameter, a definite risk of perforation exists even in the absence of mechanical obstruction.
    b. Nasointestinal intubation with decompression remains the only effective proven therapy.
    c. Passage of flatus and/or a bowel movement herald the end of the ileus.
    d. Neostigmine is a very effective and safe therapeutic intervention without any recognized side effects.

15. Inadequate blood flow and impaired oxygenation have deleterious effects on the bowel. True statements regarding these physiological derangements include:
    a. In the small bowel, O_2 delivery is least to the tip of the villi.
    b. Inability to absorb glucose has been reported for several months in infants who have sustained severe anoxia at birth.
    c. Impaired blood flow with subsequent dilatation of bowel loops is associated with bacterial overgrowth which is known to lead to fat malabsorption.
    d. All of the above.

16. A 5-year-old boy who was admitted to the PICU over 1 week ago is recovering from multiple organ dysfunction syndrome. He has had frequent diarrheal stools throughout the day. From a therapeutic standpoint, which of the following would be the most appropriate initial diagnostic test?
    a. Stool culture for corona virus.
    b. Eliza test for rotavirus.
    c. *Clostridium difficile* toxin assay.
    d. Small bowel radiographic imaging series.
    e. Sigmoido-colonoscopy with biopsy.

17. Which of the following most accurately describes the laboratory findings in acute pancreatitis?
    a. The degree of elevation of serum amylase closely correlates with the severity of acute pancreatitis.
    b. Serum lipase levels tend to be elevated for a shorter period than serum amylase levels.
    c. Pancreatic trypsinogen serum levels rise early in the course of pancreatitis and remain elevated for up to 5 days.
    d. One of the ominous prognostic signs is hypercarbia.
    e. All of the above.

18. Which of the following symptoms is least likely to be associated with Reye's Syndrome?
    a. Bleeding.
    b. Cerebral edema.
    c. Coma.
    d. Jaundice.

19. Patients who develop fulminant hepatic failure as a result of Hepatitis B infection when compared with patients who do not develop hepatic failure have which of the following serological characteristics?
    a. Later appearance of antibodies to the Hepatitis B surface antigen.
    b. Later appearance of antibodies to the Hepatitis E antigen.
    c. More rapid clearance of Hepatitis B antigen.
    d. All of the above.

20. With regard to management of fulminant hepatic failure with coma, all of the following statements describe the appropriate clinical picture and management except:
    a. A single toxicology screening test on admission should be obtained to rule out other treatable causes of encephalopathy with coma.
    b. Hyponatremia because of an antidiuretic hormone-like effect and hypokalemia resulting from hyperaldosteronism are recognized electrolyte abnormalities that require meticulous correction.
    c. Arterial ammonia levels are useful in confirming a hepatic origin to the coma.
    d. Fatty acid emulsion should be used liberally to provide calories and help clear the encephalopathy.

Questions 21–23: A 3-year-old boy with history of biliary atresia and Kassai procedure is admitted to the PICU with vomiting of fresh blood of 20 minutes' duration. Examination reveals a diaphoretic child with tachycardia. He has vomited several ounces of fresh blood during the period of time that he was being admitted to the PICU.

21. Appropriate therapeutic interventions for this patient include all of the following except:
    a. Saline gastric lavage.
    b. Fresh frozen plasma.
    c. Volume expanders.
    d. Because sodium retention may lead to anasarca, saline administration should be withheld in these patients in spite of marginal blood pressure.

22. If the bleeding in this patient persists, the next step in the management process would be:
    a. Portosystemic anastomosis.
    b. Variceal banding.
    c. Endoscopy.
    d. Vagotomy.

23. The above patient underwent sclerotherapy. Potential complications include:
    a. Rebleeding from gastric varices.
    b. Fever.
    c. Ulceration.
    d. Stricture.
    e. All of the above.

24. Hypoxia is observed in up to 40% of patients with hepatic failure. Factors that contribute to hypoxia include all of the following except:
    a. Neurogenic pulmonary edema.
    b. An antidiuretic hormone-like effect leading to fluid overload.
    c. Intrapulmonary shunting.
    d. Patent foramen ovale.

Questions 25–27: An 8-year-old male with cirrhosis of the liver caused by congenital biliary atresia is on the waiting list for liver transplantation.

25. Prolonged use of ibuprofen in this patient results in:
    a. Water retention.
    b. Dilutional hyponatremia.
    c. Ascites resistant to diuretics.
    d. All of the above.

26. The patient develops oliguria with urine output decreasing to 300 mL/day. Central venous pressure is 8 mmHg. Blood urea nitrogen is 60 mg% and urinalysis does not show red blood cell or while blood cell casts. Urine electrolytes: sodium level is 9 mEq/L, potassium is 5.8 mEq/L, and chloride is 10 mEq/L. Urine osmolality is 310 mOsmol/L. The most likely diagnosis is:
    a. Prerenal azotemia as a result of hypovolemia.
    b. Hepatorenal syndrome.
    c. Acute tubular necrosis.
    d. Acute cortical necrosis.
    e. None of the above.

27. Preventive measures that have been shown to be helpful for the clinical condition described in Question 26 include all of the following measures except:
    a. Avoiding large volume paracentesis.
    b. Avoiding use of potent diuretics.
    c. Use of dopamine at 6 mg/kg/minute.
    d. In the event that this diagnosis is suspected, intravascular volume expansion suing salt-poor albumin to raise the central venous pressure to 10 mmHg is a helpful preventative measure.
    e. Avoiding use of prostaglandin antagonists.

28. Which of the following statements pertaining to hepatic encephalopathy is most accurate?
    a. All patients with hepatic encephalopathy have elevated serum ammonia levels.
    b. The height of ammonia correlates with the grade of encephalopathy.
    c. Arterial and venous ammonia correlate equally with the degree of encephalopathy.
    d. Plasma octopamine levels have been shown to always inversely correlate with the degree of encephalopathy.
    e. None of the above.

29. A 10-month-old boy with end-stage liver disease from biliary atresia (that was not recognized in early infancy) is admitted to the PICU with lethargy. Appropriate intervention that is expected to improve the clinical status of the patient include:
    a. Reduction of protein intake.
    b. Use of oral lactulose.
    c. Use of oral neomycin.
    d. Use of hypertonic glucose.
    e. All of the above.

30. A 7-year-old with fulminant hepatic failure is admitted to the PICU because he has become progressively more difficult to arouse. Physical examination reveals a child who responds to painful stimuli by moaning. Increased tone in the extremities is noted, and pupils are dilated and react sluggishly to light. Correct statements pertaining to this patient include all of the following except:
    a. Inappropriate pathological cerebral vascular tone and altered permeability of the blood–brain barrier are contributing to this patient's symptomatology.
    b. Intracranial pressure monitoring will facilitate management of this patient.
    c. A PCO_2 of more than 25 torr is associated with cerebral vasodilation and the level of consciousness correlates with the degree of respiratory alkalosis.
    d. Steroids have been shown to decrease mortality in this setting.
    e. If the patient progresses to decorticate posturing and becomes ventilator dependent, it is usually too late to initiate liver transplantation.

31. Statements pertaining to patients in fulminant hepatic failure that are true include:
    a. Rapid deterioration in the clinical course is an indication to contemplate liver transplantation.
    b. Patients with poor prognosis with chronic hepatitis secondary to hepatitis C should be considered for liver transplantation earlier.
    c. Patients with acetaminophen-induced fulminant hepatic failure have a better prognosis than fulminant hepatic failure because of viral hepatitis.
    d. Hemoperfusion is known to temporarily reverse coma in these patients.
    e. All of the above.

32. Match the following drug with its appropriate description:

a.	Cyclosporin.	d.	FK506.
b.	Azathioprine.	e.	Corticosteroids.
c.	OKT$_3$.		

_____ Inhibits purine nucleotidase.
_____ Selectively inhibits T-helper lymphocytes.
_____ A macrolide antibiotic.
_____ Pulmonary edema.
_____ Direct lymphocytotoxicity.

33. In which of the following clinical situations is right hemidiaphragmatic paralysis seen more often than left hemidiaphragmatic paralysis?
    a. Liver transplantation.
    b. Palliative repair of congenital heart disease.
    c. Both.
    d. Neither.

34. An 8-year-old boy who underwent liver transplantation last month from an ABO-compatible, non-identical recipient is admitted to the PICU for right lower lobe pneumonia. His hemoglobin is 5.4 g%, and the total bilirubin is 8 mg% (from 2 mg% 8 days ago). The alanine transaminase and aspartate transaminase are 38 IU/L and 48 IU/L, respectively. The reticulocyte count is 5%. Correct statements regarding this clinical situation include all of the following except:
    a. Serial reticulocyte counts are the most useful tool in following the progression of this patient's hematological problem.
    b. Haptoglobin is a valuable and useful test for this hematological problem.
    c. The patient should receive type O blood when transfusion is contemplated.
    d. This hematological condition usually resolves spontaneously in 2–4 weeks.
    e. Hemoglobinuria is a recognized feature.

35. Regarding hepatic clearance of medications, adjustment of drug dosage, and liver disease, true statements include all of the following except:
    a. Liver disease is usually homogenous and affects drug metabolism equally.
    b. In acute hepatic disease, clearance is more likely to affect drugs that undergo oxidation rather than those that undergo conjugation.
    c. In treating patients with liver disease, preference should be given to drugs that are metabolized through glucuronidation.
    d. Changes in protein binding are not likely to be clinically important when the bound fraction of the drug is less than 80%.
    e. For drugs that undergo efficient hepatic biotransformation, clearance of the drug is proportionate to liver blood flow.

36. Which of the following statements is least accurate with regard to nutritional support in children in the ICU?
    a. Hepatic cholestasis associated with parenteral nutrition responds favorably to providing some enteral nutrition.
    b. Glutamine, when added to parenteral nutrition, improves structure and function of the intestine towing to its trophic effects.
    c. Branched chain amino acids always resolve hepatic encephalopathy regardless of the etiology.
    d. Trophamine with 100 mg/kg body weight of L-lysine allows more of the calcium and phosphorus to be in solution, which is clinically relevant.
    e. Carbohydrate administration in excess of 14 mg/kg/minute exacerbates hepatic steatosis.

37. Serum proteins can be used as biochemical markers for nutritional status. Match the following markers with its approximate half-life.

a.	Albumin.	c.	Transferrin.
b.	Prealbumin.	d.	Retinal binding protein.

_____ 20 days.   _____ 8 days.
_____ 10 hours.   _____ 2 days.

38. The difference between medium-chain triglycerides (MCTs) and long-chain fat is that MCTs:
    a. Inhibit gastric emptying more so than long-chain fat.
    b. Are absorbed at a slower rate than long-chain fat.
    c. Are converted into energy faster than long-chain fat.
    d. Are absorbed via the lymphatic lacteals.
    e. None of the above.

39. Which of the following is true regarding nutrition in the critically ill child?
    a. Disaccharidase activity may be diminished after acute injury.
    b. Predigested protein (hydrolysates) formulas are the principal formulas recommended for critically ill infants.
    c. The presence of reducing substances in the stool indicates appropriate carbohydrate absorption.
    d. Long chain triglycerides are preferred over MCTs because of their faster absorption from the intestine.
    e. A and B only.

40. Stress ulcers are usually located in:
    a. The body of the stomach.
    b. The fundus of the stomach.
    c. The antrum of the stomach.
    d. The pylorus of the stomach.

41. All of the medications listed below will decrease gastric pH and its concentration except:
    a. Ranitidine.
    b. Famotidine.
    c. Sucralfate.
    d. Proton pump inhibitors.

42. A 15-year-old female is admitted to the PICU with severe hematemesis and hemodynamic instability. Immediate management should be:
    a. Intravenous normal saline followed by room temperature normal saline via gastric lavage.
    b. Prompt resuscitation of circulation with normal saline followed by ice-cold normal saline gastric lavage.
    c. Prompt resuscitation of circulation with normal saline followed by intravenous Ranitidine infusion.
    d. All of the above.

43. The major cause of death in patients with fulminant hepatic failure is:
    a. Sepsis.
    b. Variceal hemorrhage.
    c. Cerebral edema.
    d. The initial cause of fulminant hepatic failure.
    e. None of the above.

44. Complications of acute pancreatitis include all of the following except:
    a. Pancreatic necrosis.
    b. Glomerulonephritis.
    c. Adult respiratory distress syndrome.
    d. Pancreatic pseudocyst.

45. Toxic megacolon is most likely a complication of:
    a. Crohn's colitis.
    b. Pseudomembranous enterocolitis.
    c. Ischemic colitis.
    d. Ulcerative colitis.

46. A 15-year-old male with a known diagnosis of HIV is admitted to the PICU with severe abdominal pain, bloating sensation, fever, neutropenia and thrombocytopenia. Radiographical analysis shows a dilated cecum. Immediate medical treatment includes all of the following except:
    a. Nothing per mouth.
    b. Aggressive fluid management followed by total parenteral nutrition.
    c. Antibiotics.
    d. Colonoscopy.

9 Immunology

The following chapter will focus on immunology. Pertinent questions, answers, and rationale will be reviewed. Answers for this chapter can be found beginning on page 140.

Key Words: T-cell; B-cell; immunity; bacteria; complement; antibiotics.

1. Which of the following statements least accurately describes the pattern of immunoglobulins (Igs) in the fetus, infant, and child?
   a. The level of IgG in premature infants is directly proportional to gestational age in the preterm infant.
   b. IgG levels fall during the first 4 months of extrauterine life.
   c. Adult IgG levels are reached by 4–6 years of age.
   d. By 10 weeks of intrauterine life, the fetus is capable of producing IgM.
   e. IgA levels peak in children at 1 year of age.

2. Which of the following statements is true regarding the immunological system of the neonate?
   a. T- and B-cell immunity are intact in the neonate.
   b. Phagocytosis of the full-term newborn is normal.
   c. Bacterial killing by neutrophils is intact in otherwise healthy newborns.
   d. Complement activation products are sufficient in premature infants.

3. Match the following complement component with its corresponding activity.
   _____ C3a.   a. Anaphylatoxin.
   _____ C5b-C9.   b. Cell lysis by attacking the cell membrane.

4. Drugs and disease processes can affect immune function. Select whether the following statements are true or false.
   _____ a. Nitrous oxide (N_2O) suppresses both T- and B-cell functions.
   _____ b. Halothane enhances phagocytosis.
   _____ c. Pentobarbital decreases the circulating granulocyte count.
   _____ d. Morphine depresses leukocyte chemotaxis.
   _____ e. Creation of a surgical wound dramatically increases circulatory neutrophil count.
   _____ f. B- and T-lymphocyte blood levels increase in response to surgical stress.

5. Many viral infections produce less of a stress on the neonate compared with bacterial infections. However, some of the respiratory viral agents, such as respiratory syncytial virus and infectious diarrhea, remain prevalent throughout infancy. Which of the following statements most accurately explains this phenomenon?
   a. High IgM production by the neonate.
   b. Deficient secretory IgA.
   c. A tremendous ability of the neonate to localize infection.
   d. High ability of the infant to produce antibodies against polysaccharides.
   e. All of the above.

6. Which one of the following does not increase in response to major trauma?
   a. Prostaglandin E_2
   b. Primary response to immunization.
   c. Interleukin (IL)-6.
   d. Tumor necrosis factor-α.
   e. Transforming growth factor-β.

From: *Pediatric Critical Care Review*
Edited by: R. A. Hasan and M. D. Pappas © Humana Press Inc., Totowa, NJ

7. Both trauma and surgery can compromise the host, and make the host susceptible to bacterial overgrowth and infection. All of the following statements regarding infection in postsurgical patients are true except:
   a. Anaerobic Gram-negative organisms are the most common nosocomial infections.
   b. Majority of infections in trauma victims are nosocomial.
   c. Prophylactic antibiotics are of most benefit in injuries involving the large and small bowel, and in soft tissue crush injuries and extremity avulsion injuries.
   d. When colonic contamination is possible, recommended antibiotics are aminoglycoside and clindamycin.
   e. Ampicillin provides an effective coverage against enterococci.

8. Which of the following statements is most accurate regarding the immunological changes and management of burn victims?
   a. Chemotaxis, opsonization, phagocytosis, and bacterial killing are all enhanced.
   b. Ig levels are increased.
   c. High prevalence of T-helper lymphocytes.
   d. Colonization of the burn wound in 5–7 days post-injury is predominately with Gram-negative bacteria.
   e. Early enteral feeding with a diet high in arginine and low in ω-6 fatty acid is very beneficial.

9. Match the following organism with its appropriate clinical burn wound infection/sepsis:

   > a. *Candida albicans.*
   > b. *Staphylococcus aureus.*
   > c. *Pseudomonas aeruginosa.*

   _____ Insidious course, leukocytosis, disorientation, wound granulation dissolution, and relatively low mortality rate.
   _____ Sudden hypotension, severe ileus, leukopenia, rapid course, patchy black wound necrosis.
   _____ High mortality, severe ileus, normal–low temperature, orientation intact, dry flat yellow-orange granular wound.

10. An 8-year-old child who is a victim of multiple traumas has survived the initial post-injury period and has been admitted to the pediatric intensive care unit. From this point, he is most likely to die from:
    a. Shock.   d. Hemorrhage.
    b. Starvation.   e. Air embolism.
    c. Infection.

11. Select whether the following statements regarding malnutrition are true or false.
    _____ a. Marasmus and kwashiorkor primarily affect cell-mediated immunity.
    _____ b. Children with kwashiorkor have enlarged thymus glands that can be detected radiographically.
    _____ c. Seroconversion in malnourished children in response to diphtheria and tetanus toxoids is normal.

12. Administration of glucocorticoids to patients in the intensive care unit is likely to be associated with all of the following except:
    a. Increased circulating pool of T-lymphocytes.
    b. Impaired ability of monocytes to kill bacteria and fungi.
    c. Reduced IL-1 and IL-2.
    d. Maturation of macrophages is inhibited.
    e. Antigen processing by lymphocytes is inhibited.

13. Match the immunosuppressive agent with its anticipated effect:
    _____ Cyclosporin.   a. Renal failure, systemic hypertension.
    _____ Azathioprine.   b. Decreases purine synthesis.

14. Which of the following statements regarding asplenia is not true?
    a. Predisposition to infection and sepsis by *Pneumococcus* and *Haemophilus influenzae.*
    b. Prophylaxis with daily oral penicillin is recommended.
    c. Pneumococcal vaccine should be administered 2 weeks prior to splenectomy in children older than 2 years of age.
    d. Infants with congenital asplenia have associated major bony deformities.

15. A 12-year-old boy who is a victim of multiple traumas with cerebrospinal fluid otorrhea develops a high fever associated with nuchal rigidity. Cerebrospinal fluid reveals elevated levels of polymorphonuclear leukocytes and protein. The most likely bacterial pathogen in this patient is:
    a. *H. influenzae* Type B.
    b. *Escheria coli.*
    c. *Pneumococcus.*
    d. *H. influenzae* non-typable.
    e. Serratia.

16. Match the following immunodeficiency disorder with its clinical presentation:

    > a. Pancreatic exocrine deficiency with neutropenia.
    > b. Partial albinism, photophobia with abnormality at cytotoxic granules in phagocytic cells.
    > c. IgA deficiency with diminished T-cell response; associated with lymphosarcoma.
    > d. Eczema, thrombocytopenia, decreased IgM, increased IgA, and increased IgE.
    > e. Autosomal-recessive and X-linked pattern of inheritance, associated with catalase-positive bacteria.

    _____ Wiskott-Aldrich Syndrome.
    _____ Ataxia–telangiectasia.
    _____ Chronic granulomatous disease of childhood.
    _____ Chediak-Higashi Syndrome.
    _____ Schwachman-Diamond Syndrome.

17. All of the following may be indicative of an immunodeficiency except:
    a. Recurrent serious bacterial infection.
    b. Unusual clinical present with common microbe.
    c. Recurrent skin infections.
    d. Chronic diarrhea.
    e. Recurrent or persistent meningoencephalitis with only one bacterial source identified.

18. AIDS has become a disease presence that has greatly affected childhood morbidity and mortality. All of the following statements are true except:
    a. Worldwide, it is estimated that more than 500,000 children are HIV positive.
    b. Vertical transmission is the most common mode of infection in infants with AIDS.
    c. Childhood sexual abuse comprises 25% of all pediatric AIDS cases.

    d. A finite risk of HIV-infected blood products remains.
    e. The enzyme-linked immunosorbent assay is the primary screening test for HIV infection.

19. All of the following statements regarding childhood AIDS are true except:
    a. Perinatal HIV transfusion can occur before, during, or after delivery.
    b. The lymphocyte and macrophage are the primary cells of HIV transmission.
    c. Most children undergo an acute "flu-like" illness and primary viremia.
    d. The HIV immune deficiency is manifested by the decline in CD4 T-lymphocytes.

20. State whether the following statements regarding childhood AIDS are true or false.
    _____ a. The earliest manifestations in HIV-infected children include lymphadenopathy, hepatosplenomegaly, and skin infections.
    _____ b. The presence of HIV antibodies can usually be detected within 6–12 weeks of the primary infection.
    _____ c. The Western blot is the primary screening test for HIV.
    _____ d. It may take up to 15 months for maternal antibodies to disappear from the fetal circulation in an infant born to an HIV-positive mother.
    _____ e. Polymerase chain reaction permits amplification of HIV antibody, making it more specific than enzyme-linked immunosorbent assay.
    _____ f. A common laboratory abnormality to suggest HIV infection is hypogammaglobulinemia.

21. *Pneumocystis carinii* is an opportunistic organism which can devastate the immunocompromised host. Which of the following statements regarding *P. carinii* is true?
    a. The organism attaches to type I alveolar cells.
    b. Reactivation of the organism in older children and adults most likely accounts for their infection.
    c. Fever, cough, dyspnea, and tachypnea are the prominent clinical manifestations.
    d. Bronchoalveolar lavage is, at present, the most commonly used method of obtaining fluid for diagnosis of *P. carinii* pneumonia (PCP).
    e. All of the above.

22. Match the drugs for treatment of *P. carinii* with the following common side effects.

> a. Trimethoprim/sulfamethoxazole.
> b. Pentamidine.

_____ Cutaneous eruptions.
_____ Pancreatitis.
_____ Azotemia.

23. All of the following statements regarding the treatment of PCP are true except:
    a. Trimethoprim-sulfamethoxazole is the initial drug choice combination for treatment.
    b. Corticosteroids may be used as an adjunct to antimicrobial therapy.
    c. Aerosolized pentamidine is as effective as intravenous administration.
    d. PCP can be prevented by antimicrobial chemoprophylaxis.
    e. If untreated, the mortality rate approaches 100%.

24. All of the following statements regarding viral or bacterial pneumonia in children with HIV are true except:
    a. *Respiratory syncytial virus* is more likely to cause pneumonia than bronchiolitis.
    b. Measles has a self-limiting, benign respiratory course.
    c. Cytomegalavirus can cause severe visceral disease.
    d. Ribavirin demonstrates in vitro activity against the measles virus.
    e. The most common bacterial causes of pneumonia in children with AIDS are *Streptococcus pneumonia*, *H. influenza*, and *P. aeruginosa*.

25. All of the following statements regarding renal disease in HIV and AIDS in children are true except:
    a. Approximately 30–55% of HIV-infected children eventually develop renal disease.
    b. Focal segmental glomerulosclerosis is the most common histological finding in HIV children with kidney disease.
    c. High-dose steroids may alter the course of glomerulosclerosis in children with HIV.
    d. Hypernatremia is the most common electrolyte disorder in persons with AIDS.
    e. Children with HIV nephropathy generally do not follow the rapid loss of renal function as do adults.

26. Select whether the following statements are true or false regarding children with HIV and AIDS.
    _____ a. HIV encephalopathy is present in greater than 75% of HIV-infected children.
    _____ b. The most common intracranial mass lesion in HIV-infected children is the lymphoma.
    _____ c. Intravenous Ig may decrease bacterial infections.
    _____ d. *Mycobacterium tuberculosis* and *Mycobacterium avium*-intracellular complex are the most important myobacterial infections in HIV-infected children.
    _____ e. Oral ketoconazole is the treatment for candidal esophagitis.
    _____ f. The risk of acquiring HIV secondary to a needle stick is less than 1%.
    _____ g. Blood is the single most infectious medium for HIV in the medical care setting.

27. Which of the following statements is true regarding the production of lymphokines with antigenic challenge?
    a. Antigen is processed by the macrophage with presentation to the T-cell (vesting) to produce J-interferon, interleukins, and B-cells differentiating factor.
    b. The B-cell is activated by antigen to secrete antibody-secreting cells.
    c. T-cells comprise 55–75% of the lymphocyte population.
    d. IgG and IgM are potent bacterial organ opsonins which activate complement via the classical pathway.
    e. All of the above.

28. All of the following statements regarding immune system physiology are true except:
    a. The alternative pathway is activated by bacterial cell wall components via interaction with C3b.
    b. C3a and C5a are chemotactic for neutrophils.
    c. C5 is important in fungal infection control.
    d. C6–9 are necessary for control of *Neisseria* infections.
    e. A selective lack of B-cells is seen in DiGeorge Syndrome.

10 Metabolic Disorders

The following chapter will focus on metabolic disorders. Pertinent questions, answers, and rationale will be reviewed. Answers for this chapter can be found beginning on page 144.

Key Words: Acidosis; alkalosis; defect; encephalopathy; blood gas.

1. Match the metabolic abnormalities listed (A–D) with the specific corresponding disorder below.

	Metabolic acidosis	Ketosis	Hyperammonemia	Lactic acidemia
a.	–	–	+++	–
b.	++	+	+	–
c.	+	+	–	–
d.	+++	+	–	+++

____ Organic acidemia.
____ Maple syrup urine disease.
____ Urea cycle defect.
____ Congenital lactic acidosis.

2. All of the following statements regarding hyperammonemia in infants are true except:
   a. In children, cytotoxic cerebral edema and increased intracranial pressure may occur.
   b. Its toxicity is reversible.
   c. Ammonia is normally detoxified in astrocytes by glutamate dehydrogenase and glutamine synthetase.
   d. The pronounced depletion of adenosine triphosphate in the brain reticular activating system accounts for the altered level of consciousness.
   e. There is an active urea cycle within the brain.

3. A newborn baby girl was a product of a full-term spontaneous vaginal delivery after an uneventful pregnancy and is noted to have recurrent intractable clonic and myoclonic seizures that have been resistant to therapy. The baby has been breast fed only twice and has been afebrile. Sepsis work-up has been negative so far. Arterial blood gases, blood glucose and blood ammonia and serum urine ketones have all been within normal limits. At this juncture, one should think about

   a. Ornithine transcarbamylase deficiency.
   b. Methylmalonic acidemia.
   c. Nonketotic hyperglycinemia.
   d. Maple syrup urine disease.
   e. Congenital lactic acidosis.

4. All of the following statements are accepted hypotheses of hepatic encephalopathy except:
   a. Synergistic effects of accumulation of toxins with coma-producing potential.
   b. The false transmitter hypothesis.
   c. The neural inhibition of γ-aminobutyric acid.
   d. Professor Mertz revelation.

5. All of the following statements are true regarding the neuropathology of metabolic encephalopathy except:
   a. Infarction is usually present with hypoglycemia.
   b. Hypoglycemia causes superficial cortical layer necrosis.
   c. Proliferation of the protoplasmic astrocyte (Alzheimer type II astrocyte) occurs.
   d. Degenerative changes of cortical layers 5 and 6 develop.

6. Match the following therapeutic interventions with the corresponding disorder it is intended for.

a. Arginine hydrochloride.	d. Thiamine.
b. Biotin.	e. Riboflavin.
c. Vitamin B_{12}.	

____ Multiple carboxylase deficiency.
____ Hyperammonemia because of urea cycle defects.
____ Methylmalonic acidemia.
____ Maple syrup urine disease.
____ Multiple acyl-coenzyme A dehydrogenase deficiency.

From: *Pediatric Critical Care Review*
Edited by: R. A. Hasan and M. D. Pappas © Humana Press Inc., Totowa, NJ

7. A 13-year-old female with a history of chronic adrenal insufficiency presents to the pediatric intensive care unit with a blood pressure of 60/30 mmHg and a heart rate of 125 beats per minute. All of the following suggest adrenocortical insufficiency except:
   a. Hyperkalemia.
   b. Hyponatremia..
   c. Hyperglycemia.
   d. Hypercalcemia.
   e. Anemia

8. Diabetic ketoacidosis is associated with insulin deficiency with elevation of all of the following hormones except:
   a. Growth hormone.
   b. Glucagon.
   c. Somatostatin.
   d. Epinephrine.
   e. Glucocorticoids.

9. Match the following answers with their correct descriptions:

	pH	PCO_2	PaO_2	HCO_3
a.	7.38	66	45	35
b.	7.04	18	120	5
c.	7.25	15	124	7
d.	7.15	78	60	26
e.	7.35	80	35	35

_____ A 16-year-old female with new onset diabetic ketoacidosis.

_____ A 12-year-old with cerebral palsy having severe scoliosis and excessive emesis as a result of bowel obstruction

_____ A 15-year-old male presenting with paresis after eating strawberry jam that is more than 1 year old.

_____ A 16-year-old female who recently separated from her boyfriend and came to the emergency room with nausea, vomiting, tinnitus, abdominal pain, and agitation.

10. All of the following statements regarding the rapid adrenocorticotropic hormone stimulation test are true except:
    a. A blunted cortisol response can be a result of primary or secondary adrenocortical insufficiency.
    b. This test is only a screening procedure.
    c. A normal response eliminates the possibility of primary adrenocortical insufficiency.
    d. A normal response eliminates the possibility of secondary adrenocortical insufficiency.

11. In sick euthyroid syndrome, all of the following statements are true except:
    a. There is a decrease in serum T3 levels.
    b. 30–50% have low T4 levels.
    c. There is a high thyroid stimulating hormone level.
    d. There is an increase in reverse T3 level.

11 Pain Management

The following chapter will focus on pain management. Pertinent questions, answers, and rationale will be reviewed. Answers for this chapter can be found beginning on page 146.

Key Words: Pain management; classes; fibers; receptor; μ, χ; δ; σ.

1. All of the following statements regarding pain neurophysiology are true except:
   a. A-δ fibers are associated with sharp localized pain, whereas C fibers are associated with dull diffuse pain.
   b. Substance P, a peripheral pain transmitter, can increase the responsiveness of peripheral nociceptors to pain.
   c. The underlying principle of transcutaneous electrical nerve stimulation is such that large diameter peripheral nerves are stimulated, effectively blocking nociceptive information from the periphery.
   d. The neuroanatomic pathways for pain transmission develop at 4 months of age.
   e. Pain may be relieved by altering the patient's emotional responses to it.

2. Which of the following statements is true regarding opioids and opioid receptors?
   a. The opioids most commonly used in the management of pain are κ agonists.
   b. The receptor μ_1 involves respiratory depression, and the μ_2 receptor involves supraspinal analgesia.
   c. μ_2-Receptor stimulation causes tachycardia.
   d. The μ_2 receptors are more abundant at birth and may account for the increased risk of opioid-induced respiratory depression in infants.

3. Match the pain receptor with its anticipated effect or prototype agonist.

a. μ Receptor.	c. δ Receptor.
b. κ Receptor.	d. σ Receptor.

   _____ Dysphoria/hallucinations.
   _____ Inhibition of antidiuretic hormone release.
   _____ Inhibits gastrointestinal motility.

   _____ Phencyclidine.
   _____ Methadone.

4. Match the opioid with its effect.

a. Seizures in newborns.
b. Catastrophic interaction with monoamine oxidase inhibitors.
c. Chest wall and glottic rigidity.

   _____ Meperidine.
   _____ Fentanyl.
   _____ Morphine.

5. Which of the following statements is true regarding the commonly used μ-agonist drugs?
   a. Meperidine produces tachycardia.
   b. Morphine causes histamine release.
   c. Fentanyl minimizes hemodynamic effects.
   d. Codeine can only be administered orally.
   e. All of the above.

6. Which of the following statements is true regarding fentanyl?
   a. Fentanyl is less potent than morphine.
   b. Fentanyl is largely devoid of hypnotic and sedative activity.
   c. Sufentanil is less potent than fentanyl.
   d. Fentanyl is highly bound to α-1 acid glycoprotein.

7. Which of the following statements is true regarding meperidine?
   a. It is 10 times more potent than morphine.
   b. It effectively stops shivering in low doses.
   c. The metabolite normeperidine prevents central nervous system excitation.
   d. It may be used safely in combination with monoamine oxidase inhibitors.

From: *Pediatric Critical Care Review*
Edited by: R. A. Hasan and M. D. Pappas © Humana Press Inc., Totowa, NJ

8. Which of the following statements is true regarding methadone?
   a. The half-life is approximately 19 hours.
   b. Clonidine may be used concomitantly to treat opiate withdrawal.
   c. It has poor gastrointestinal tract bioavailability.
   d. None of the above.

9. Which of the following is true regarding hydromorphone?
   a. Rapid onset with a 4- to 6-hour duration.
   b. Less potent than morphine.
   c. Less sedating than morphine.
   d. None of the above.

10. Which of the following ise true regarding intrathecal and epidural opioid analgesia?
    a. Morphine will have a greater latency and duration of action than fentanyl.
    b. Hydrophilic agents produce more segmental analgesia with less rostral spread than lipid-soluble agents.
    c. Both light touch and proprioception are preserved.
    d. All of the above.

11. All of the following statements are true regarding naloxone except:
    a. It is an opioid antagonist.
    b. Very small doses may alleviate the respiratory depression effect of opioids without affecting their analgesic effects.
    c. It is rapidly metabolized in the liver.
    d. Produces sedation in patients who have not received opioids.
    e. May induce withdrawal symptoms in chronic opioid abusers.

12. All of the following statements regarding ketamine are true except:
    a. Loss of consciousness is heralded by nystagmus.
    b. Nightmares are more common in children than adults.
    c. Cerebral metabolism and cerebral blood flow increase.
    d. Mean arterial pressure, heart rate, and cardiac output increase.
    e. Profound hypotension may occur in patients with depleted catecholamine stores.

13. Select whether the following statements are true or false regarding ketamine.
    _____ a. It is a ventilatory depressant.
    _____ b. Laryngeal reflexes are generally lost.
    _____ c. Increases pulmonary compliance.
    _____ d. Highly lipid-soluble.
    _____ e. Redistribution explains its short duration of action.
    _____ f. Reduction in liver blood flow prolongs half life.

14. Which of the following statements is true regarding local anesthetics?
    a. There are two types, amides and esters, which are both weak bases.
    b. The nonionized (base) form crosses the nerve membrane.
    c. Acidosis and hypercapnea increase their toxicity.
    d. Because of the lower Cm (minimum concentration necessary to block a nerve impulse), less local anesthetic is necessary to block pain than produce paralysis.
    e. All of the above.

15. Rank the following by order of highest to lowest regarding absorption of anesthetic administration— 1 = highest, 5 = lowest.
    _____ a. Distal peripheral.
    _____ b. Caudal/epidural.
    _____ c. Brachial plexus.
    _____ d. Subcutaneous.
    _____ e. Intercostal/intratracheal.

16. All of the following regarding benzodiazepines are true except:
    a. γ-Aminobutyric acis is the major neuroinhibitory neurotransmitter within the brain.
    b. Binding to α-sites facilitates binding to β-sites, which causes hyperpolarization.
    c. Tidal volume is decreased.
    d. Produces preload and afterload reduction.
    e. Midazolam increases coronary sinus blood flow and myocardial oxygen consumption.

17. Benzodiazepines can effectively treat anxiety in children. Select whether the following statements are true or false.
    _____ a. Midazolam is four times more potent than diazepam.
    _____ b. Midazolam is painful when administered intravenously.

_____ c. When midazolam is used for more than 7 days and is acutely stopped, withdrawal symptoms may present.

18. Match the following barbiturate with its associated effect.

> a. Pentobarbital.   b. Thiopental.

_____ Effect terminated by redistribution from the brain to other body compartments.
_____ Sleep induced in 10–15 minutes.

19. Select whether the following statement is true or false.
    _____ a. The incident rate of cardiac arrest with anesthesia in children is 1:700.

20. Match the American Society of Anesthesiology physical status classification with the appropriate descriptive.

> a. Class I.   d. Class IV.
> b. Class II.   e. Class V.
> c. Class III.

_____ Moribund patient with little chance of survival.
_____ Severe systemic disease.
_____ No organic, physiologic, biochemical, or psychiatric disturbance.
_____ Mild-moderate systemic disturbance.
_____ Severe systemic disorder which is life-threatening and not always correctable by the operative procedure.

21. Which of the following drugs stimulate histamine release?
    a. Morphine.   d. Latex.
    b. Protamine.   e. All of the above.
    c. Barbiturates.

22. Select whether the following statements are true or false regarding inhalational anesthetics.
    _____ a. Most common pediatric inhalational anesthesia involves halothane, enflurane, and isoflurane usually in conjunction with an oxygen/nitrous oxide mixture.
    _____ b. Minute ventilation and inspired concentration determine the rate of removal of the agent from the alveolus.
    _____ c. Nitrous oxide achieves a steady state within 5–10 minutes.

23. All of the following statements regarding succinyl choline are true except:
    a. Intragastric, intraocular, and intracranial pressure are increased.
    b. Metabolism is by plasma and hepatic pseudo-cholinesterase.
    c. Hepatic dysfunction, hypermagnesemia, and pregnancy prolong emergence.
    d. Severe bradycardia may occur.
    e. A decrease in potassium accompanies administration.

24. Which of the following statements is true regarding nondepolarizing neuromuscular blockers?
    a. They represent false transmitters.
    b. Residual effects can be characterized by an unsustained response to a tetanic stimulation of 50 Hz at 2.5 seconds.
    c. Hypokalemia, respiratory acidosis, hypermagnesemia, and a decreased body temperature can result in failure to reverse their effects.
    d. Calcium channel blockers, nitroglycerin, and high dose corticosteroids potentiate their neuromuscular blockade.
    e. All of the above.

12   Pharmocology and Toxicology

The following chapter will focus on pharmacology and toxicology. Pertinent questions, answers, and rationale will be reviewed. Answers for this chapter can be found beginning on page 148.

Key Words: Overdose; antidote; hemoperfusion; hemodialysis; lavage; coma; poison.

1. Presumptive, quantitative adjustments of drug regimens in order to compensate for anticipated variations in volume of distribution are usually not practical except with:
   a. Congestive heart failure.
   b. Iatrogenic volume expansion such as septic shock.
   c. Ascites.
   d. Obesity.

2. A loading dose of a drug is necessary when:
   a. Drug accumulation is not expected but there is a need for rapid acquisition of a therapeutic level.
   b. The dosing interval/half-life is more than three, and there is a need to get a therapeutic level rapidly.
   c. The dosing interval/half-life is less than three, but rapid acquisition of a therapeutic level is needed.
   d. None of the above.

3. A 12-month-old child (weight = 10 kg; length = 75 cm) with a serum creatinine of 1.2 needs amikacin for a Gram-negative bacterial infection. The usual dose for amikacin is 15 mg/kg/day and amikacin is 98% excreted in the urine unchanged. Based on the information provided, the most appropriate dose is:

$$\left(\text{Clearance} = \frac{\text{Length} \times K}{\text{S. creatinine}}\right.$$

   where $K = 0.45$ for infants)

$$(D_r = D_n \times (1 - [f (1 - RI)])$$

   where f is 0.98 for amikacin*
   a. 10 mg/kg/day.
   b. 8 mg/kg/day.

---

*Note: RI, Renal index; Dr, Dose in renal failure; Dn, Dose with normal renal function.

  c. 4.5 mg/kg/day.
  d. 2.5 mg/kg/day.
  e. Cannot be calculated from the data given.

4. Regarding steroid replacement treatment in children who have been on long-term steroid therapy and admitted to the pediatric intensive care unit:
   a. Sepsis or major trauma necessitates administration of 3–4 times the maintenance dose.
   b. When in doubt, the clinician could reasonably give 100–200 mg/m²/day of hydrocortisone as a continuous infusion or in divided doses.
   c. High-dose hydrocortisone should be started 1–2 days prior to surgery at 4 times the maintenance dose, and weaned over 5–7 days.
   d. When converting to oral maintenance, the dose should be double the maintenance dose wing to inactivation by gastric acidity.
   e. All of the above

5. The most selective α adrenergic blocker is:
   a. Phenoxybenzamine.   c. Phentolamine.
   b. Prazosin.   d. Atenolol.

6. Which of the following is not true regarding cocaine metabolism?
   a. Cocaine is quickly metabolized to benzoylecgonine, which is excreted in the urine within 24 hours.
   b. Most urine drug screens detect benzoylecgonine.
   c. Metabolism of cocaine in the liver is by ester hydrolysis by pseudocholincoterase as well as nonenzymatic hydrolysis.
   d. Cocaine is absorbed from the bladder and vagina.
   e. Cocaine is excreted in the urine unchanged and is detected by most drug screening tests in this form.

From: *Pediatric Critical Care Review*
Edited by: R. A. Hasan and M. D. Pappas © Humana Press Inc., Totowa, NJ

7. Which of the following statements is true regarding
    deferoxamine?
    a. Efficacy of deferoxamine is related entirely to
        the actual excretion of the amount of iron
        ingested in a setting of iron poisoning.
    b. It inhibits virulence of *Yersinia enterocolitis*.
    c. Lack of color change in urine after administra-
        tion of deferoxamine is an indication for dis-
        continuing therapy.
    d. Deferoxamine administration interferes with sub-
        sequent laboratory determination of iron levels.
    e. Children usually require more than 72 hours of
        deferoxamine therapy.

8. Regarding diagnosis of amphetamine overdose,
    choose the most accurate statement:
    a. Diagnosis by history is rarely reliable.
    b. There is no readily available serum analysis.
    c. The qualitative urine test is not valuable in the
        acute setting.
    d. High degree of suspicion along with clinical
        judgment may be helpful in diagnosis.
    e. All of the above.

9. Which of the following statements is true regarding
    evaluation of a patient suspected of amphetamine
    abuse?
    a. Hyperthermia requires immediate attention.
    b. Delirium and agitation are treated with benzodi-
        azepine.
    c. Neuroleptics lower seizure threshold, alter tem-
        perature regulation, and may cause dystonia in
        patients with cocaine intoxication that is diffi-
        cult to differentiate from amphetamine abuse.
    d. Death from amphetamines results from dys-
        rhythmias and intracerebral hemorrhage.
    e. All of the above.

10. The most valuable time to assess serum iron level
    after ingestion (when tablet breakdown is com-
    plete but iron has not been completely distributed
    to tissue) is:
    a. 2–4 hours.   d. 8–10 hours.
    b. 4–6 hours.   e. None of the above.
    c. 6–8 hours.

11. Properties of iron that help promote toxicity include:
    a. First order absorption with poor excretion.
    b. Zero order absorption, but rapid excretion.
    c. Zero order absorption, but slow excretion.
    d. None of the above.

12. In a patient with iron poisoning who is receiving
    deferoxamine, the most accurate method for meas-
    urement of iron is:
    a. Calorimetric method.
    b. Radioimmune assay method.
    c. Atomic absorption spectrophotometric method.
    d. All these methods are equally accurate.

13. A true statement about use of deferoxamine in iron
    poisoning is:
    a. Iron that is bound to various proteins is avidly
        chelated by deferoxamine.
    b. Efficacy of deferoxamine is related entirely to the
        actual excretion of the amount of iron ingested.
    c. Deferoxamine prevents toxicity by making iron
        unavailable for cellular binding through forma-
        tion of furoxamine (FA).
    d. Cytochrome-bound iron is complexed by defer-
        oxamine.
    e. Deferoxamine is very well absorbed from the
        gut when given enterally.

14. In a setting of iron poisoning, gastric lavage is indi-
    cated in all of the following circumstances except:
    a. Chewable tablet forms of iron are ingested.
    b. Pill fragments are seen in the emesis.
    c. Pill fragments are seen on the chest or abdomi-
        nal radiograph.
    d. Any patients with iron poisoning should under-
        go gastric lavage regardless of type of tablets or
        time of presentation.

15. Activated charcoal is ineffective in the setting of
    iron poisoning. Which of the following lavage solu-
    tions have been shown to dramatically decrease
    absorption of and the toxicity resulting from iron?
    a. Phosphate lavage solution.
    b. Bicarbonate lavage solution.
    c. Deferoxamine lavage solution.
    d. None of the above.

16. Regarding management of a child with iron inges-
    tion/overdose:
    a. Any conscious child who has ingested more
        than 20 mg/kg of elemental iron and who has
        not vomited spontaneously may be given syrup
        of ipecac at home and brought to the hospital.
    b. When two children are found sharing a bottle of
        iron pills, the smaller child would have the
        greater risk of toxicity.

c. If gastrointestinal symptoms do not develop within 6 hours of ingestion, the child may be discharged home safely.

d. The presence of tachycardia, tachypnea, and hypoperfusion necessitates immediate chelation regardless of dose/concentration of Fe^{++}.

e. All of the above.

17. Match the pathway with its correct description.

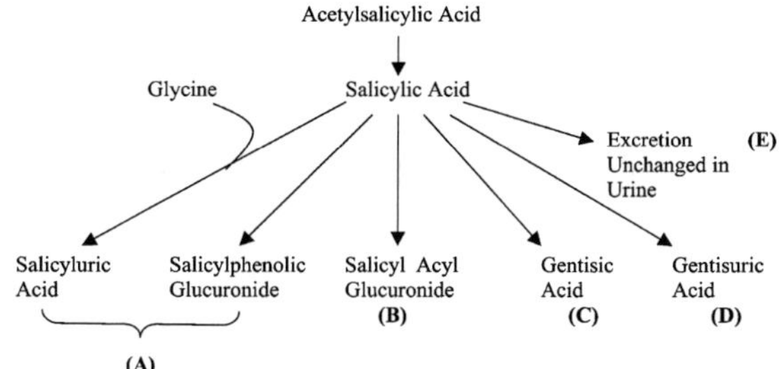

_____ Major metabolic pathway for elimination when therapeutic doses are used.

_____ Becomes of paramount importance during salicylate intoxication.

_____ Follows the Michaelis-Menten Kinetics (saturable kinetics) with overdose of salicylate.

18. The half-life of salicylates at therapeutic doses is 2–4 hours. This may be as long as 20 hours in a setting of overdose because:

a. At high concentration two of the dominant metabolic pathways follow the Michaelis-Menten Kinetics.

b. Protein binding increases.

c. Volume of distribution decreases.

d. pKa changes.

19. The Done nomogram used in salicylate poisoning does not take into consideration which of the following?

a. A single acute ingestion of nonenteric coated tablets.

b. Urinary pH.

c. Blood pH.

d. Use only 6 hours or more after ingestion.

e. Development in a largely pediatric population.

20. Which of the following statements is correct regarding evaluation and management of patients with possible poisoning or overdose?

a.Respiratory acidosis is a recognized feature of salicylate toxicity.

b. Alterations in mental status and the presence of metabolic derangements confirm the diagnosis of acetaminophen overdose.

c. Elevation of temperature directly resulting from salicylate toxicity is seen in mild cases.

d. In children, the respiratory alkalosis is transient and metabolic acidosis predominates with salicylate overdose.

21. Which of the following statements is least accurate regarding salicylate overdose?

a. Aspirin is the leading cause of childhood poisoning today.

b. A urine ferric chloride test that turns purple suggests salicylate ingestion.

c. In an obtunded patient who requires endotracheal intubation, hyperventilation to maintain alkalemia is of paramount importance in salicylate poisoning.

d. Repeated dose activation charcoal possibly works by preventing desorption of salicylate from charcoal.

e. Ketonuria is a recognized abnormality in urinalysis.

22. Which of the following statements regarding management of salicylate poisoning is true?

a. Following endotracheal intubation, rapid normalization of plasma pH should be attempted.

b. Renal excretion of salicylate depends to a significant degree on urinary flow, making forced diuresis a remarkably beneficial intervention.

c. Concomitant alkalinization of blood and urine is not recommended.

d. Acetazolamide, although less popular, has the same efficiency and safety in maintaining urinary alkalinization as bicarbonate.

e. The presence of a respiratory acidosis warrants evaluation for another toxin or pulmonary edema.

23. When it is difficult to achieve an adequate urinary alkalinization in salicylate poisoning, one should suspect all of the following except:

a. Hypokalemia.

b. Hypovolemia.

c. Hyperkalemia.

d. Excretion of organic acids.

24. In the setting of acetaminophen overdose, *N*-acetyl-cysteine should be withheld in which of the following situations?
    a. When acetaminophen levels will be available, but not until 12 hours after ingestion.
    b. Toxic acetaminophen levels documented, but 26 hours after ingestion.
    c. Toxic acetaminophen levels documented, but patient is already in fulminant hepatic failure.
    d. None of the above.

25. Which of the following would be an effective therapy for prevention of hepatic injury following severe acetaminophen overdose?
    a. *N*-acetylcysteine.
    b. Hemoperfusion.
    c. Hemodialysis.
    d. Peritoneal dialysis.
    e. All of the above.

26. Poor prognostic factors in a patient with acetaminophen overdose and consideration for early referral for possible liver transplantation include:
    a. A rise in prothrombin time to 1.8 times control on day 3, grade III (encephalopathy and an admission serum creatinine more than 3.3 mg%, all combined.
    b. Admission pH of less than 7.3.
    c. An increase in the ratio of Factor VIII to Factor V.
    d. All of the above.
    e. None of the above.

27. Which of the following statements is most accurate regarding management of acetaminophen toxicity?
    a. Gastric lavage is useful within the first 24 hours of ingestion.
    b. Activated charcoal is effective within 48 hours of ingestion.
    c. If an acetaminophen level will not be available within 8 hours of ingestion, a dose of *N*,acetyl-cysteine should be given regardless of the amount ingested.
    d. Patients on anticonvulsants should be treated with *N*-acetylcysteine at a higher level of acetaminophen.

28. Mechanisms of action of *N*-acetylcysteine for acetaminophen overdose, when administered within the first 8 hours after ingestion, do not include which of the following?
    a. A precursor for glutathione replenishment.
    b. A precursor for sulfate replenishment.
    c. A glutathione substitute to directly conjugate *N*-acetylbenzoquinoneimine.
    d. Redirection of *N*-acetylbenzoquinoneimine back to acetaminophen.
    e. An antioxidant.

29. Mechanisms responsible for the beneficial effects of late administration (>8 hours) of *N*-acetylcysteine for acetaminophen overdose include all of the following except:
    a. Possibly a precursor for endothelium-derived relaxing factor.
    b. Decreased neutrophil accumulation.
    c. Improved microcirculatory changes.
    d. Improved tissue O_2 delivery or extraction.
    e. Redirection of *N*-acetylbenzoquinoneimine back to acetaminophen.

30. Which of the following statements is least accurate regarding the overdose with and toxicity from acetaminophen?
    a. Peak plasma levels almost always occur 4 hours after ingestion.
    b. Hepatotoxicity is produced only by products of metabolism through P-450 mixed function oxidase system.
    c. Hepatotoxicity is periportal with centrilobular sparing.
    d. Children appear to be less vulnerable than adults to the toxic effects of acetaminophen.
    e. Patients on anticonvulsants who develop acetaminophen toxicity have higher mortality rate.

31. Regarding acetaminophen toxicity in overdose settings:
    a. In a younger child with extremely high levels, hypotension, hypothermia, apnea, and metabolic acidosis occur.
    b. Liver function tests should be repeated every 24 hours for 4 days.
    c. Acetaminophen level analyzed by calorimetric method is unreliable in the presence of elevated bilirubin, renal failure, or salicylism.
    d. All of the above.

32. Indications for oral *N*-acetylcysteine in an acetaminophen overdose include:
    a. Serum acetaminophen in the toxic range on Rumack-Matthew nomogram.
    b. Initial aspartate amino transaminase and prothrombin time that are increased at the time of presentation.
    c. Prior or present vomiting with ingestion of more than 140 mg/kg.

    d. History of a large acetaminophen ingestion at an unknown time.

    e. All of the above.

33. Pharmacological properties of theophylline that are pertinent to the management of a patient who presents with theophylline overdose do not include which of the following?

    a. Theophylline overdose is associated with release of epinephrine and norepinephrine.

    b. Theophylline toxicity is associated with cyclic adenosine monophosphate production via β-adrenergic receptor stimulation.

    c. Theophylline toxicity is associated with decreased cyclic adenosine monophosphate degradation via inhibition of phosphodiesterase.

    d. Hypotension is owing to peripheral vasodilation secondary to stimulation of B_2 receptors.

    e. At very high serum levels, theophylline blocks B_2 receptors.

34. All of the following are true regarding cardiovascular manifestations of theophylline toxicity except:

    a. If the patient does not have tachycardia, the diagnosis of theophylline overdose is suspect.

    b. β-adrenergic stimulation is responsible for the electrolyte and acid–base disturbances.

    c. Antiemetics with anticholinergic activity are preferred.

    d. If a pressor is needed to treat blood pressure, a pure α-adrenergic agent is preferred.

    e. The cardiovascular toxicity is because of release of epinephrine and norepinephrine.

35. Which of the following is the most potent opioid?

    a. Morphine sulfate.

    b. Meperidine.

    c. Morphine-6-β-glucuronide.

    d. Codeine.

36. Seizures developing in a setting of opioid overdose is usually a result of hypoxia, except when overdose is because of:

    a. Fentanyl.

    b. Meperidine.

    c. Morphine sulfate.

    d. Methadone.

    e. Codeine.

37. Match the drug with its correct dosing specifications.

a. Sodium nitrite.	c. Both.
b. Sodium thiosulfate.	d. Neither.

    ____ Dose needs to be adjusted for hemoglobin concentration.

    ____ Dose needs to be adjusted for body weight.

    ____ Efficacy can be increased by coadministration of 100% O_2.

38. The combustion of which of the following materials may produce cyanide?

    a. Wool and silk.   d. Nitrocellulose.

    b. Synthetic rubber.   e. All of the above.

    c. Polyurethane.

39. A 15-year-old white female who had ingested a bottle full of sustained release theophylline tablets has been admitted to the PICU, where she has been receiving supportive measures and multidose activated charcoal every hour with intravenous metoclopramide to combat vomiting. In spite of these aggressive measures, theophylline levels have failed to decline over the last 6 hours. The most appropriate next step is:

    a. Upper gastrointestinal tract radiography or endoscopy.

    b. Charcoal hemoperfusion.

    c. Hemodialysis.

    d. Peritoneal dialysis.

    e. None of the above.

40. In a patient with acute theophylline overdose, which of the following laboratory data is least expected?

    a. Respiratory alkalosis.   d. Leukocytosis.

    b. Hyperglycemia.   e. Metabolic acidosis.

    c. Hyperkalemia.

41. Regarding intensive care management of significant theophylline toxicity, all of the following are true except:

    a. Agitation should be evaluated for hypoglycemia.

    b. A vasopressor with predominantly α-adrenergic activity is preferred to treat hypotension unresponsive to intravenous fluid administration.

    c. Hypotension poorly responsive to fluid and pressors is an indication for hemoperfusion.

    d. Repeated dose activated charcoal should be discontinued during hemoperfusion.

    e. When hemoperfusion and hemodialysis are used in series, the electrolyte abnormalities are easier to correct.

42. Which of the following opioids is most likely to cause intraventricular conduction defect, heart block, and bigeminy:
    a. Heroin.
    b. Morphine sulfate.
    c. Propoxyphene.
    d. Meperidine.
    e. None of the above.

43. Hypotension in association with opioid overdose is the result of:
    a. Bradycardia.
    b. Histamine release.
    c. Inhibition of the central adrenergic response to bradycardia leading to vasodilation and hypotension.
    d. All of the above.

44. A 16-year-old was found comatose at home with a heart rate of 45 beats per minute (bpm) and a respiratory rate of 3 bpm with central cyanosis; pupils were pinpoint. En route to the hospital, he had two episodes of seizures. The electrocardiogram (ECG) monitor shows second-degree heart block, a heart rate of 43 bpm with evidence of intraventricular conduction defect. He is given multiple doses of naloxone up to 15 mg, which lead to improvement in his mental status, but the ECG changes persist. The most likely explanation is:
    a. Propoxyphene overdose.
    b. Heroin overdose.
    c. Tricyclic overdose.
    d. Phenothiazine overdose.
    e. Meperidine overdose.

45. When patients develop addiction to opioids, tolerance does not develop to which of the following side effects:
    a. Euphoria.
    b. Sedation.
    c. Miosis.
    d. Constipation.
    e. None of the above.

46. Regarding gastrointestinal decontamination following opioid overdose, all of the following statements are true except:
    a. The benefits of gastric lavage are greater than expected because opioids delay gastric emptying
    b. Use of activated charcoal is contraindicated in "body packers."
    c. Gastric lavage should be followed by activated charcoal.
    d. Elimination of propoxyphene and diphenoxylate is enhanced by multiple-dose-activated charcoal.

47. Acute respiratory failure is a recognized complication of opioid overdose. A true statement regarding this complication is:
    a. Acute respiratory distress syndrome (ARDS) is not seen following overdose with heroin and methadone.
    b. When ARDS develops following opioid overdose, it is always present on admission to the hospital.
    c. Pulmonary edema develops following subcutaneous and intravenous abuse, as well as following insufflation of opioids.
    d. None of the above.

48. A 16-year-old is suspected of having opioid overdose. He shows a definite, but only partial, response to naloxone. He should be evaluated for:
    a. Hypoglycemia.
    b. Hypoxia from ARDS leading to encephalopathy.
    c. Exposure to 3-methylfentanyl.
    d. Postictal phase.
    e. All of the above.

49. With methanol intoxication, which of the following factors has been shown to correlate best with a poor outcome:
    a. Degree of hyperventilation.
    b. Delay of toxic symptoms for more than 10 hours.
    c. Degree of headache.
    d. Elevation of blood glycolic acid levels.

50. With methanol intoxication, the most characteristic finding and the one that correlates best with the degree of metabolic acidosis is:
    a. Dilated pupils with poor response to light and accommodation, and hyperemia of optic disc.
    b. Oxalaturia.
    c. Elevated levels of glycolic acid.
    d. Hyperventilation.
    e. None of the above.

51. Regarding therapy of ethylene glycol poisoning with ethanol:
    a. When dialysis is initiated, the dose of ethanol should be reduced by 50%.
    b. A concentration of 80–100% should be used for oral route.
    c. Only a 5–10% concentration should be used intravenously to avoid phlebitis.
    d. 100-proof whiskey would equal 100% v:v ratio.
    e. None of the above.

52. Match the poisoning with the correct response.

> a. Ethylene glycol poisoning.
> b. Methanol poisoning.
> c. Both.
> d. Neither.

    _____ Alkalinization is advantageous.
    _____ Charcoal hemoperfusion is indicated.
    _____ Peritoneal dialysis indicated.
    _____ 50 mg of pyridoxine intravenously every 6 hours converts the metabolism of this substance to a less harmful end product.
    _____ 100 mg of thiamine intravenously every 6 hours produces the harmless substance α-*OH–b* ketoadipic acid.
    _____ Folic acid 50 mg intravenously every 6 hours enhances the elimination of toxic byproducts of this toxin.

53. A true statement regarding use of naloxone for opioid overdose in an adolescent is:
    a. The typical initial dose of naloxone should be 0.1 mg intravenously.
    b. If the first dose fails to reverse symptoms, then no additional doses are necessary.
    c. Blind sublingual naloxone injection may be life saving if the patient is hypotensive and intravenous access cannot be established.
    d. In a setting where there is no ventilatory insufficiency, high-dose naloxone is still recommended.

54. When a patient responds to a naloxone bolus, pharmakokinetic studies indicate that _______ of the initial dose that caused reversal of the respiratory depression, administered each hour is adequate to prevent recurrence of symptoms:
    a. One-third.   d. Two times the dose.
    b. One-half.   e. None of the above.
    c. Two-thirds.

55. A 15-year-old white female who recently had a fight with her boyfriend was found comatose after having ingested a full bottle of amitriptyline. The least appropriate initial investigation is:
    a. 12-lead ECG.
    b. Electrolytes.
    c. Acetaminophen levels.
    d. Tricyclic antidepressant levels.

56. Seventy minutes after arrival in the emergency department, the patient in Question 55 develops wide complex tachycardia at 160 bpm with a blood pressure of 70/40 mmHg. All of the following statements are true except:
    a. This effect is caused by slowing of sodium influx into the myocardial cells during phase 0 of depolarization.
    b. This adverse effect can be attended by hyperventilation to a pH of 7.55.
    c. Hypotension should be treated aggressively because lactic acidosis enhances binding of the ingested medication to sodium channels in the myocardium.
    d. Lidocaine may be effective in treating this dysrhythmia.
    e. Hypertonic saline is as effective as Na HCO_3 to treat this dysrrhythmia.

57. The same patient began to develop generalized tonic clonic seizure activity. After securing an adequate airway, the following should be done:
    a. Phenytoin should be the drug of choice.
    b. Flumazenil is likely to have some synergic effects in controlling seizure activity.
    c. Benzodiazepines should be avoided.
    d. If the seizure is prolonged, adequate hydration, and monitoring of renal function is essential.
    e. All of the above.

58. True statements regarding the patient referenced in Question 55 include:
    a. This patient should have received ipecac soon after ingestion.
    b. Unlikely amitriptyline, second generation cyclic antidepressant are uniformly less toxic than the first generation.
    c. Multiple-dose-activated charcoal enhances elimination.
    d. Physostigmine is a helpful therapeutic modality in this patient if the anticholinergic symptoms are severe.
    e. All of the above.

59. Drugs that should be avoided in the patient in Question 55 include:
    a. Class IA and IC antiarrhythmics.
    b. Phenytoin.
    c. Flumazenil.
    d. Propranolol and verapramil.
    e. All of the above.

60. Match the clinical features and medical management to the corresponding drug or toxin in a setting of overdose.

a. Paraldehyde.	d. Isopropyl alcohol.
b. Toluene.	e. None of the above.
c. Isoniazid.	

    _____ Mild metabolic acidosis with ketonuria.
    _____ High anion gap metabolic acidosis or nonanion gap renal tubular acidosis.
    _____ Seizure responsive to Vitamin B_6.
    _____ Ketonemia, ketonuria in the absence of metabolic acidosis, but with hyperosmolality.

61. Regarding organophosphate poisoning, all of the following are true except:
    a. Sweating and fasciculation may precede other symptoms after cutaneous exposure.
    b. Severely poisoned patients are comatose, weak, and hypotensive.
    c. The odor of garlic on the breath can be a prominent finding.
    d. Tachycardia and hypertension are virtually never seen.
    e. An electroencephalogram is useful in differentiating severe fasciculations from true seizures.

62. Pralidoxime is an acetylcholinesterase reactivator and is the only such drug available in the United States for use in patients with organophosphate/pesticide poisoning. Which one of the following statements is true?
    a. The benefits of pralidoxime is least striking at the nicotinic receptors.
    b. Weakness and muscle fasciculations are contraindications to use of pralidoxime.
    c. Improvement in strength may be observed within 10 minutes of administration.
    d. To be effective, the drug needs to be given within 4 hours of exposure to organophosphates.
    e. Is contraindicated in patients with carbomate poisoning.

63. Regarding management of organophosphate insecticide poisoning:
    a. Manifestations occur even if only 5% of cholinesterase is inhibited.
    b. Plasma cholinesterase level is lowered by administration of morphine or codeine.
    c. The end point of atropinization is maximum pupillary dilation.
    d. Tachycardia is a contraindication to the use of atropine.
    e. All of the above.

64. Which of the following factors is least likely to influence the efficacy of hemoperfusion:
    a. Rate of flow.
    b. Affinity of the adsorbent for the drug.
    c. Rate of equilibrium of the drug from peripheral tissue to the blood.
    d. Lipid solubility.
    e. Volume of distribution.

65. Complications of hemoperfusion include all of the following except:
    a. Hypoglycemia.   d. Hypotension.
    b. Hyperthermia.   e. Hypocalcemia.
    c. Thrombocytopenia.

66. Repeated-dose-activated charcoal is not recommended for overdose with which of the following drugs:
    a. Phenobarbital.   d. Theophylline.
    b. Carbamazepine.   e. Ferrous sulfate.
    c. Digitalis.

67. Match the poison with its correct action.

a. Carbamates.	c. Both.
b. Organophosphates.	d. Neither.

    _____ Temporary inactivation of acetylcholinesterase.
    _____ Does not penetrate the central nervous system.
    _____ Only atropine is indicated as an antidote.

68. Drugs with a low P_{Ka} (3–7) that are amenable to alkaline diuresis are:
    a. Phenobarbital.   d. All of the above.
    b. Isoniazid.   e. None of the above.
    c. Salicylates.

69. A 3-year-old with severe salicylate overdose is in the pediatric intensive care unit being treated with supportive care and HCO_3 infusion. However, you have not been able to establish an alkaline urine pH. The most helpful intervention would be:
    a. Administration of large doses of furosemide.
    b. Saline loading.
    c. Increase the dose of HCO_3.
    d. Potassium supplementation.
    e. Initiate acetazolamide.

70. Drugs that are easily dialyzable are characterized by all of the following except:
    a. Have a small volume of distribution (<2 L/kg).
    b. Are highly water-soluble.
    c. Are poorly protein bound (<90%).
    d. Have a small molecular weight.
    e. Have a large volume of distribution.

71. The clinical usefulness of hemoperfusion is most dependent on which of the following features of a drug or toxin:
    a. Water solubility.
    b. Protein binding.
    c. Molecular weight.
    d. Lipid solubility.
    e. Volume of distribution.

72. Match the clinical sign with the correct drug.

a. Fasciculations.	c. Both.
b. Myoclonus.	d. Neither.

    ____ Organophosphate poisoning.
    ____ Anti-cholinergic overdose.
    ____ Phenothiazine overdose.
    ____ Haloperidol overdose.

73. A 4-month-old who presented with cyanosis and lethargy is noted to have an 88% saturation on pulse oximetry. PaO_2 is 70 torr and the measured O_2 saturation (by the co-oxymeter) is 76%. A possible etiological agent is:
    a. Benzocaine.
    b. Nitrates.
    c. Nitrites.
    d. Carbon monoxide.
    e. All of the above.

74. Which of the following drugs and toxins does not have the tendency to form concretions in the stomach?
    a. Ferrous sulfate.
    b. Salicylates.
    c. Slow-release tablets of theophylline.
    d. Acetaminophen.
    e. Barbiturates.

75. In treating children with poisoning, use of repeated-dose-activated charcoal for a prolonged period of time is contraindicated in cases of ingestion with:
    a. Enteric coated preparation.
    b. Corrosives.
    c. Anticholinergics with ileus.
    d. Mineral acids.
    e. All of the above.

76. Hypotension in a poisoned child is most closely associated with:
    a. Myocardial depression.
    b. Hypoalbuminemia.
    c. Hypovolemia.
    d. Electrolyte imbalance.
    e. None of the above.

77. Dysrhythmias associated with tricyclic antidepressants are best treated with:
    a. Procainamide.
    b. Quinidine.
    c. Na HCO_3.
    d. Epinephrine.
    e. None of the above.

78. Hypertension is a prominent feature of intoxication with:
    a. Amphetamine.
    b. Dimetab™.
    c. Phencyclidine.
    d. Cocaine.
    e. All of the above.

79. Match the following drugs and toxins to the corresponding odor it is most closely associated with:

a. Garlic.	d. Pears.
b. Bitter almonds.	e. Rotten eggs.
c. Shoe polish.	

    ____ Arsenic.
    ____ Cyanide.
    ____ Nitrobenzone.
    ____ Chlorohydrate.
    ____ Hydrogen sulfide.

13 Traumatology

The following chapter will focus on traumatology. Pertinent questions, answers, and rationale will be reviewed. Answers for this chapter can be found beginning on page 155.

Key Words: Hemorrhage; consciousness; seizure; burns; injury.

1. Motor vehicle accidents are the most contributing factor in childhood trauma. All of the following statements are true except:
   a. Multisystem trauma accounts for 50% of deaths occurring in children older than 1 year of age.
   b. Baroreceptors in the carotid sinus and aortic arch inhibit sympathetic events to the heart and blood vessels via the vagus and glossopharyngeal nerves.
   c. Tissue injury and local ischemia stimulate the nociceptive receptors, which in turn can cause profound systemic effects.
   d. Following hemorrhage in humans, the rise in osmolality is directly related to the intravascular influx of sodium.
   e. Sympathetic activity favors precapillary vasoconstriction.

2. The "flight or fight" catecholamine response occurs in traumatic events. Which of the following statements is true?
   a. Catecholamines produce hypoglycemia and hypokalemia.
   b. α-Stimulation increases insulin and glucagon secretion.
   c. β-Stimulation increases insulin and glucagon secretion.
   d. The overall effect of catecholamines on the islet cells is to increase glycogen and increase insulin secretion.
   e. Cortisol increases the peripheral utilization of glucose.

3. Select whether the following statements regarding endocrine physiology are true or false.
   _____ a. Insulin is produced in the β-cell of the pancreas.
   _____ b. Glycogen is produced in the α-cell of the pancreas.
   _____ c. Diuresis is stimulated by α-adrenergic receptors.
   _____ d. Angiotension II is a weak vasoconstrictor.
   _____ e. Aldosterone decreases Na^+ reabsorption.
   _____ f. Angiotension may cause ischemic renal tubular necrosis.
   _____ g. β-Endorphin potentiates release of growth hormone, antidiuretic hormone, and adrenocorticotropic hormone.

4. All of the following statements regarding trauma are true except:
   a. Sodium citrate raises gastric pH, thereby reducing consequences of aspiration.
   b. Denitrogenation or preoxygenation is one of the primary steps of rapid sequence intubation.
   c. Open operative cricothyroidotomy is an acceptable method for airway maintenance when conventional intubation fails.
   d. Reversal of nondepolarizing muscle relaxants can be achieved with anticholinesterases and antimuscarinics.
   e. Children younger than 6 years of age do not fasciculate when given succinyl choline.

From: *Pediatric Critical Care Review*
Edited by: R. A. Hasan and M. D. Pappas © Humana Press Inc., Totowa, NJ

5. Match the following most commonly used fluid replacement with its most descriptive choice:

> a. 6% Hydroxyethyl starch.
> b. 5% Albumin.
> c. Lactated ringers.

_____ Intravascular half-life = 24 hours.
_____ Elimination half-time = 17 days.
_____ Chloride similar to plasma chloride.

6. Hemorrhage sustained as a result of severe trauma may require volumes of blood products. All of the following statements are true except:
   a. Blood must be administered to trauma patients who comprise advanced trauma life support Class III and IV.
   b. Type O, Rh-negative blood may be used when type specific blood is unavailable.
   c. Most coagulation factors in banked blood are unstable.
   d. Specific consideration of fresh frozen plasma (FFP) administration must at least begin when 200% of the calculated circulating blood volume has been replaced with crystalloid and red cell concentrates.
   e. Consideration of platelet administration begins when 100–150% of calculated circulating blood volume has been replaced with crystalloid and red cell concentrates.

7. A 10-year-old boy is struck by a car while riding his bike. He is dragged approximately 30 feet and suffers a large blood loss and multiple fractures. Which of the following statements is true regarding this situation?
   a. Weil's "5–2" or "7–3" rule is based on changes from fluid boluses in pulmonary capillary wedge pressure and central venous pressure, respectively.
   b. With compartment pressures of 20 cm H_2O in muscle compartment syndrome, immediate fasciotomy is indicated.
   c. In flail chest, the nearer the defect is located to the diaphragm, the more serious the effect is on ventilation.
   d. Cardiac tamponade may present with "paradoxical pulse" and hypertension.
   e. Pulmonary hematoma takes 3–4 weeks to resolve.

8. Select whether the following statements regarding childhood trauma are true or false.
   _____ a. Rupture of the diaphragm is more common on the right side.
   _____ b. Aortic rupture most frequently occurs near the attachment of the ligamentation arteriosum.
   _____ c. Traumatic asphyxia results from sudden intense compression of the chest wall with the glottis closed.
   _____ d. Urgent thoracotomy may be necessary when blood loss greater than 100 mL/hour occurs via a chest tube.
   _____ e. Pulmonary compliance increases with adult respiratory distress syndrome.
   _____ f. The spleen and liver are the most commonly injured solid organs in pediatric blunt trauma.
   _____ g. An intravenous pyelogram is contraindicated in a trauma victim experiencing gross hematuria with physical evidence of renal injury.
   _____ h. Peritoneal lavage can irritate the peritoneum for 24–48 hours and obscure subsequent abdominal evaluations.
   _____ e. Abuse is the most common cause of head injury in children younger than 1 year.

9. All of the following are criteria for skull films after head trauma except:
   a. Age younger than 1 year.
   b. Loss of consciousness up to 2 minutes.
   c. Palpable scalp hematoma.
   d. Cerebrospinal fluid from nose or ear.
   e. Battle's sign.

10. Head and spinal cord injury are the most severe results of childhood trauma. All of the following statements are true except:
    a. Late posttraumatic epilepsy occurs at least one week after head injury.
    b. The overall incidence of posttraumatic seizures is approximately 7–10%.
    c. Following traumatic impact of the spinal cord, small flame hemorrhages are observed on the gray matter and pia arachnoid.
    d. The release of lysosomal enzymes following spinal cord injury may predispose patients to traumatic paralysis.
    e. Increased perfusion following spinal cord trauma produces tissue necrosis and ischemia.

11. Select whether the following statements regarding spinal cord injury are true or false.
    _____ a. Succinylcholine induced hyperkalemia begins 3 days after injury and may persist for as long as 1 year following injury.
    _____ b. Urolithiasis may occur secondary to immobility after spinal cord injury.
    _____ c. Urinary tract infection is one of the major causes of mortality in patients with spinal cord injury.

12. All of the following statements regarding child abuse are true except:
    a. Incidence is approximately 6–10:1,000 within a population.
    b. Children are usually older than 2 years of age.
    c. Large head and weak neck muscles contribute to "shaking" injuries of the infant brain.
    d. Child risk factors include chronically ill children.
    e. Parental risk factors include poor self-esteem.

13. All of the following regarding the pathophysiology of thermal injury are true except:
    a. Edema is maximal at 24 hours and gradually resolves over 3–5 days.
    b. Osmotic pressure in burned tissue increases.
    c. Low cardiac output is secondary to decreased circulating blood volume.
    d. Hypertension occurs in up to 60% of pediatric patients.
    e. The mechanism of hypertension appears not to be secondary to hypervolemia.

14. Which of the following is true regarding pulmonary dysfunction in patients with major burns?
    a. Extravascular lung water does not contribute to plasma colloid osmotic pressure-pulmonary artery pressure wedge gradient, despite weight gain and peripheral edema.
    b. Thermal injury does not cause an increase in pulmonary capillary permeability.
    c. Inhalation injury does not appear to cause significant interstitial edema directly.
    d. Sepsis-induced pulmonary capillary membrane injury is the principle cause of pulmonary edema after thermal injury.
    e. All of the above.

15. Select whether the following statements are true or false regarding thermal injury.
    _____ a. Renal blood flow is decreased immediately following thermal injury.
    _____ b. Glomerular filtration rate is increased with the onset of the postburn hypermetabolic state.
    _____ c. Hepatic dysfunction occurs in less than 5% of patients.
    _____ d. Thrombocytosis occurs in the first several days followed by thrombocytopenia.
    _____ e. Factors V and VIII increase with fibrinogen levels.
    _____ f. Septic bone marrow suppression is likely with generalized bleeding and thrombocytopenia.
    _____ g. Red blood cell (RBC) mass increases.
    _____ h. Hypoxia is the most common cause of encephalopathy in the first 48 hours.
    _____ i. Acalculous cholecystitis is manifested by fever, abdominal distention, and jaundice.
    _____ j. Severe burn injury is associated with immunocompromise.
    _____ k. Refractory anemia is present until the wound is closed.

16. Match the following type of burn with its clinical characteristics:

| a. 1st degree. | c. 3rd degree. |
| b. 2nd degree. | d. 4th degree. |

    _____ Extends to hypodermic fat.
    _____ Deep injury to bone, joint, or muscle.
    _____ Restricted to epithelial cells.
    _____ Usually occurs secondary to high voltage electrical injury.
    _____ "Full thickness injury."
    _____ Surgical closure is indicated.
    _____ Erythema and pain;mild blistering.
    _____ Viable dermal papillae separated by intervals smaller than 1 mm are seen within a few days.

17. A child suffers a severe burn that includes his entire left arm, right leg, and back. What percentage of body surface area (BSA) has been affected based on the "rule of 9s"?
    a. 52%.
    b. 45%.
    c. 12%.
    d. 23%.
    e. 92%.

18. Match the following term with its appropriate definition:

> a. Minor burn.
> b. Moderate burn.
> c. Severe burn.

_____ Involves 5–15% of BSA.
_____ Presence of smoke inhalation.
_____ No significant involvement of hands, feet, or perineum.

19. All of the following statements are true regarding burns and inhalation injury except:
    a. More house fire mortality occurs from smoke inhalation than tissue damage from flames.
    b. Sites of chemical burns should be flushed with copious amounts of isopropyl alcohol.
    c. Any patient whose immunization series is uncertain should receive age-appropriate toxoid and intramuscular tetanus immunoglobulin.
    d. The home is the most common place of pediatric burn accidents.
    e. Scalding is the most common type of burn in the pediatric population.

20. Which of the following would require referral to a burn center by the American Burn Association guidelines?
    a. Electrical burns
    b. Third-degree burns covering more than 5% of BSA in any age patient.
    c. Partial-thickness and third-degree burns involving face, eyes, ears, hands, feet, genitalia, perineum, and major joints.
    d. Partial-thickness and third-degree burns involving more than 10% of BSA in patients younger than 10 years of age.
    e. All of the above.

21. Select whether the following statements are true or false regarding thermal injury.
    _____ a. Massive catecholamine release results in normotension despite hypovolemia.
    _____ b. Children with burns over less than 5% of BSA always require intravenous resuscitation.
    _____ c. Muscle relaxants or sedation is contraindicated prior to tracheal intubation in children displaying upper airway obstruction.

_____ d. Succinyl choline is contraindicated 7 days after injury.
_____ e. The wound initially is colonized by airborne Gram-positive bacteria followed by endogenous Gram-positive flora.

22. Match the following drug with its associated effect.

> a. Silver sulfadiazine.
> b. Mafenide.
> c. Aqueous Na nitrate.
> d. Iodophors.
> e. Topical bacitracin cream.

_____ Rapid eschar penetration.
_____ Contraindicated in pregnancy.
_____ Rapid resistance.
_____ Painful.
_____ Carbonic anhydrase inhibitor.

23. Which of the following is true regarding the Parkland formula?
    a. First 24 hours: 4 mL/kg/BSA burned percentage + maintenance fluid of lactated Ringers to maintain urine output greater than 0.5 mL/kg/hour.
    b. First 24 hours: 4 mL/kg/BSA + 1/2 maintenance lactated Ringers to maintain urine output greater than 0.5 mL/kg/hour.
    c. Second 24 hours: maintenance fluid of glucose-containing hypotonic fluid, colloid to maintain urine output, and albumin to treat hypoalbuminemia.
    d. A and C.
    e. B and C.

24. Select whether the following statements are true or false regarding burns.
    _____ a. *Enterobacter cloacae* and *Staphylococus aureus* are commonly resistant to silver sulfadiazine.
    _____ b. Silver nitrate may induce methemoglobinemia.
    _____ c. 10 organisms per gram of tissue constitutes burn wound sepsis.
    _____ d. Surgical excision and closure should be performed more than 1 month after presentation.
    _____ e. The principal form of wound coverage is autografting.

25. Which of the following statements are true regarding nutrition in pediatric burn victims?
    a. Dietary lipid content should be more than 25% of total diet kcals.
    b. Parental feeds appear to have a benefit over enteral feeds.
    c. Very early (4 hours after injury) institution of enteral nutrition may lead to early achievement of positive nitrogen balance.
    d. Patients with burns more than 10% BSA are recommended to receive 20% total cals from protein: nonprotein kcal/nitrogen ratio 100:1, or 2.5 g/kg/day of amino acids.
    e. C and D.

26. All of the following statements are true regarding smoke inhalation injury except:
    a. Thermal injury from smoke inhalation is usually limited to the supraglottic airway.
    b. Carbon monoxide (CO) accounts for approximately one-half of all fatal poisonings in the United States.
    c. The largest source of CO is generated from incomplete combustion of carbon-containing compounds.
    d. When examination of the mouth and pharynx reveals erythema or blistering, tracheal intubation is recommended.
    e. Inhalation injury accounts for a small (10–15%) mortality associated with major burns.

27. All of the following statements are true regarding CO poisoning except:
    a. The P_{50} is 0.10 mmHg.
    b. Leftward shift of the oxyhemoglobin dissociation curve occurs.
    c. There is an effect on the cytochrome-oxydase system.
    d. A CO hemoglobin (Hb) value within normal limits rules out recent CO poisoning.
    e. The PO_2 is frequently normal.

28. Which of the following is true regarding organ responses to CO?
    a. Heart rate and coronary blood flow increase.
    b. Pulmonary edema occurs in 10–30% of cases.
    c. Cerebral blood flow increases.
    d. Cherry-red skin color is commonly encountered.
    e. A, B, and C.

29. Select whether the following statements are true or false regarding CO poisoning.
    _____ a. Renal failure may occur secondary to myoglobinuria.
    _____ b. Hypoamylasemia occurs commonly.
    _____ c. Mild acidosis should be corrected if present.
    _____ d. The half-life when breathing room air is 5–6 hours.
    _____ e. The half-life when breathing 100% is 1.5 hours.
    _____ f. The half-life when breathing 100% at 2.5 atmosphere is one-half hour.
    _____ g. The level of consciousness at admission and the development of neuropsychiatric sequelae are directly related.
    _____ h. Hyperbaric oxygen treatment is recommended for CO Hb greater than 25%.

30. Match the following CO concentration with its symptom:

    | a. 0.007 (CO Hb – 10%). |
    | b. 0.022 (CO Hb – 30%). |
    | c. 0.195 (CO Hb – 80%). |

    _____ Rapidly fatal.
    _____ Shortness of breath with vigorous exercise.
    _____ Disturbed judgment.

31. Which of the following statements is true regarding smoke injury victims?
    a. Cyanide poisoning from smoke commonly occurs in the absence of CO toxicity.
    b. The treatment of smoke inhalation respiratory injury is supportive.
    c. Arterial blood gases may be normal for the first 12–24 hours in pulmonary inhalation injury.
    d. Smoke injury increases ciliary functions.
    e. B and C.

32. All of the following statements are true regarding electrical injury except:
    a. Joule's law, $P = I^2R$ (where P = power [heat], I = amperage, and R = resistance) explains why tissue damage is greatest in high-resistant tissues (e.g., bone and fat).
    b. Surface burns result from ignition of clothing.
    c. Arc burns may reach 3000°C.
    d. At low voltage, direct current is more dangerous than alternating current.
    e. Ohm's law states $V = I \times R$ (where I = flow, V = voltage, and R = resistance).

33. Select whether the following statements are true or false regarding electrical burns.
    _____ a. Water content and a thinner stratum corneum raise skin resistance in children compared with adults.
    _____ b. Tissue injury is directly proportional to current intensity.
    _____ c. Ventricular fibrillation can be caused by current passing through the chest at approximately 100 mA.
    _____ d. Tetanic spasm of respiratory muscles occur at 10 mA.
    _____ e. Neurological findings are uncommon.
    _____ f. Nearly two-thirds of people struck by lightening die.
    _____ g. Transient arrhythmias occur in approximately 30% of patients.

34. Regarding the pathophysiology of head injury, all of the following are true except:
    a. Blood pressure autoregulation is maintained better than CO_2 autoregulation.
    b. CO_2 autoregulation has prognostic value in that outcome is better in patients with intact CO_2 vasoresponsivity.
    c. Low cerebral blood flow in the frontoparietal cortex suggests the likelihood of poor neurological outcome.
    d. Cerebral O_2 consumption is directly related to the cerebral O_2 content difference.
    e. Brain stem evoked potentials persist even during profound barbiturate coma.

35. Regarding blood transfusion in trauma patients, all of the following statements are true except:
    a. To eliminate serious hemolytic reactions, it is best to obtain at least an ABO-Rh type and partial cross-match when using uncross-matched blood.
    b. ABO-Rh-type-specific and cross-matched blood is preferable to type O, Rh-negative cross-matched blood.
    c. Type O, Rh-negative, cross-matched, packed RBCs should be used in preference to type O, Rh-negative, whole blood.
    d. The immediate phase cross-match (partial cross-match) will fail to detect a major portion of clinically significant antibodies.
    e. With packed RBCs, one gains double the Hb per unit of blood as is found in a whole unit of blood.

36. Which of the following regarding clinical management of hemostatic defects in patients with trauma is inaccurate?
    a. A rapid drop in platelet count to 50,000/mm^3 is more relevant than a slow drop to 10,000/mm^3 in a patient with leukemia.
    b. Dilutional coagulopathy is easily and rapidly correctable if perfusion is satisfactory.
    c. FFP administration is appropriate when a volume of fluid equivalent to twice the blood volume of the patient has been administered.
    d. Platelet administration should be considered when 150% of the circulatory blood volume has been replaced with crystalloid solutions.
    e. FFP yields only 10% of the equivalent clotting factors of a single unit of fresh whole blood.

37. A constant finding in compartment syndrome is:
    a. Paresthesia.
    b. Weakness.
    c. Pain with passive motion.
    d. Loss of distal pulses.
    e. Loss of sensation and proprioceptive functions distally.

38. In a patient with multiple traumas, which of the following statements would be least accurate?
    a. An oral gastric tube should be passed in all patients with abdominal trauma.
    b. If a pelvic fracture is suspected, a rectal examination should be done.
    c. If a genitourinary injury is suspected, urinary catheterization should be avoided.
    d. With refractory hypotension and a presence of a normal peripheral perfusion, spinal cord injury is highly suspect.
    e. Pain on passive motion is a constant finding with compartment syndrome.

39. Chest trauma in children is usually seen in a setting of multiple traumas involving other organs. Characteristics of chest trauma unique to children do not include which one of the following?
    a. Serious intrathoracic injury may be present in the absence of obvious external chest wall injury.
    b. There is a low incidence of great vessels and airway injury because of the mobility of the mediastinum.
    c. The excessive mediastinal shift contributes to the rapid development of cardiovascular and ventilatory compromise.

d. Almost all deaths from thoracic trauma in children occur at the scene.

e. Penetrating trauma in children is very unusual.

40. In children with multiple traumas, when cardiac arrest develops from one trauma it results from:
    a. Hypovolemia.
    b. Aortic rupture.
    c. Aortic dissection.
    d. Cardiac tamponade.
    e. None of the above.

41. Which of the following statements is least accurate in regard to flail chest in children?
    a. Frequently associated lung contusion.
    b. Thoracic radiograph frequently shows rib fractures.
    c. It is rarely seen in children.
    d. Initial therapy should include humidified oxygen and limitation of crystalloid solutions.
    e. Definitive therapy involves positive pressure ventilation, with positive end expiratory pressure.

42. The least common occult and potentially serious injury to the chest of a child with multiple traumas is:
    a. Pulmonary contusion.
    b. Pulmonary laceration.
    c. Pulmonary hematoma.
    d. Tracheobronchial tear.
    e. Esophageal rupture.

43. A 2-year-old white male who was a victim of a motor vehicle accident with multiple traumas, is noted to have diffuse opacification of the entire right lower lobe of the lung, associated with blunting of the right costophrenic angle. After endotracheal intubation, blood is retrieved during suctioning of the endotracheal tube. Which of the following statements would be considered inaccurate regarding the diagnosis in this child?
    a. Persistent air leak at the chest tube insertion for pneumothorax is consistent with parenchymal lung injury.
    b. Radiographical changes of opacification tend to disappear into the sixth day.
    c. Overhydration, particularly with crystalloids, may ameliorate some of the respiratory symptoms in this child.
    d. Empyema and lung abscess are recognized complications.
    e. Acute respiratory distress syndrome is a recognized complication.

44. Approximately 150,000 individuals die world-wide per year as a result of submersion injuries. All of the following statements regarding submersion injuries in the United States are true except:
    a. Overall incidence of drowning is approximately 6 per 100,000 population.
    b. Twenty-five percent of deaths as a result of drowning are secondary to exhaustion while swimming.
    c. More than half of drowning cases are not resuscitated.
    d. The majority of all drowning victims are males less than 20 years of age.
    e. Eighty percent of drowning accidents occur in the spring.

45. Which of the following statements regarding drowning and near drowning is true?
    a. The majority of accidental drownings occur in the Northeastern United States.
    b. Sunday is the most common day of the week for drowning accidents.
    c. Bathtubs are the most common site for submersion accidents in children.
    d. Childhood drowning rates are highest in Caucasians.
    e. Bathtub drownings occur most frequently in infants who are being supervised by a sibling generally less than 4 years of age.

46. Select whether the following statements pertinent to drowning and near drowning are true or false.
    _____ a. Drowning refers to death from submersion within 24 hours of the occurrence.
    _____ b. Most human drowning victims aspirate greater than 25 mL/kg of fluid.
    _____ c. Fresh water causes wash-out and dilution of surfactant, whereas saltwater inactivates surfactant.
    _____ d. Pulmonary function tests demonstrate hyperreactive airways in children who have recovered from near drownings, but who did not require mechanical ventilatory support.

47. The pathophysiology of submersion injury can include which of the processes below:
    a. Asphyxia.
    b. Fluid overload.
    c. Pulmonary injury.
    d. Hypothermia and the diving reflex.
    e. All of the above.

48. Hypothermia can present as a complicating factor in a submersion injury. Which of the following statements is true regarding hypothermia?
    a. Therapeutic hypothermia has been shown to improve outcome after near-drowning.
    b. Moderate hypothermia (32–35°C) causes cessation of shivering, with a decrease in heart rate, blood pressure, and oxygen consumption.
    c. Resuscitation of a drowning victim should continue until the core temperature is 28°C before the patient is declared dead.
    d. Coagulopathies occur frequently with hypothermia.
    e. Pupillary dilatation occurs at core temperatures higher than 33°C.

49. Select whether the following statements are true or false regarding drowning and near drowning.
    _____ a. Positive pressure ventilatory support is indicated when PaO_2 is less than 100 mmHg despite FiO_2 of .40.
    _____ b. Chest radiograph findings correlate well with clinical outcome.
    _____ c. Cardiopulmonary resuscitation in the emergency room, pH less than 7.0, coma, and ventilatory support when combined, predict a high mortality in children with submersion injuries.
    _____ d. Glasgow Coma Scale less than 6 predicts a high probability of mortality in submersion victims.
    _____ e. Positive end expiratory pressure is the cornerstone of therapy.
    _____ f. Steroids are useful for treating cerebral edema following ischemic or anoxic insults.
    _____ g. Intracranial pressure monitoring after submersion injury is highly recommended.
    _____ h. Victims swallow large amounts of water prior to loss of consciousness and before aspiration occurs.

50. Which of the following is true regarding brain death?
    a. In the premature infant, the electroencephalogram (ECG) is not a reliable diagnostic tool for brain death.
    b. Contrast medium, when used in cerebral angiography, can cause reactive hypotension.
    c. Radionuclide flow studies have been noted to show cerebral blood-flow, despite clinical brain death and electrocerebral silence on the ECG.
    d. Analysis of evoked response potentials are not suppressed by sedative anesthetic drugs.
    e. All of the above.

51. All of the following statements regarding the *Report of the Task Force for Determination of Brain Death in Children* are true except:
    a. Brain death cannot be diagnosed in infants less than 7 days of age.
    b. Two examinations and an ECG separated by 48 hours are necessary in brain death cases of children from 7 days to 2 months of age.
    c. Two examinations and an ECG separated by 24 hours are necessary in brain death cases of children from 2 months to 1 year of age; however, repeat examination/ECG is not necessary if a radionuclide brain flow study demonstrates absent perfusion.
    d. Two examinations 12 hours apart in a child less than 1 year of age with irreversible brain damage requires corroborative testing.

52. Stereotyped movements of the extremities and extensor posturing in patients with brain death are called the:
    a. Lazarus sign.
    b. Spinal sign.
    c. Brainstem reflex.
    d. Reflex sign.
    e. Mertz sign.

53. Brain death is a necessity in order for organ donation to occur. Select whether the following statements are true or false regarding brain death.
    _____ a. Hemodynamically, there should not be a cardiac acceleration response to atropine in brain dead patients.
    _____ b. A hypertensive response to a surgical incision in brain dead organ donors in the absence of vasopressor agents or volume administration has been described.
    _____ c. Cerebral blood flow may be depressed as much as 40% during barbiturate coma.
    _____ d. It frequently requires 1–2 days for family members to gather and absorb the reality of death in another family member.

14   Statistics

The following chapter will focus on statistics. Pertinent questions, answers, and rationale will be reviewed. Answers for this chapter can be found beginning on page 161.

Key Words: Sample size; null; data; error; percentage; deviation.

1. When conducting research, type 1 errors (α-errors) occur for all of the following reasons except:
   a. Small sample size.
   b. Too many analyses.
   c. Analyzing data too often and stopping the study when a significant difference is found.
   d. Too few subgroups.
   e. Too many variables.

2. A study was conducted to evaluate the efficacy of a new medication in lowering the pulmonary hypertension that is seen postoperatively after repair of congenital heart defects compared with the "traditional approach." The α-error was set at 0.05, β-error at 0.2, and the authors were looking at a 25% improvement. At the conclusion of the study, no difference was found between the new drug and the traditional therapy. A true statement regarding this study includes:
   a. There is a 50% chance that the null hypothesis was accepted when there was a difference.
   b. The power of the study is 20%.
   c. The p value was set at 0.5 in this study, and there is an 80% chance that an improvement in response to the new drug was missed.
   d. There is an 80% chance that the authors did not miss a 25% difference between the two treatments.

3. The number of groups is not a factor in the selection of a statistical test in which of the following type of data?
   a. Nominal data.
   b. Ordinal data.
   c. Continuous data.

   d. None of the above.
   e. All of the above.

4. True statements regarding correlation include all of the following except:
   a. How strong the correlation is depends on the slope of the line.
   b. With a larger sample size, one is more likely to get statistical significance with the same correlation coefficient.
   c. For ordinal (ranked) data, Spearman's rho or Kendall's tau are used instead of Pearson correlation coefficient for continuous data.
   d. When one is interested in correlations using nominal data, such correlations are obtained with odds ratio or relative risk determination.
   e. Correlation does not make judgments as to whether one variable affects or predicts another.

5. A study is being conducted to evaluate the effect of the presence of an attending physician looking over the shoulder of the fellow while he is performing a procedure, in terms of complications related to the procedure. At the end of the study, relative risks are calculated. True statements include:
   a. A relative risk value of 0.35 indicates that the presence of an attending physician is associated with lower complications.
   b. A relative risk value of 1 means that the presence of an attending physician doesn't make any difference.
   c. A relative risk value of 5 indicates that the presence of the attending physician increased the risk of complication five times.
   d. None of the above.
   e. A, B, and C.

From: *Pediatric Critical Care Review*
Edited by: R. A. Hasan and M. D. Pappas © Humana Press Inc., Totowa, NJ

6. A study is being conducted to evaluate the following: Does dressing change by the nurse in the pediatric intensive care unit increase the risk of wound infection? One thousand children are enrolled. Of the dressings changed by the nurse, 75 did develop wound infection while 25 did not. Of the dressings changed by the primary surgical attending, 125 developed wound infection, whereas 775 did not. The relative risk value of the nurse changing the surgical dressing in this case is closest to:
   a. 1.
   b. 5.
   c. 10.
   d. 0.035.
   e. 7.

7. True statements pertaining to standard error of the mean include all of the following except:
   a. Standard error of the mean measures the dispersion of a number of sample means around the true population mean.
   b. Standard error of the mean represents the precision with which a sample mean estimates the true population mean.
   c. Standard error of the mean is usually larger than standard deviation.
   d. There is a 95% chance that the true mean of the population from which the samples were obtained lies within ± 1.96 standard error of the mean of the sample mean.
   e. When you say "with 95% confidence, 86% ± 5% of the people find this journal useful," the ± 5% represents ± 1.96 standard error of the mean.

8. Match the following with its correct association.

   ┌─────────────────────────────────┐
   │ a. Standard deviation.   │
   │ b. Standard error of the mean. │
   │ c. Mean.   │
   │ d. α-Error.   │
   │ e. β-Error.   │
   └─────────────────────────────────┘

   ____ Quantifies the variability (dispension) of the individual values from the mean within a sample.
   ____ Provides the confidence interval of the population mean.
   ____ Should not be used as a measure of central tendency for ranked data.
   ____ Wide variability of the data is associated with this.
   ____ When conducting a research project, the more variables we look at, the greater the chance of producing the item listed above.

9. Lidocaine is being infused at 20 mg/kg/minute into a patient who has a volume of distribution for lidocaine of 1.1 L/kg. If the half-life of lidocaine is 100 minutes at a steady state, the lidocaine concentration would be:
   a. 1.6 mg/mL.
   b. 2.6 mg/mL.
   c. 0.6 mg/mL.
   d. 8.6 mg/mL.
   e. None of the above.

10. In Question 9, without a bolus, the steady state will be reached in:
   a. 6.7 hours.
   b. 5.7 hours.
   c. 8.7 hours.
   d. 3.7 hours.
   e. None of the above.

11. It is necessary to compare data from two groups by nonparametric tests when:
   a. There are fewer than 10 data points in each group.
   b. The two groups are not of equal size.
   c. The data are expressed as ranks.
   d. The data are expressed as ratios.
   e. The two groups have different standard error of the mean.

15 Ethics

The following chapter will focus on ethics. Pertinent questions, answers, and rationale will be reviewed. Answers for this chapter can be found beginning on page 162.

Key Words: Consent; informed; doctrine; guardian; parental; care; legal.

1. The process of informed consent involves that the patient or the patient's surrogate:
   a. Is/are competent.
   b. Have comprehensible information about the medical situation and treatment.
   c. Have information about alternative treatments and their consequences, and have an understanding of what they have learned.
   d. All of the above.
   e. Only A and B.

2. Children who can make their own decisions and give consents for medical treatment separate from their parents include:
   a. Children who are pregnant or are already parents.
   b. Children who graduated from high school.
   c. Children who have joined the armed forces.
   d. Children who live separately and independent from their parents.
   e. All of the above.

3. Appropriate statements pertaining to the mature minor doctrine include all of the following except:
   a. A minor (child) should have the opportunity to accept or decline life-sustaining treatment, such as mechanical ventilation or dialysis.
   b. The child may refuse a blood transfusion that might otherwise be essential for appropriate medical care, if this is because of long-standing, well-thought beliefs, such as those held by adolescents who are Jehovah's witnesses.
   c. The law does recognize that some children have legitimate independent claims regarding their medical care that may differ from the expressed wishes of their parents.
   d. This legal entitlement means that the proposed decision maker is actually competent.
   e. Physicians must assess the decision-making capacity of patients or their surrogates.

4. In order to give an informed consent, the patient or legal guardian must possess a decision-making capacity. This capacity has several features and elements that include all of the following except:
   a. The patient or surrogate does not need to have the ability to manipulate the information provided to them.
   b. Capacity includes the ability to deliberate about alternative options.
   c. Capacity to make medical decisions involves specific determinations for each significant decision.
   d. Capacity involves the ability to understand and communicate about the medical situation.
   e. Capacity involves the ability to make a choice among alternatives.

5. You are involved in the treatment of a critically ill child with sepsis and multiple organ dysfunction syndrome at a university children's hospital. In this situation, all of the following actions and statements are true except:
   a. Parental religious beliefs should not prevent this child from receiving a clearly beneficial therapy.
   b. The best interest of the child should remain the guiding principle in most cases where there is any dispute with the parents.
   c. Treatment can go forward with permission from only one parent.
   d. When parents refuse involvement of trainees in the care of their child, the best course of action is to remind them that this is a teaching institution and proceed with the care with your trainees.
   e. Children may receive treatment by court approval over and against parental wishes, when the therapy constitutes the standard of care.

From: *Pediatric Critical Care Review*
Edited by: R. A. Hasan and M. D. Pappas © Humana Press Inc., Totowa, NJ

6. In order for a patient to succeed in a claim for damages, he/she must prove:
   a. That the physician failed to meet the standard of care.
   b. That the physician's error led to legally recognized injuries.
   c. That the physician's error approximately caused the patient to suffer legally recognizable damage.
   d. All of the above.
   e. A only.

7. Regarding the doctor–patient relationship involved in a malpractice suit, which of the following statements is true?
   a. It is illegal to alter patient's medical records at a later time even when a reason for an addition is indicated.
   b. It can be hard to deny charges that inappropriate care was provided when the medical record has little or no information.
   c. When a physician treats a patient with a chronic medical problem, he/she is liable for the entire problem even after one encounter.
   d. Most jurisdictions state that the physician is responsible for the patient's noncompliance.
   e. All of the above.

8. In the United States, a 14-year-old who is healthy without any significant past medical history is most likely to die from:
   a. Suicide.
   b. Homicide.
   c. Leukemia.
   d. Accident.
   e. Brain tumor.

9. "Baby Doe" regulations include that health care providers cannot withhold medically beneficial treatment from a child on the basis of a handicap. An exceptions includes:
   a. If the infant is imminently dying.
   b. The treatment would be inhumane.
   c. The infant is permanently comatose.
   d. All of the above.
   e. A and B only.

10. You are called to the pediatric intensive care unit (PICU) as soon as possible because the parents of a 6-month-old child with Down's syndrome and atrioventricular canal defect in congestive heart failure are very angry at the staff, and are expressing dissatisfaction with the care provided to their child. Upon your arrival, you notice the father is indeed very angry and is asking to transfer his child to another institution. All of the following would be appropriate responses except:
    a. Listening to their concerns is one of the most effective interventions in dealing with this family.
    b. A team meeting with this family should be promptly convened.
    c. You should remind the parents that you and the staff were up all night taking care of this child, and at this point, everybody on the team is somewhat tired and exhausted.
    d. Accept the emotional outburst of the father calmly.
    e. Assure the parents that their child is being appropriately cared for and comforted.

11. Measures that can be taken to prevent hostility among parents, such as the ones in Question 10, include:
    a. Orientation to policies of the PICU as soon as possible after the admission of the child.
    b. Introduction of the staff soon after admission.
    c. If there is evidence that the parents are showing signs of dissatisfaction with the care, a team meeting with the family should be promptly convened.
    d. Family education to alleviate any knowledge deficit.
    e. All of the above.

12. A 12-month-old baby of a single mother, who was apparently being watched by the mother's boyfriend, was admitted to your PICU for persistent seizures. Physical examination was significant for the presence of multiple retinal hemorrhages, and the computed tomography scan revealed intracerebral hemorrhage and a subdural hematoma. Correct statements pertaining to this case include all of the following except:
    a. A complete copy of the medical record is extremely helpful during the initial investigation.
    b. If you are asked to testify in court regarding this case, a monitory compensation is expected.
    c. Accidental injury, other than a car accident, rarely causes intracranial injury in infants.
    d. Remind your staff that the parents of this child should be treated in the same professional and supportive manner that is employed with the parents of any other critically injured child.
    e. In discussing this case with one of your residents who will be testifying in court, it is crucial to remember that most physicians are unprepared by training and experience to go to court as expert witnesses.

16 Answers

The following chapter includes the answers and rationale to each of the questions listed in Chapters 1–15. References are included for each answer.

CHAPTER 1: RESPIRATORY SYSTEM

1. E The Murphy eye side hole does not provide protection against obstruction of the endotracheal tube. The incidence of tube obstruction is approximately 5% in the pediatric population, and approximately 80% of tube obstructions occur in endotracheal tubes that are 3.5 mm in diameter or smaller. The channel on the straight blade is the visual pathway for the person performing the intubation. (Rogers MC, et al. *Textbook of Pediatric Intensive Care*, 3rd Edition; pp. 59–64.)

2. A Subglottic stenosis occurs in 2–6% of pediatric patients following tracheal intubation. (Parkin JL, et al. Ann Otolaryngology, 1976; 85:673.)

3. E All are true. (Rogers MC, et al. *Textbook of Pediatric Intensive Care*, 3rd Edition; pp. 65–76)

4–5. D, E Postextubation croup occurs in approximately 5% of intubated children and usually resolves in 24 hours. It is more common in patients with frequent coughing episodes and in patients who move more frequently while intubated. It has been shown to be more prevalent in children 1–4 years or age, particularly in association with any type of surgery in the head/neck area. (Kemper, et al. Crit Care Med, 1991; 19:352.)

6–8. E, E, E The mortality rate for tracheostomy is 1–3%. The mortality rate and complications are highest in infants. Following tracheostomy, there appears to be an increase in airway secretions for 24–48 hours during which time the patient will need frequent suctioning. The patient will also need to be evaluated for possible air leak, such as subcutaneous emphysema or pneumomediastinum, and monitoring for postoperative bleeding. (Zeifouni A, et al. J Otolaryngology, 1993; 22:431-434; Crysdale, WS. Ann Otorhinolaryngology, 1988; 97:493.)

9. C The tracheostomy tubes, in fact, may measure 0.5 mm larger than the previously used endotracheal tube, because the site of insertion is below the cricoid cartilage. The initial change of the tracheostomy tube must be done with the surgeon in attendance as a precaution against complications. (Rogers MC, et al. *Textbook of Pediatric Intensive Care*, 3rd Edition; pp. 72–73.)

10. A This is a rare complication of prolonged tracheostomy, and it is most likely a result of erosion of the innominate artery. Under these circumstances, a cuffed tracheostomy tube should be passed beyond the site of bleeding and immediately inflated. (Crysdale WS. Ann Otorhinolaryngology, 1988; 97:493–499.)

11. B An anterior (and not a posterior) tracheal flap at the operation site for tracheostomy is one of the etiologies of obstruction following decannulation. Other etiologies include: fusion of vocal cords, granuloma, and temporary adductor failure. (Carter P, et al. Ann Otorhinolaryngology, 1983; 92:398–401; Sasaki CT, et al. Ann J Dis Child, 1978; 132:266–269.)

12. D Tracheostomy tubes are not plugged prior to decannulation, as this may increase the airway resistance significantly, and a tracheostomy stoma is usually left to heal on its own. Plastic tracheostomy tubes have been associated with less evidence of stricture and subsequent tracheal stenosis. Tracheostomy tubes are placed below the cricoid cartilage. (Sasaki CT. Am J Dis Child, 1978; 132:266–269.)

From: *Pediatric Critical Care Review*
Edited by: R. A. Hasan and M. D. Pappas © Humana Press Inc., Totowa, NJ

13.   T, T   The same principles applied for tracheal intubation in a patient with closed head injury should be applied here. (Rogers MC, et al. *Textbook of Pediatric Intensive Care*, 3rd Edition; pp. 65–68.)

14.   D   Contraindications to nasotracheal intubation include bleeding diatheses and suspicion of basilar skull fracture. (Rogers MC, et al. *Textbook of Pediatric Intensive Care*, 3rd Edition; pp. 65–68.)

15.   C   In a patient with closed head injury, one should avoid ketamine because it increases intracranial pressure, possibly through a cholinergic mechanism. In a setting of hypotension and shock, thiopental, particularly in the usual dose of 2–4 mg, should be avoided because it may potentiate hypotension, which might be detrimental to the patient. Vecuronium seems to cause minimal hemodynamic disturbances, and therefore, in combination with lidocaine and low-dose (1–2 mg/kg) thiopental would be the most appropriate combination in this patient. (Rogers MC, et al. *Textbook of Pediatric Intensive Care*, 3rd Edition; pp. 63–70.)

16.   A   In a patient with hypovolemia or shock, ketamine seems to be the most appropriate choice because it is a cardiovascular system stimulant, along with vecuronium, which is associated with minimal hemodynamic disturbances would be most the most appropriate combination. (Rogers MC, et al. *Textbook of Pediatric Intensive Care*, 3rd Edition; pp. 63–70.)

17.   D   With turbulent airflow, the resistance to airflow is proportionate to density. A helium–O_2 (HeliOx) mixture has a lower density than an O_2–nitrogen mixture. This leads to a reduced resistance to airflow. Use of an oxyhood is not recommended because helium tends to separate as a layer at the top of the oxyhood. It usually is given through a tight-fitting face mask. The ventilator transducer is calibrated with an air–O_2 mixture, and therefore, with a HeliOx mixture, the tidal volume may not be accurate unless it is measured directly. (Kemper KJ. Crit Care Med, 1991; 19:356; Ellean C. J Pediatrics, 1993; 122:132–135.)

18.   E   The theory is that increased negative interstitial pressure is a contributing factor to the development of pulmonary edema in association with upper airway obstruction. To further review theories that explain the development of pulmonary edema in children with croup and epiglottitis, *see* the following ref-

erences. (Travis KW, et al. Pediatrics 1977; 59:695; Lichtenstein S. Fed Proc 1975; 34:436.)

19,20.   E, E   Children who develop hyaline membrane disease or have pulmonary hypoplasia owing to a wide variety of reasons including diaphragmatic hernia, children with tracheoesophageal fistula, and those who develop early neonatal infections resulting from, but not limited to, group B streptococcal infection, ureaplasma, respiratory syncytial virus, or cytomegalovirus, seem to be at a higher risk of developing bronchopulmonary dysplasia. Other risk factors include male sex, white race, and a birth-weight of less than 750 g. (Kennedy KA. Semin Perinatol, 1993; 17:247.)

21.   D   Negative, rather than positive, pleural pressure has a tendency to promote formation of pulmonary edema. All other factors in the question tend to promote pulmonary edema. (Robin ED. N Engl J Med, 1973; 288:239.)

22.   E.   Refer to answers 19–20.

23–24.   E, D   Air within the connective tissue sheath leads to compression of the surrounding peripheral airway with subsequent increased airway resistance and hyperinflation. Impaired lymphatic drainage promotes pulmonary edema. Once extra-alveolar air develops, it may dissect into the subcutaneous space and mediastinum. Further extension into the pericardium and peritoneum may occur. The primary event appears to be epithelial necrosis. (Watts, JL. Pediatrics 1977; 60:273; Hansen TN. Clin Perinatol 1984; 11:653.)

25.   D   Infants with bronchopulmonary dysplasia (BPD) have been shown to have a blunted arousal response to hypoxia. Increased chest wall compliance places these infants at a mechanical disadvantage, particularly during periods of decreased or low intercostal muscle activity, such as during rapid eye movement during sleep. The peripheral chemoreceptors are intact in these babies. Prolonged ventilatory support may lead to disuse atrophy of respiratory muscles. (Gray M. Pediatrics 1988; 82:59; Knosely AS. J Pediatr 1988; 113:1074.)

26.   E   Normally, the blood flow through the right coronary artery occurs during both diastole and systole, as opposed to the blood flow through the left coronary artery, which occurs primarily during diastole. In infants with bronchopulmonary dysplasia, with the development of pulmonary hypertension and particularly with progressive pulmonary hypertension, the blood flow through the right coronary artery becomes limited to diastole as right ventricular pressure and volume increase. (Berman W. Pediatrics, 1982; 70:708.)

27. A Infants with BPD have been shown to develop a significant reduction in pulmonary vascular resistance in response to low flow oxygen therapy. Acute, recurrent hypoxia precipitated by a variety of factors such as handling, feeding, or infection may precipitate pulmonary hypertension or pulmonary hypertensive crises with sudden death. (Long, LA. Pediatrics, 1980; 65:203. Grag M. Pediatrics, 1988; 81:635.)

28–30. C, C, C Improved mucociliary clearance is a recognized effect of β_2-agonists. Methylxanthines increase chemoreceptor sensitivity to carbon dioxide and induce hyperthermia rather than hypothermia. (Santa-Cruz R. Am Review of Resp Dis 1974; 109:458; Aranda JV. Clin Perinatol, 1979; 6:87.)

31–32. D, D Diuretics cause decreased transvascular efflux of fluid in the lung, and have been associated with improved survival in patients with BPD. Recognized side effects of furosemide include chloride depletion, metabolic alkalosis, renal calcification, and ototoxicity. Some of these factors have been implicated in poor growth and poor outcome in infants with BPD. (Perlman JM. Pediatrics, 1986; 77:212; Hurnagle KG. Pediatrics, 1982; 70:360.)

33–35. E, D, D Respiratory acidosis, hyperinflation, disuse atrophy from prolonged mechanical ventilation, and tracheal intubation have been associated with decreased respiratory muscle capacity. Advantages of tracheostomy include a stable airway with more freedom of mobility and oral stimulation. Tracheostomy decreases anatomic dead space, and therefore is unlikely to lead to elevation of carbon dioxide. It also decreases work of breathing partly through the same mechanism. (Rogers MC, et al. *Textbook of Pediatric Intensive Care*, 3rd Edition; pp. 183–186.)

36. D Use of pulmonary vasodilators would lead to ventilation–perfusion mismatch which is likely to increase the dead space. Allowing the patient's spontaneous respiratory rate to have a higher contribution to the total ventilatory support while on mechanical ventilation will decrease dead space, as does tracheostomy. (Rogers MC, et al. *Textbook of Pediatric Intensive Care*, 3rd Edition; pp. 183–186.)

37. B Self-explanatory. (Rogers MC, et al. *Textbook of Pediatric Intensive Care*, 3rd Edition; pp. 97–98.)

38. A Diffusion defect as the only cause of gas exchange abnormalities is extremely rare. (Rogers MC, et al. *Textbook of Pediatric Intensive Care*, 3rd Edition; pp. 97–98.)

39. D Diaphragmatic hernia, if not detected and corrected before 16 weeks of gestation, will lead to irreversible changes in the lung; in this case, the left lung, which is expected to remain hypoplastic. (Rogers MC, et al. *Textbook of Pediatric Intensive Care*, 3rd Edition; pp. 105–106.)

40. E Canals of Lambert do not develop until approximately 6 years of age. (Rogers MC, et al. *Textbook of Pediatric Intensive Care*, 3rd Edition; pp. 105–106.)

41. A, B The intra-alveolar Pores of Kohn do not develop until after 2 years of age. (Rogers MC, et al. *Textbook of Pediatric Intensive Care*, 3rd Edition; pp. 105–106.)

42. E Dead space ventilation = alveolar ventilation × (alveolar CO_2 – exhaled CO_2) ÷ alveolar CO_2. (Rogers MC, et al. *Textbook of Pediatric Intensive Care*, 3rd Edition; pp. 107–108.)

43. C Dead space ventilation = (arterial CO_2 – exhaled CO_2) ÷ arterial CO_2 × alveolar ventilation. (Rogers MC, et al. *Textbook of Pediatric Intensive Care*, 3rd Edition; pp. 107–108.)

44. B The normal ratio of dead space ventilation to alveolar ventilation is 0.3 or less. (Rogers MC, et al. *Textbook of Pediatric Intensive Care*, 3rd Edition; pp. 107–108.)

45–47. A, B, C Expiratory braking refers to the increase in airway resistance in the upper airway during exhalation, which leads to an increase in end expiratory lung volume. This would lead to an increase in functional residual capacity (FRC). It is decreased during active sleep because it is arousal-dependent. Specific compliance and specific conductance are the same for adults and children. (Kosch PC, Stark AR.J Appl Physiol, 1984; 57:1126–1133.)

48.   B   Time constant = resistance × compliance. Whenever one of the components of the time constant (i.e., either the resistance or the compliance) increases, the movement of air from one lung unit to another would be prolonged, leading to an increase in the time constant. Therefore, applying these principles in the diagram, because the resistance in the airway leading to unit A is increased, and the compliance of unit C is also increased, these two units will contain less volume of gas when inflation is interrupted prematurely. (Rogers MC, et al. *Textbook of Pediatric Intensive Care*, 3rd Edition; pp. 104–106.)

49.   B   Diaphragmatic hernia adversely affects the pulmonary vasculature and lead to pulmonary hypoplasia if it is not corrected before 16 weeks of intrauterine life. (Please *see* Answer 40.)

50.   C   Regional or localized hypoxic pulmonary vasoconstriction does not increase pulmonary vascular resistance significantly. (Rogers MC, et al. *Textbook of Pediatric Intensive Care*, 3rd Edition; pp. 106–112.)

51.   E   All statements are examples of a shunt. (Rogers MC, et al. *Textbook of Pediatric Intensive Care*, 3rd Edition; pp. 110–112.)

52.   D   The alveolar air exchange equation makes all of the above assumptions. (Rogers MC, et al. *Textbook of Pediatric Intensive Care*, 3rd Edition; pp. 110,111.)

53.   D   Cardiac output equals oxygen consumption divided by arteriovenous oxygen content difference, and therefore, if oxygen consumption increases for a constant cardiac output, the mixed venous oxygen content must decrease. (Rogers MC, et al. *Textbook of Pediatric Intensive Care*, 3rd Edition; pp. 108,109.)

54.   D   This is the major mechanism (i.e., low perfusion/ventilation [V/Q] segments) in adults. (Rogers MC, et al. *Textbook of Pediatric Intensive Care*, 3rd Edition; pp. 111,112.)

55.   E   Transfer factor decreases with age. (Rogers MC, et al. *Textbook of Pediatric Intensive Care*, 3rd Edition; pp. 112,113.)

56.   D   Hemoglobin (Hb)-F is more easily oxidizable compared to Hb-A. (Martin H, et al. Nature, 1963; 200:898–900.)

57.   D   Neonates and young infants are more susceptible to the development of methemoglobinemia because (1) the iron in Hb-F is oxidized more readily; and (2) the young infant is relatively deficient in the enzyme, met-Hb reductase. When the levels of met-Hb exceed 30–40%, cyanosis and symptoms of decreased O_2 transport are noted. (Rogers MC, et al. *Textbook of Pediatric Intensive Care*, 3rd Edition; pp. 114–116.)

58.   D   Resting oxygen consumption in a 1-week-old infant is three times that of an adult based on the body weight per kilogram. (Rogers MC, et al. *Textbook of Pediatric Intensive Care*, 3rd Edition; pp. 118.)

59.   C O_2 consumption $(VO_2) = \dfrac{\text{Cardiac Output}}{CaO_2 - CVO_2}$

Where CaO_2 = arterial O_2 content.
CVO_2 = mixed venous O_2 content.
O_2 delivery $(DO_2) = Q \times CaO_2$
Q = Cardiac Output
CaO_2 = Hb (grams%) × 1.34 × O_2 saturation
        + PaO_2 × 0.003

Therefore alterations in cardiac output or peripheral circulatory disturbances (that alter blood flow at the capillary level) will affect O_2 consumption. P_{50} affects the unloading of O_2 from Hb. The higher the P_{50}, the more the unloading of O_2 to tissue. (Rogers MC, et al. *Textbook of Pediatric Intensive Care*, 3rd Edition; p. 118.)

60.   B   Peripheral chemoreceptors respond to a falling oxygen saturation in a linear fashion by increasing the inspired minute ventilation. There is an exponential increase in minute ventilation as PaO_2 falls, particularly at PaO_2 less than 60 torr. (Berger AJ, et al. N Engl J Med, 1977; 297:194–198.)

61.   D   Laryngeal and bronchial receptors respond to increasing CO_2 in a linear fashion. (Berger AJ, et al. N Engl J Med, 1977; 297:194–198.)

62. D The carbon dioxide response curve which relates alveolar CO_2 to alveolar ventilation is shifted to the left in the neonate. (Rigatto H. Apnea. Pediatr Clin North Am, 1982; 29:1105.)

63. D Preterm infants have a characteristic breathing pattern referred to as periodic breathing (i.e., pauses in respirations lasting 5–10 seconds). Owing to the higher O_2 demand, newborn infants compensate by having a higher minute ventilation and a shift in the CO_2 response curve to the left. The carotid bodies are present in preterm infants. (Rigatto H. Pediatr Clin North Am, 1982; 29:1105.)

64. D Total respiratory system compliance equals lung compliance plus chest wall compliance. With age, there is a progressive reduction in chest wall compliance which accounts for a reduction in the total respiratory system compliance. (Sharp JT, et al. J Appl Physiology, 1970; 29:775–780.)

65–67. D, D, C Closing capacity (CC) is the lung volume below the FRC where alveoli in dependent lung regions have a tendency to collapse.

In infants, CC is often equal to or greater than FRC, and therefore, tidal breathing often takes place in the range of CC. This phenomenon is a result of the very low elastic recoil of the chest, and it increases the risk of atelectasis. (Smith CA. *The Physiology of the Newborn Infant*. Springfield, IL, 1976; pp. 206–207.)

68–69. D, D This may result in ischemia of respiratory muscles at a high respiratory rate. Low levels of sarcoplasmic reticulum in the fetal diaphragmatic muscle have been observed. (Maxwell LC, et al. J Appl Physiol, 1983; 54:551.)

70. B Babies who were born prematurely continue to be at high risk of apnea postoperatively (following general anesthesia) and therefore, should be monitored for 24–48 hours after anesthesia. Aminophylline will increase breathing without significantly altering the CO_2 and pH around the respiratory center. It appears to increase the sensitivity of the respiratory center to carbon dioxide. Patients with adenotonsillar hypertrophy who undergo surgical resection may be admitted to the pediatric intensive care unit (ICU) because of airway obstruction from postoperative edema or sometimes owing to decreased ventilatory drive after anesthesia. The increased opioid activity

found in the spinal fluid in these patients may be a contributing factor to decreased ventilatory drive noted perioperatively. (Kurth CD, et al. Anesthesiol, 1987; 66:483; Gislason T, et al. Chest 1989; 96:250; Lavaher S. Thorax, 1989; 44:121.)

71. E Work of breathing is increased because of chest wall distortion secondary to instability of the chest wall. (Robotham JL. Crit Care Med, 1979; 7:563.)

72. D The more compliant chest wall of the young child contributes to the clinical manifestation of diaphragmatic paralysis. (Rogers MC, et al. *Textbook of Pediatric Intensive Care*, 3rd Edition; pp. 123, 247.)

73. C The upper airway contributes, to a much higher degree, to total respiratory resistance in children than in adults. This may mask the physiologically more important airway resistance. (Cook LD, et al. J Clin Invest, 1957; 36:440)

74. B, A The relationship between alveolar ventilation and both PaO_2 and $PaCO_2$ are nonlinear, as depicted on the graph. (Benumof J. In: Miller RD. *Anesthesia*, Churchill, Livingstone, NY 1981; pp. 699.)

75. B West Zone I occurs when ventilation is wasted. Alveolar pressure remains constant, whereas pulmonary artery pressure tends to increase from apex to base in the erect posture. Hyperinflation, pulmonary embolus, and shock all lead to a decrease in pulmonary blood flow, with consequent wasting of ventilation. (Benumof J. *Anesthesia*, Churchill, Livingstone, NY 1981; pp. 699.)

76. C The so-called West Zone 4 of the lung develops when there is interstitial edema, and under those circumstances, there will be less transduction of fluid across the capillary membrane. (Benumof J. *Anesthesia*, Livingstone, NY 1981; pp. 699.)

77. A Pressure = Flow × Resistance (i.e., mean pulmonary pressure = CO × pulmonary vascular resistance). (Rogers MC, et al. *Textbook of Pediatric Intensive Care*, 2nd Edition; pp. 138.)

78. A, B Regional hypoxic pulmonary vasoconstriction does not result in significant elevation of pulmonary artery pressure, and it seems to be a protective mechanism for the host. (Fishman AP. Civ Res, 1976; 38:221.)

79,80. B, E Compliance of the chest wall is described in option D. Bronchiolitis primarily affects the airway and, unless associated with significant pneumonia, it does not increase the elastic recoil of the lungs. (Rogers MC, et al. *Textbook of Pediatric Intensive Care*, 2nd Edition; pp. 138,139.)

81. B Dynamic compliance is smaller than static compliance because dynamic compliance is equal to the change in volume divided by peak inspiratory pressure minus positive end expiratory pressure (PEEP), as opposed static compliance, which equals volume divided by plateau pressure minus PEEP. Because peak inspiratory pressure is greater than the plateau pressure, the dynamic compliance would be smaller than the static compliance. (Rogers MC, et al. *Textbook of Pediatric Intensive Care*, 2nd Edition; pp. 138,139.)

82. B All other conditions are associated with decreased compliance. (Rogers MC, et al. *Textbook of Pediatric Intensive Care*, 2nd Edition; pp. 138,139.)

83. A In fact, airway resistance accounts for more than 80% of nonelastic resistance. (Rogers MC, et al. *Textbook of Pediatric Intensive Care*, 2nd Edition; pp. 140–142.)

84. B Time constant is the product of compliance (C) and resistance (R). Mathematically, 63% of lung inflation or deflation occurs with one time constant. (Rogers MC, et al. *Textbook of Pediatric Intensive Care*, 2nd Edition; pp. 105,106.)

85. B Hyperinflation leads to increased physiological dead space. (Rogers MC, et al. *Textbook of Pediatric Intensive Care*, 1992; pp. 142,143.)

86, 87. E, B Pulmonary edema is more likely to lead to a decrease in functional residual capacity rather than an increase in closing capacity. Elimination of secretions and use of effective bronchodilators are useful strategies to improve closing capacity.

88. A Because blood flow falls more dramatically than ventilation from the base of the lung toward the apex of the lung, the ventilation perfusion ratio increases exponentially as one moves up the lung.

(West JB. *Ventilation/Blood Flow and Gas Exchange*, 3rd Edition; Oxford, Blackwell Scientific, 1977; p. 30.)

89, 90. B, D A significant portion of the tidal volume dissipates when the compliance of the ventilatory circuit is high. Patient's compliance and resistance also affects the actual delivered tidal volume. The exhalation valve is usually kept close to the airway opening in order to minimize the circuit volume. (Rogers MC. *Textbook of Pediatric Intensive Care*, 2nd Edition; pp. 147–150.)

91–93. A, B, D In clinical medicine, carbon monoxide (CO) poisoning is probably the most common application of hyperbaric O_2 therapy. The half-life of CO is actually decreased to 23 minutes at 3.0 atmospheric pressure, as opposed to 180 minutes with 100% oxygen at the normal atmospheric pressure. Sixty to 90 minutes of hyperbaric oxygen at 2 to 2.5 atmospheric pressure seems to be safe, without significant central nervous system (CNS) toxicity, although other side effects mentioned in the question are possible. (Rogers MC, et al. *Textbook of Pediatric Intensive Care*, 2nd Edition; pp. 156,157.)

94. E With turbulent airflow, the resistance to airflow is proportionate to density (as opposed to viscosity with laminar flow). Because helium is not as dense as nitrogen, it has a beneficial role in patients with upper airway obstruction, such as croup. More recently, the HeliOx mixture has also been shown to improve gas exchange in patients with acute asthma with or without ventilatory support. HeliOx mixture minimizes work of breathing by altering the resistance to airflow. HeliOx mixture is most beneficial at 80:20 or 70:30 ratios. (Rogers MC, et al. *Textbook of Pediatric Intensive Care*, 2nd Edition; p. 157.)

95. A The flow through the ventilator circuit is set at 8 L/minute. Therefore, $8000 \div 60 \times 0.5 = 66 \div 6 = 11$ mL/kg.

96. C Most of gas exchange takes place during exhalation. (Rogers MC, et al. *Textbook of Pediatric Intensive Care*, 2nd Edition; pp. 156–159.)

97–99. D, A, A The inspiratory pressure relief valve is housed in the expiratory limb of the circuit in these ventilators. Actually, in order to minimize work of breathing, the inspiratory gas flow in the continuous flow circuit should meet the patient's inspiratory flow rate demand. (Rogers MC, et al. *Textbook of Pediatric Intensive Care*, 2nd Edition; pp. 156–159.)

100. **A** In the pressure support mode of ventilation, the length of the cycle, as well as depth and flow characteristics, are determined by the patient. (Rogers MC, et al. *Textbook of Pediatric Intensive Care*, 2nd Edition; pp. 156–159.)

101, 102. **D, E** All three options are methods of providing an inverse ratio ventilation, which has been used successfully to improve oxygenation and ventilation at a reduced peak inspiratory pressure. During inverse ratio ventilation, the tidal volume is a function of multiple factors, some of which are enumerated in the question. (Tharralt RS, et al. Chest, 1988; 94:755.)

103. **C** The decrease in oxygen delivery associated with elevation of PEEP is usually responsive to adequate fluid resuscitation and inotropic support, unless one is using extremely high levels of PEEP. (Rogers MC, et al. *Textbook of Pediatric Intensive Care*, 3rd Edition; pp. 297–300.)

104. **D** Please *see* Rogers MC, et al. *Textbook of Pediatric Intensive Care*, 3rd Edition; pp. 184.

105. **E** All of these factors are operative when it comes to the adverse hemodynamic effects of PEEP. (Rogers MC, et al. *Textbook of Pediatric Intensive Care*, 2nd Edition; pp. 186.)

106. **E** Unless they progress to a tension pneumothorax or a tension pneumoperitoneum, none of the manifestations of barotrauma mentioned are usually clinically significant (i.e., do not require immediate intervention). (Rogers MC, et al. *Textbook of Pediatric Intensive Care*, 2nd Edition; pp. 186–188.)

107. **B** During tension pneumothorax, the intrapleural pressure is consistently higher than the atmospheric pressure. (Rogers MC, et al. *Textbook of Pediatric Intensive Care*, 3rd Edition; pp. 307–309.)

108. **B** Veno-venous extracorporeal life support (ECLS) usually requires a higher rate of flow because of the recirculation of the previously oxygenated blood. This is true when the pulmonary bed is totally non-

functional. (Rogers MC, et al. *Textbook of Pediatric Intensive Care*, 3rd Edition; pp. 317,318.)

109. **B, A, A** veno-venous ECLS maintains pulmonary blood flow with oxygenated blood, but it does not assist the systemic circulation. On the other hand, veno-arterial ECLS) does assist the systemic circulation and it also tends to decrease the pulmonary artery pressure. (Rogers MC, et al. *Textbook of Pediatric Intensive Care*, 3rd Edition; pp. 317,318.)

110. **C** The oxygen saturation that is obtained using pulse oximetry is called a functional saturation, and the pulse oximetry obtains the ratio of oxy-Hb divided by the total Hb. (Rogers MC, et al. *Textbook of Pediatric Intensive Care*, 3rd Edition; pp. 333–336.)

111. **C** Methylene blue absorbs light maximally at 668 nm. The pulse oximeter interprets this extra absorbance as reduced Hb, and therefore a lower oxygen saturation is obtained. The oxygen saturation obtained by the pulse oximetry could drop dramatically within 30 seconds of an intravenous administration of methylene blue, and it remains reduced for approximately 2 minutes. (Scheller M. Anesthesiology, 1986; 65:550.)

112. **A** Carboxy-Hb and met-Hb produce these findings. (Barker SJ. Anesthesiology, 1987; 66:677.)

113. **D** With an increase in met-Hb concentration, the saturation on the pulse oximeter decreases and plateaus at approximately 85%. Met-Hb absorbs light significantly at both 660 nm and 940 nm wavelengths, thereby confusing the pulse oximeter photo detector into believing that both oxy-Hb and reduced Hb are increased. This results in increases in both the denominator and numerator. As this happens, the microprocessor-driven algorithm of the red absorbance and infrared absorbance approaches unity and this gives rise to a saturation of approximately 85% on the calibration curve. Hyperbilirubinemia does not interfere with reading of the pulse oximetry. (Barker SJ, et al. Anesthesiology, 1988; 68:279.)

114, 115. **D, E** In the presence of normal oxygen extraction and utilization by the tissue, an increase in oxygen delivery will not result in decreased mixed-venous oxygen saturation. Increased oxygen consumption leads to a decrease in mixed venous oxygen saturation, and not vice versa. (Rogers MC, et al. *Textbook of Pediatric Intensive Care*, 2nd Edition; pp. 210,211.)

116. D This capnogram reveals irregularity in the pattern of the exhalation of the CO_2 which most likely reflects irregularity in the pattern of breathing of this patient. Adding 20 cmH_2O of pressure support will decrease the work of breathing by overcoming the work that is necessary to open the demand valve mechanism that is operating in this ventilator. It will also help to overcome some of the resistance of the endotracheal tube. (Carlon G, et al. Crit Care Med, 1988; 16:550.)

117. E Hypoventilation is likely to lead to a gradual increase in the level of end tidal CO_2. All other clinical conditions indicated in the question lead to a sudden decline in end tidal CO_2 levels. (Carlon G, et al. Crit Care Med, 1988; 16:550.)

118. A The presence of a gas bubble in a syringe will usually affect the PaO_2. The effect on the PaO_2 will depend on the amount of oxygen that is inspired by the patient. In patients on room air, this will lead to a false elevation of PaO_2 (atmospheric PO_2 is usually higher than alveolar PO_2). On the other hand, in patients who are receiving a high fraction of inspired oxygen and have normal lungs, the presence of an air bubble in a syringe may spuriously lower the PaO_2. Excess heparin does lead to a drop in $PaCO_2$, but usually there are no changes in the pH level because it is neutralized by the acidity of heparin. (Rogers MC, et al. *Textbook of Pediatric Intensive Care*, 3rd Edition; pp. 353–359.)

119. E Reticulocytes and band forms are highly metabolic immature cells that are most likely to lead to a change in the blood gas results. (Rogers MC, et al. *Textbook of Pediatric Intensive Care*, 3rd Edition; pp. 355–359.)

120. D Aspirin, especially with overdose, is likely to lead to high anion gap metabolic acidosis (HAGMA). All other drugs do not. (Rogers MC, et al. *Textbook of Pediatric Intensive Care*, 3rd Edition; p. 361.)

121. D Other abnormalities of the CNS, esophagus, and cardiovascular system have been reported in association with choanal atresia. Therefore, evaluation for possible other anomalies should be done in patients with posterior choanal atresia. (Rogers MC, et al. *Textbook of Pediatric Intensive Care*, 2nd Edition; pp. 231–233.)

122. D Nasal obstruction is usually seen when the mass is located at the base of the brain. (Rogers MC, et al. *Textbook of Pediatric Intensive Care*, 2nd Edition; pp. 231–233.)

123. E All are features of angiofibroma. (Rogers MC, et al. *Textbook of Pediatric Intensive Care*, 2nd Edition; pp. 231–233.)

124. A, A, B, B Vocal cords in infants are concave, the anterior attachment to the trachea is lower, and the glottis is located higher in the neck compared with an adult. (Rogers MC, et al. *Textbook of Pediatric Intensive Care*, 2nd Edition; pp. 231–233.)

125. C At 4–6 months of age, the epiglottis loses contact with the soft palate and assumes a more erect posture, allowing oral (mouth) breathing. The lateral diameter of the newborn glottis is only about 4–5 mm, and at birth the trachea is approximately 5–7 cm in length. The glottis assumes the adult location at C6 by about 12 years of age. (Rogers MC, et al. *Textbook of Pediatric Intensive Care*, 2nd Edition; pp. 231–233.)

126. A (Rogers MC, et al. *Textbook of Pediatric Intensive Care*, 2nd Edition; pp. 231–232.)

127. B $\pi R^2 = 16 \pi$ when the diameter is 8 mm which gives rise to a radius of 4 mm. With a uniform 1 mm reduction in the size of the airway, this will decrease the diameter from 8 to 6 mm, and decrease the radius from 4 to 3 mm. Now $\pi R^2 = 9 \pi$, $9 \div 16 = 54\%$, which means that the diameter of the airway has been decreased by 44%. (Rogers MC, et al. *Textbook of Pediatric Intensive Care*, 2nd Edition; pp. 231–233.)

128. E All of these are measures that may be needed to intervene with laryngospasm. (Rogers MC, et al. *Textbook of Pediatric Intensive Care*, 2nd Edition; pp. 233–234.)

129. B Congenital anomalies are the most common cause of chronic stridor in children less than 2 years of age. (Rogers MC, et al. *Textbook of Pediatric Intensive Care*, 2nd Edition; pp. 235–238.)

130. **C** Please *see* Rogers MC, et al. *Textbook of Pediatric Intensive Care*, 2nd Edition; pp. 235–238

131. **C** Laryngotracheomalacia is characterized by normal voice. (Rogers MC, et al. *Textbook of Pediatric Intensive Care*, 2nd Edition; p. 236.)

132. **C, C** Both laryngomalacia and airway or subglottic hemangioma usually present with symptoms before 6 months of age. In both cases, the treatment is conservative because in most cases, the problem resolves spontaneously by the end of the 2nd birthday. (Rogers MC, et al. *Textbook of Pediatric Intensive Care*, 2nd Edition; pp. 235–238.)

133. **E** All of these conditions pose difficult airway management. (Rogers MC, et al. *Textbook of Pediatric Intensive Care*, 2nd Edition; pp. 235–238.)

134. **D** All of the choices are complications that may be noted in the postoperative period following repair of cleft lip and cleft palate. Occasionally, bronchospasm is also seen. (Rogers MC, et al. *Textbook of Pediatric Intensive Care*, 2nd Edition; pp. 235–238.)

135. **C** Both these conditions are characterized by macroglossia with a short neck, which combine to produce a difficult airway. Both of these conditions belong to the mucopolysaccharidoses. (Rogers MC, et al. *Textbook of Pediatric Intensive Care*, 2nd Edition; p. 241.)

136. **E** Please *see* Rogers MC, et al. *Textbook of Pediatric Intensive Care*, 2nd Edition; p. 241.

137. **A** The typical age for this condition is younger than 3 years. It is important to obtain inspiratory radiographs to evaluate the thickness of the retropharyngeal soft tissue. Measurement of this soft tissue is important in the diagnosis of the retropharyngeal abscess. (Rogers MC, et al. *Textbook of Pediatric Intensive Care*, 2nd Edition; p. 242.)

138. **B** In fact, frequent tracheal suctioning is necessary in these patients to prevent airway obstruction because the infection/inflammation induces an increase in airway secretions. (Rogers MC, et al. *Textbook of Pediatric Intensive Care*, 2nd Edition; pp. 242–245.)

139. **D** These are the indications for extubation in a patient with a viral croup. (Rogers MC, et al. *Textbook of Pediatric Intensive Care*, 2nd Edition; pp. 244–246.)

140. **D** The amount of subcutaneous emphysema of the neck area does not correlate with the severity of airway injury. Nasotracheal intubation should be avoided in patients with midfacial fractures, and also in patients suspected of having a fracture of the base of the skull. (Rogers MC, et al. *Textbook of Pediatric Intensive Care*, 2nd Edition; pp. 245–248.)

141. **A** Seventy to eighty percent of subglottic stenosis occurs following endotracheal intubation. (Rogers MC, et al. *Textbook of Pediatric Intensive Care*, 2nd Edition; pp. 245–248.)

142. **E** The accepted duration of time for intubation to prevent subglottic stenosis is unknown. (Rogers MC, et al. *Textbook of Pediatric Intensive Care*, 2nd Edition; pp. 245–248.)

143. **D** A HeliOx mixture in various combinations has been shown to be effective in the management of postextubation stridor and burn victims with significant stridor. (Rogers MC, et al. *Textbook of Pediatric Intensive Care*, 2nd Edition; p. 245.)

144. **D** Most of these airway papillomas resolve by the teenage years. (Rogers MC, et al. *Textbook of Pediatric Intensive Care*, 2nd Edition; p 252.)

145. **A** These patients respond to relatively low concentrations of inspired oxygen. (Rogers MC, et al. *Textbook of Pediatric Intensive Care*, 2nd Edition; pp. 258–260.)

146. **D** High antidiuretic hormone (ADH) levels in association with elevation of renin has been reported in patients with bronchiolitis. (Gozal D, et al. Pediatr Res, 1990; 27:204–209.)

147. **C** High ADH in association with high aldosterone levels has been reported in patients with respiratory syncytial virus bronchiolitis. Because of this combination of hormonal abnormalities, there is a decrease in urine output associated with a normal urine sodium concentration. (Gozal D, et al. Pediatr Res, 1990; 27:204–209.)

148–151. A, A, E, B Maximum mid-expiratory flow rate is one of the flow volume parameters that demonstrates the most severe decrease during an attack of asthma. This is also the parameter that is the last to improve following treatment for acute asthma. Patients with asthma, particularly those that are in status asthmaticus, have an increased residual volume. (Rogers MC, et al. *Textbook of Pediatric Intensive Care*, 2nd Edition; pp. 264–270.)

152, 153. D, D Transmural pressure = intraluminal pressure – extraluminal pressure. With higher negative inspiratory pressure, as seen with status asthmaticus, there is an increase in afterload during inspiration with a subsequent decrease in left ventricular output, which is followed by a sharp increase in left ventricular output during subsequent expiration. This leads to the phenomenon of pulsus paradoxus (PP). A decrease in PP may indicate an improvement in the patient's condition (i.e., a smaller fall in pleural), but it may also indicate the patient's fatigue and worsening clinical condition. Another factor that contributes to PP is ventricular interdependence, which can be exaggerated by the pulmonary hypertension, as it may be seen with severe status asthmaticus. The hypoxia that is seen during status asthmaticus results from V/Q mismatch, excessive O_2 requirement secondary to increased metabolic demand, and a degree of interstitial edema. (Rogers MC, et al. *Textbook of Pediatric Intensive Care*, 2nd Edition; pp. 268–270.)

154. A The degree of hypoxemia does not correlate with the degree of airway obstruction as assessed by the reduction in forced expiratory volume in 1 second (FEV_1). (McFaden ER, et al. N Engl J Med, 1968; 278:1029.)

155. D As the FEV_1 drops below 20% predicted, PCO_2 rises, hypoxemia occurs, and pulsus paradoxus is present in almost all of these patients. (McFaden ER, et al. N Engl J Med, 1968; 278:1029.)

156. B   0.3 liters $\longrightarrow$ 1 PSI

χ liters $\longrightarrow$ 1100 PSI

therefore:

$$\chi = \frac{1100 \times 0.3}{1} = \frac{330 \text{ L}}{4 \text{ L/minute}} = 82.5 \text{ minutes}$$

157. B Both V/Q increase as one moves from the apex of the lungs toward the base of the lung. However, perfusion increases more than ventilation. Therefore, apical regions are underperfused with a V/Q of approximately 3, whereas basal regions of the lungs are underventilated in relation to perfusion with a V/Q of approximately 0.6. (West JB. *Ventilation/Blood Flow and Gas Exchange*, 3rd Edition. Oxford, Blackwell Scientific, 1977; pp. 30,31.)

158. C The major indication for tracheostomy in early burn management is upper airway obstruction which may be owing to edema, a foreign body, or laryngeal trauma such that an endotracheal tube cannot be passed. (Carvajal HF, Parks DM. *Pediatric Burn Management*, Yearbook Medical Publishers, Inc., 1988; pp. 167,168.)

159. D In the human, there are five stages of lung development:

1. Embryonal (Day 26–Day 52): characterized by development of trachea and major bronchi.
2. Pseudoglandular (Day 52–Week 16): characterized by development of remaining tracheobronchial tree.
3. Canalicular (Week 17–Week 28): characterized by development of vascular bed and framework of acinus.
4. Saccular (Week 29–Week 36): characterized by increased complexity of saccules.
5. Alveolar (Week 26–Term): characterized by development of alveoli.

The lungs emerge as a bud from the pharynx at day 26 following conception. This bud elongates, separates from the esophagus, and continues to divide to form the main bronchi. Extensive subdivision in the pseudoglandular stage leads to formation of the conducting airway, the most peripheral of which are the terminal bronchioles, which give rise to respiratory bronchioles and alveolar ducts during the canalicular stage. During this later stage, the acinus is formed. An acinus is the gas exchange unit associated with a single-terminal bronchiole, and will eventually contain three orders of respiratory bronchioles: alveolar ducts, alveolar sacs, and alveoli.

The Saccular stage was formerly thought to be the last stage of lung development prior to birth. However, because alveoli form before birth, the termination of this period is now arbitrarily set at 35–36 weeks' gestation. At the beginning of this phase (28 weeks' gestation) the terminal structures are call saccules. They are cylindrical structures with a smooth wall. They become subdivided by ridges called secondary crests. Further subdivision between crests results in small spaces termed subsaccules. Exactly when these subsaccules can be termed alveoli is a matter of debate. The range of timing is between 29–36 weeks' gestation. Most of postnatal formation of alveoli occurs over the first 1–1.5 years of life. Pores of Kohn are not established until several years after birth. (Langston C, Kida K, Reed M, et al. Am Rev Resp Dis, 1984; 129:607.)

160.　B　$PaO_2 = PiO_2 - \dfrac{PaCO_2}{RQ}$

$$= \dfrac{(747 - 47) \times 0.4 - 40}{0.8}$$

$$= 280 - 50 = \mathbf{230}$$

Alveolar arterial O_2 gradient $= PAO_2 - PaO_2$

$$= 230 - 100$$

$$= \mathbf{130}$$

(Kandra TG, Rosenthal M.Int Anesthesiol, 1993; 31:119–121.)

161.　B　Please *see* Jodka PG, Heard SO. Int Anesthesiol, 2000; 35:1–10.

162.　E　Bronchopleural fistulae (BPF) can result from blunt trauma, barotraumas, or inflammatory diseases of the lung. Patients with BPF can present acutely because of pulmonary flooding or tension pneumothorax, or subacutely with an insidious clinical course. A persistent air leak without evidence of technical problem in the pleural drainage apparatus also indicates a BPF. Several techniques can be employed using bronchoscopy to localize the proximal endobronchial site of the fistulous tract. Occasionally, air bubbles can be seen emanating from the segmental bronchus. Washing the suspected segment with saline and coughing may accentuate the bubbling. Techniques for obliteration of the fistula bronchoscopically have also been described. (McManigle JE, et al. Chest, 1990; 97:1235–1238.)

163.　C　After a delay of 2–8 minutes, intramuscular ketamine (4–8 mg/kg) produces anesthesia for 20–40 minutes. More than 90–92% of ketamine is absorbed after an intramuscular injection. (White PF, Way WL, Trevor AJ. Anesthesiology, 1982; 56:119.)

164.　D　The cellular proliferative phase, after alveolar injury, is characterized by type II cellular hyperplasia, which appears to be a reparative process. These cuboidal cells may virtually cover the entire alveolar surface. They will later transform into the thin, type I alveolar epithelial cells. (Royall JA, Matalon S. In: Fuhrman BP, Zimmerman JJ. *Pediatric Critical Care*, Mosby Yearbook 1992, pp. 445–456.)

165.　A　Tachypnea is the earliest sign of respiratory muscle fatigue. As a compensation for the decrease in efficient tidal volume, the respiratory rate increases in an attempt to maintain minute ventilation. (Nunn JF. *Applied Respiratory Physiology*, 3rd Edition. Boston: Butterworth, 1987, p. 109.)

166.　C　CO_2 binds with deoxy-Hb to form carbamino-Hb, which is one of the forms in which CO_2 is transported in the blood. However, only 10% of CO_2 in blood is transported in this form. Myoglobin approaches full saturation at a PO_2 of 15–30 mmHg, which is the level pertaining to voluntary muscle. The bulk of its oxygen may be released only at very low O_2 tension. 2,3-Diphosphoglycerate decreases the affinity of O_2 for Hb, and thus, facilitates release of O_2 to tissues and so does carbon dioxide. This latter phenomenon is also known as the Bohr effect. O_2 binds to one of the six coordination bonds of the iron atom. Hydrogen binds to the imidazole ring of histidine on the globin chains of the Hb molecule. (Nunn JF. *Applied Respiratory Physiology*, 4th Edition; pp. 273–275; Guyton AC. *Textbook of Medical Physiology*, 8th Edition; pp. 440–442.)

167.　E　Increasing PEEP will diminish left-to-right shunting by increasing the pulmonary vascular resistance. All other measures stated in the question would increase left-to-right shunt flow. (Meliones JN, et al. *Respiratory Support in Infants & Children*; p. 352.)

168.　D　Linoleic acid is the primary precursor of arachidonic acid. (Abman S, Stenmark K. Am J Physiology, 1992; 262: L214.)

169.　C　O_2 delivery $(DO_2) =$ Cardiac output (CO) $\times$ Arterial O_2 Content (CaO_2)

$CaO_2 = $ Hb (gm%) $\times 1.34 \times O_2$ Sat $+ PaO_2 \times 0.003$

In this case, increasing the Hb from 9 to 14 gm% will increase O_2 delivery the most. (Fahey JT, Lister G. In:

Fuhrman BP, Zimmerman *JJ. Pediatric Critical Care,* 2nd Edition; pp. 235–240.)

170. **A** J receptors act to stimulate breathing.

171. **C** Pulmonary capillary endothelial damage is one of the earliest changes in ARDS. Capillary congestion occurs with intraluminal aggregation of platelets, fibrin, and neutrophils. Pulmonary capillary endothelial cells undergo swelling and focal necrosis with destruction of mitochondria, endoplasmic reticulum, and ribosomes during the first few hours of ARDS. (Rogers MC, et al. *Textbook of Pediatric Intensive Care*, 2nd Edition; pp. 297,298.)

172. **A** The Mapleson D breathing circuit (shown in figure below) can be described as a T-piece with an expiratory limb. The fresh gas inlet is located near the patient, and the expiratory pressure release valve is near the reservoir bag. The pressure release valve opens as pressure increases during expiration and a portion of the expired gas along with fresh gas is released into the atmosphere. During the next inspiration, the patient receives a combination of fresh gas and the exhaled gas. The content of this inspired gas is determined by:

1. Rate of fresh gas flow: A fresh gas flow more than two times the minute ventilation prevents rebreathing.
2. Patient's tidal volume: the amount of rebreathing increases as the tidal volume increases.
3. Duration of expiration: a short expiratory pause provides inadequate time to flush the alveolar gas (occurs with faster respiratory rate); this allows rebreathing.

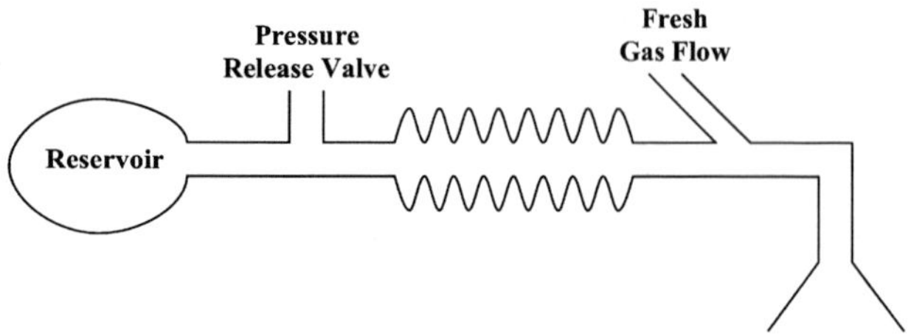

(Barash PG, Cullen BF, Stoelting RK. *Clinical Anesthesia*, 2nd Edition; pp. 654.)

173. **C** When peak airway pressure is allowed to increase to a level beyond that which is necessary to maximally distend the lungs, barotrauma and lung injury result. Because regional differences in lung resistance and compliance often coexist, maintaining a constant tidal volume may overdistend areas of the lung that are aerated if the remainder of the lung is collapsed. Similarly, maintaining a constant inspiratory flow pattern when regional differences in lung units exist will selectively increase distention of lung units with lower resistance. (Haake R, et al. Chest, 1987; 1:608.)

174. **D** Pulmonary conditions associated with decreased compliance, such as pulmonary fibrosis and ARDS or increased airway resistance such as bronchial asthma and chronic obstructive pulmonary disease (COPD), have the potential for being homogenous. This homogeneity can result in regional overdistention during positive pressure ventilation. Hyperinflation secondary to airway narrowing or collapse, such as seen with auto-PEEP, increases end-expiratory lung volume, but does not result in lung expansion of the hyperinflated lung units until airway pressure exceeds the level of auto-PEEP. Although the work of breathing during spontaneous breathing is increased by auto-PEEP, end-inspiratory lung volumes do not increase. (Bone RC, Stober G. Med Clin Noth Am, 1983; 67:599.)

175. **D** Changes in intrathoracic pressure correlate highly with changes in lung volume. Changes in intrathoracic pressure are independent of lung compliance. An increase in respiratory rate with lung conditions associated with increased expiratory airway resistance will result in dynamic hyperinflation, because there is inadequate time for exhalation. Examples are COPD, asthma, and other causes of intrathoracic airway obstruction. Thus, overdistention is possible with a fixed tidal breath or tidal volume. Because regional lung compliance, even in healthy individuals, is different under all conditions, uniform expansion of all lung units by positive pressure ventilation at any setting probably never occurs. (Marini JJ. In: Pinsky MR, Dhainaut JFA, Ed. *Pathophysiologic Foundations of Critical Care*, 1993; pp. 453–471.)

176. **B** Please *see* Marini JJ. In: Pinsky MR, Dhainaut JFA, eds. *Pathophysiologic Foundations of Critical Care*, 1993; pp. 453–471.

177. **A** Nitric oxide is synthesized from the amino acid arginine by the action of the enzyme nitric oxide synthetase. (Nichols DG, et al. *Critical Heart Disease in Infants and Children.* Mosby, 1995; pp. 36, 78, 111, 206.)

178. D Systemic-to-pulmonary shunt is often created in neonates and infants with an underlying cardiac defect in order to improve pulmonary blood flow and oxygenation. Examples are the (modified) Blalock-Taussig shunt that connects the subclavian artery to the pulmonary artery using a synthetic material, and the aortic to pulmonary window, which usually connects the ascending aorta to the pulmonary artery. Conditions that lead to a reduction in pulmonary artery pressure and pulmonary vascular resistance would increase the flow across the shunt with an increase in left-to-right shunt. Examples include: alkalosis, vasodilators such as hydralazine and nitroprusside, an increase in the concentration of inspired oxygen, and selective pulmonary vasodilators, such as nitric oxide. Interventions that lead to an increase in pulmonary vascular resistance, such as increasing PEEP, would lead to a reduction in pulmonary blood flow and a reduction in the left-to-right shunt. (Nichols DG, et al. *Critical Heart Disease in Infants and Children*, Mosby, 1995; pp. 460.)

179. B Tachypnea in this infant would be the earliest evidence of inspiratory muscle fatigue. (Nichols DG, et al. *Critical Heart Disease in Infants and Children*, Mosby, 1995; pp. 319–332.)

180. C Nitric dioxide is the toxic by-product. The rate of formation of this toxic product is dependent on the duration of contact between oxygen and nitric oxide. (Nichols DG, et al. *Critical Heart Disease in Infants and Children*, Mosby, 1995; pp. 36, 78, 111, 206.)

181. E Please *see* Rogers MC, et al. *Textbook of Pediatric Intensive Care*, 2nd Edition; pp. 157, 245–246.

182. C Histological features of infants with BPD include squamous metaplasia of the airway epithelium (large and small airways), increased peribronchial smooth muscle with fibrosis, submucosal edema, and inflammation with hypertrophy of submucosal glands. In the parenchyma, there are areas of fibrosis with atelectasis alternating with areas of hyperinflation, which, on gross examination of the lungs, has a cobblestone appearance. In more long-standing cases,

there is diminution in alveolarization and surface area. The decrease in the number of alveoli probably reflects the onset of the insult with subsequent failure of the ability to regenerate new alveoli. This is associated with an increased number of small pulmonary arteries, which may contribute to pulmonary hypertension. The pulmonary arterial tree shows proliferation of the intima, smooth muscle hypertrophy, distal extension of smooth muscles, and adventitial thickening. (Abman SH, Groothius JR. Pediatr Clin North Am, 1994; 41, pp. 277–291.)

183. C Upper airway obstruction usually does not lead to an alveolar–arterial oxygen gradient. On rare occasions when upper airway obstruction is complicated by postobstruction pulmonary edema, this is possible. (Rogers MC, et al. *Textbook of Pediatric Intensive Care*, 2nd Edition; pp. 231–296.)

184. E The lungs have a tendency to collapse, while the chest wall has a tendency to move outward. Thus the elastic forces of the lung and the chest wall are in opposite directions. These two opposing forces are linked by the pleural surfaces and the nest pressure is the intrapleural pressure. (Rogers MC, et al. *Textbook of Pediatric Intensive Care*, 2nd Edition; pp. 145.)

185. B Bronchogenic cyst accounts for 5% of mediastinal masses. It is found in five major locations: right paratracheal region (20%); carinal region (51%); hilar region (9%); paraesophageal (14%); and pericardial/retrosternal. (Taussig LM. *Pediatric Respiratory Medicine*, 1999; p. 1118.)

186. E Hysteresis refers to the failure of a system to follow identical paths of response during application and during withdrawal of a force. In the lungs, this is due mainly to surface properties and alveolar recruitment–derecruitment. In the chest wall, this is because of muscles and ligaments, both of which exhibit hysteresis. (Taussig LM. *Pediatric Respiratory Medicine*, 1999; pp. 100–101.)

187. A Increasing the length of muscle fibers (to a limited extent) would increase the force of contraction and thus the efficiency of the diaphragm. The diaphragm is most efficient at the lung volume that corresponds to the FRC, and thus increasing the end-expiratory lung volume above this does not improve the efficiency of the diaphragm. Increasing the radius of curvature increases the efficiency of the diaphragm. The diaphragm of an infant has less radius of curvature than that of an adult, and is less efficient. (Fuhrman BP, Zimmerman JJ. *Pediatric Critical Care*, 2nd Edition; pp. 407.)

188. A Bronchoalveolar lavage in ARDS is characterized by predominance of polymorphonuclear leukocytes (PMNs), of 10 greater than 85%. (Reynolds HY. Am Rev Resp Dis, 1987; 135:250–263.)

189. B Massive hemoptysis is relatively uncommon in cystic fibrosis patients. It occurs in 10% of adolescents and adult patients with cystic fibrosis. Massive hemoptysis usually occurs from the bronchial circulation resulting from the higher systemic pressure compared with the pulmonary circulation. Often an untreated exacerbation of the disease is a triggering factor, but sometimes there is no clear cause. If hemoptysis persists, bronchial artery embolization is warranted; this requires bronchial arteriography. (Sweeney N, Fellows K. Chest, 1990; 97:1322–1326.)

190. B In infants, the continuous muscle tone of the thorax is important to maintain FRC, because the chest wall is very compliant and lacks the rigidity necessary to oppose the elastic recoil of the lung, which tends to lower FRC. With age, as chest wall compliance decreases and the chest wall becomes more rigid and capable to oppose the elastic recoil of the lungs, FRC increases. (Rogers MC, et al. *Textbook of Pediatric Intensive Care*, 2nd Edition; pp. 112–128.)

191. B A HeliOx mixture is less dense that a nitrogen–O_2 (air) mixture. With turbulent flow (seen with upper airway obstruction, such as subglottic stenosis), resistance to air flow is proportional to density. A HeliOx mixture is useful in reducing the resistance to flow and work of breathing. (Rogers MC, et al. *Textbook of Pediatric Intensive Care*, 3rd Edition; pp. 275–276.)

192. B Refer to the answer for Question 182.

193. D $PAO_2 = (BP – Vapor\ Pressure) \times FiO_2 – PaCO_2 / RQ$

Because $PaCO_2$ and RQ are assumed to remain constant, they will remain the same under both situations: $(760 – 47) \times 0.27 = 192.51$

In order to keep the PaO2 the same, and therefore compensate for the same degree of alveolar–arterial oxygen gradient as the atmospheric pressure decreases, the alveolar oxygen tension must remain the same (i.e., 192.51). Therefore,

$(632 – 47) \times$ Unknown fraction of inspired oxygen $= 192.51$

$FiO_2 = 192.51 / 632–47 = 192.51 / 585 = 0.3290$

(Rogers MC, et al. *Textbook of Pediatric Intensive Care*, 2nd Edition; pp. 116,117.)

194. B The function of this protein is to promote formation of a surfactant layer. It is, therefore, essential for effective reduction of the surface tension induced by surfactant. (Fuhrman BP, Zimmerman JJ. *Pediatric Critical Care*, 2nd Edition; pp. 382,383.)

195. E Type I alveolar cells are less in number than type II alveolar cells (which synthesize surfactant), but they cover a much larger area of the lung. Their primary function is to reduce the barrier to gas exchange. (Fuhrman BP, Zimmerman JJ. *Pediatric Critical Care*, 2nd Edition; pp. 445,446.)

196. C Forced vital capacity (FVC) is easily measured during spirometry. Data obtained from a specific patient can be compared with those from subjects who have the same height, weight, and age. FVC is highly reproducible and has a narrow range of normal values. It is affected in both obstructive and restrictive lung diseases. FVC may decline in the supine position by up to 20% in normal subjects and up to 38% in patients with underlying neuromuscular diseases. (Civeta JM, et al. *Critical Care*, 2nd Edition; pp. 565,566.)

197. A Work = Force × Distance. When it comes to the respiratory system, work is defined as the pressure that is generated by the respiratory muscle to move a particular volume of gas. (Rogers MC, et al. *Textbook of Pediatric Intensive Care*, 2nd Edition; pp. 129,130.)

198. B Alveolar O_2 tension = (Barometric Pressure – Vapor Pressure) $\times FiO_2 – PaCO_2 / RQ$

$(760 – 47) \times 0.21 – 85 / 0.8$

$713 \times 0.21 – 106.25 = 43.38$

$PAO_2 – PaO_2 = 10$

Therefore: $PaO_2 = 43 - 10 = 33$ mmHg

(Rogers MC, et al. *Textbook of Pediatric Intensive Care*, 3rd Edition; p. 90.)

199, 200.   E, A   The half-life of a drug is function of clearance (CL) and volume of distribution (Vd) according to the following formula:

Half-life = $0.693 \times$ Vd / CL

Thus half-life is affected not only by elimination, but also by Vd. For instance, during ECLS, most of the increase in the half-life is owing to an increase in the Vd, rather than a change in drug clearance. A drug's half-life can also be used to determine the time it takes for the drug to reach a steady-state concentration, a state in which the amount of drug administered equals the amount cleared by the body.

After 3 half-lives	87% of steady-state concentration is achieved.
After 4 half-lives	93% of steady-state concentration is achieved.
After 5 half-lives	97% of steady-state concentration is achieved.

(Fuhrman BP, Zimmerman JJ. *Pediatric Critical Care*, 2nd Edition; p. 1281; Behrman BE, et al. *Nelson Textbook of Pediatrics*, 15th Edition; p. 294.)

CHAPTER 2: CARDIOVASCULAR SYSTEM

1.   A   The Mueller maneuver (inspiration against closed glottis) increases afterload similar to phenylephrine. The Valsalva maneuver has the opposite effect. (Rogers MC, et al. *Textbook of Pediatric Intensive Care*, 3rd Edition; pp. 369–380.)

2.   E   The ventricular afterload is best approximated by ventricular wall stress, or the degree of stretching of the ventricular muscle. (Rogers MC, et al. *Textbook of Pediatric Intensive Care*, 3rd Edition; pp. 369–380.)

3.   D   All three mechanisms described are operative in the process of ventricular interdependence. (Rogers MC, et al. *Textbook of Pediatric Intensive Care*, 3rd Edition; pp. 369–380.)

4.   A   In the failing heart, or congestive cardiac failure, the effect of changes in intrathoracic pressure on afterload is predominant. Afterload is best approximated by ventricular wall stress. (Rogers MC, et al. *Textbook of Pediatric Intensive Care*, 3rd Edition; pp. 390,391.)

5, 6.   B, E   The right ventricle does not receive more highly oxygenated blood than the left ventricle because of the phenomenon of "streaming," wherein the blood that is returning from the umbilical vein, through the inferior vena cava, is directed to the left atrium owing to the presence of a flap in the inferior vena cava. (Nichols DG, et al. *Critical Heart Disease in Infants and Children*, Mosby, 1995; pp. 17–23.)

7.   B   After birth, because of expansion of the lungs and separation of the placenta, there is a reduction in pulmonary vascular resistance with the first breath and an increase in systemic vascular resistance resulting from loss of the low resistance placenta. (Rogers MC, et al. *Textbook of Pediatric Intensive Care*, 3rd Edition; pp. 397–411.)

8.   C   Arterioles contribute the most to the total peripheral resistance. (Rogers MC, et al. *Textbook of Pediatric Intensive Care*, 3rd Edition; pp. 409–413.)

9.   A   The major portion of oxygen consumption by the heart is directed toward the myocardial wall tension. (Rogers MC, et al. *Textbook of Pediatric Intensive Care*, 3rd Edition; pp. 420–422.)

10, 11.   D, D   Myocardial wall tension is directly proportional to intraventricular pressure and also directly proportional to the intraventricular volume. However, myocardial wall tension is inversely proportional to the myocardial wall thickness. Therefore, in a situation where the wall of the myocardium is thin, there is an increase in myocardial wall tension, and this is likely to lead to increased myocardial oxygen consumption because the majority of oxygen consumed by the heart is utilized by myocardial wall tension. A heart that is dilated (which means that there is increased intraventricular volume associated with a large preload) in the presence of a thin left ventricular wall is a heart that would be considered least efficient. (Rogers MC, et al. *Textbook of Pediatric Intensive Care*, 3rd Edition; pp. 420–422.)

12. B The diagram represents the following: area A is referred to as systolic time index, and area B is referred to as diastolic time index. Because an increase of heart rate increases myocardial oxygen consumption, tachycardia would adversely affect both of these variables, as does hypotension. Area B represents a time where the myocardium receives its blood and oxygen supply. (Rogers MC, et al. *Textbook of Pediatric Intensive Care*, 3rd Edition; pp. 420–421.)

13–15. E, E, D Ischemic heart disease in infants and children should be sought whenever there are risk factors such as those mentioned in Question 13. In the presence of these risk factors, ischemic heart disease in infants in children is not uncommon. Some of the clinical situations are enumerated in Question 15. (Rogers MC, et al. *Textbook of Pediatric Intensive Care*, 3rd Edition; pp. 422–424.)

16. A Eighty percent of infants with anomalous left coronary artery, if untreated, will die before their first birthday. There is frequently a history of screaming with feeding. History of cyanosis at birth is not a recognized feature. This condition may mimic endocardial fibroelastosis or myocarditis. (Rogers MC, et al. *Textbook of Pediatric Intensive Care*, 3rd Edition; pp. 424,425.)

17. A Kawasaki syndrome is a leading cause of ischemic heart disease in children. (Rogers MC, et al. *Textbook of Pediatric Intensive Care*, 3rd Edition; pp. 426–428.)

18. E Coronary artery involvement and cardiac abnormality are more commonly seen in children with Kawasaki syndrome, who are male, less than 1 year of age, have had a fever for longer than 2 weeks, and who have an erythrocyte sedimentation rate of more than 100 mm/hour. (Rogers MC, et al. *Textbook of Pediatric Intensive Care*, 3rd Edition; pp. 426–428.)

19. E These are recognized cardiac abnormalities in a setting of trauma. (Rogers MC, et al. *Textbook of Pediatric Intensive Care*, 3rd Edition; p. 431.)

20. B With high permeability pulmonary edema, the ratio of extravascular lung water to total lung weight increases, and the blood-free dry weight of the lung is increased because of the presence of protein in the extravascular fluid. The total dry weight of the lung is also increased. (Rogers MC, et al. *Textbook of Pediatric Intensive Care*, 3rd Edition; pp. 432–435.)

21. E K_f is the filtration coefficient. σ Is the reflection coefficient. When σ is equal to 1, there is complete restriction to passage of protein across the capillary membrane. On the other hand, when σ is equal to 0, there is no restriction to passage of protein across the capillary membrane. (Rogers MC, et al. *Textbook of Pediatric Intensive Care*, 3rd Edition; pp. 432–435.)

22. D Administration of bleomycin and cyclophosphamide, as well as radiation therapy, are known to potentiate the cardiotoxicity of anthracycline. (Rogers MC, et al. *Textbook of Pediatric Intensive Care*, 3rd Edition; pp. 436–438.)

23. C Cardiotoxicity because of doxorubicin is indeed dose-dependent, and is usually seen at doses higher than 450 mg/M^2. (Rogers MC, et al. *Textbook of Pediatric Intensive Care*, 3rd Edition; pp. 436–438.)

24. D The combination of doxorubicin and cyclophosphamide leads to cardiomyopathy with subsequent cardiac failure, which can present with pulmonary edema. (Rogers MC, et al. *Textbook of Pediatric Intensive Care*, 3rd Edition; pp. 436–438.)

25. D The lungs are the most frequently affected organs with heroin overdose. (Rogers MC, et al. *Textbook of Pediatric Intensive Care*, 3rd Edition; pp. 440–441.)

26. E All of the pulmonary vascular physiological changes listed are true. (Rogers MC, et al. *Textbook of Pediatric Intensive Care*, 3rd Edition; pp. 441–454.)

27. C It will take at least 24 hours for the levels of 2,3-diphosphoglycerate to increase in response to hypoxia. All of the other physiological responses to hypoxia are true. (Rogers MC, et al. *Textbook of Pediatric Intensive Care*, 3rd Edition; pp. 445–448.)

28. C There does not seem to be a strong correlation between the level of PaO_2 and incidence of Tet spells. All other options are true. (Rogers MC, et al.

Textbook of Pediatric Intensive Care, 3rd Edition; pp. 454–458.)

29. D Cyanosis in the face of a normal PaO_2 occurs with smoke inhalation, which is particularly associated with CO poisoning. An overdose on shoe dye leads to met-hemoglobinemia. Both these clinical conditions are characterized by a normal arterial oxygen tension, but a decreased measured oxygen saturation. Patients with a very high hematocrit also may present with cyanosis, which is usually a peripheral cyanosis in the presence of a normal PaO_2. (Rogers MC, et al. *Textbook of Pediatric Intensive Care*, 3rd Edition; pp. 456–458.)

30. D All of the three conditions mentioned benefit from a right-to-left shunt in preserving the cardiac output. (Nichols DG, et al. *Critical Heart Disease in Infants and Children*, Mosby, 1995; pp. 101–112, 755–763, 804–805.)

31. D The first priority in these patients is to obtain an echocardiogram in order to rule out any residual abnormalities that might be contributing to the abnormal cardiac output and oxygenation. (Nichols DG, et al. *Critical Heart Disease in Infants and Children*, Mosby, 1995; pp. 618–620.)

32. A Owing to pulmonary vascular endothelial dysfunction after cardiopulmonary bypass, oxygen is often not a very strong pulmonary vasodilator. With a pH greater than 7.45, it appears that the pulmonary vascular resistance decreases independent of the arterial carbon dioxide pressure ($PaCO_2$). The other options are true. (Nichols DG, et al. *Critical Heart Disease in Infants and Children*, Mosby, 1995; pp. 618–620.)

33. C These findings suggest that there is increased pulmonary blood flow, which is likely to lead to pulmonary congestion, and also a diastolic overload on the right ventricle. Use of hyperventilation and tolazoline will lead to further pulmonary congestion and may lead to deterioration of the patient's overall condition. (Nichols DG, et al. *Critical Heart Disease in Infants and Children*, Mosby, 1995; pp. 863–868.)

34–36. B, D, D Most thoracic duct injuries occur following an extrapericardial procedure, usually a pal-liative procedure such as a systemic-to-pulmonary shunt. Prior to enteral feeding, the pleural fluid may be serosanguinous. It turns into a milky color following enteral feeding. Malnutrition because of loss of protein and fat is a recognized complication, which must be managed appropriately. All are indications for surgical ligation of the thoracic duct for persistent cholothorax. (Rogers MC, et al. *Textbook of Pediatric Intensive Care*, 3rd Edition; pp. 481,482.)

37. B, A, A The purpose of the modified Fontan procedure is to eliminate the obligatory diastolic overload on the single ventricle and also to improve oxygenation. Following the Norwood procedure, a systemic-to-pulmonary shunt is created, and any situation that increases pulmonary vascular resistance leads to a decreased pulmonary blood flow, with subsequent hypoxemia. On the other hand, an increase in pulmonary vascular resistance in a patient with a modified Fontan procedure will lead to cardiogenic shock. This is owing to the fact that blood flow from the right side of the heart to the lungs is gravity-dependent because of absence of a contractile right heart. (Nichols DG, et al. *Critical Heart Disease in Infants and Children*, Mosby, 1995; pp. 868–874.)

38. C The creation of a fenestration between the upper chambers of the heart will allow shunting of the blood from the right side to the left side of the heart in a setting of increased pulmonary vascular resistance, which in turn will maintain cardiac output. It has also been shown to decrease incidence of pleural effusion and mortality. The fenestration can be closed in a cardiac catheterization laboratory at a later date. (Nichols DG, et al. *Critical Heart Disease in Infants and Children*, Mosby, 1995; pp. 881–883.)

39, 40. D, C To allow reconditioning of the left ventricle pulmonary artery binding and a Blalock-Taussing shunt are important. Focal myocardial ischemia may occur and this may affect the left ventricular function, either focally or globally. (Nichols DG, et al. *Critical Heart Disease in Infants and Children*, Mosby, 1995; pp. 825–836.)

41. A Refer to answer for Question 34.

42. D Myocardial ischemia can occur with resultant ventricular dysfunction (refer to answer for Question 40).

43. B It is usually done on the same side as the arch or the side in which the arch descends. (Nichols DG, et al. *Critical Heart Disease in Infants and Children*, Mosby, 1995; p. 746.)

44. E Ketamine is a myocardial depressant in a denervated heart. It is likely to depress the myocardial function in this setting. (Rogers MC, et al. *Textbook of Pediatric Intensive Care*, 3rd Edition; pp. 1563–1564.)

45. E A stiff myocardium with poor myocardial compliance is a recognized problem in the postoperative period following repair of Tetralogy of Fallot. Adequate volume expansion with subsequent decrease in afterload, as a result of a decrease in vasoconstriction, is likely to improve myocardial perfusion and myocardial compliance. (Nichols DG, et al. *Critical Heart Disease in Infants and Children*, Mosby, 1995; pp. 856–857.)

46. C Left ventricular stroke work index reflects contractility. (Nichols DG, et al. *Critical Heart Disease in Infants and Children*, Mosby, 1995; pp. 482–486.)

47. A Compensatory mechanisms are least efficient with shock that is cardiogenic in origin. (Rogers MC, et al. *Textbook of Pediatric Intensive Care*, 3rd Edition; pp. 577–589; Perkin RM, Levin DL. J Pediatr, 1982; 101:163.)

48. A, B In a setting of myocardial dysfunction, the effects of positive pressure ventilation on afterload predominate over the effect on preload. (Rogers MC, et al. *Textbook of Pediatric Intensive Care*, 3rd Edition; pp. 390,391.)

49. D An increased negative intrathoracic pressure associated with upper airway obstruction would increase the left ventricular afterload. (Rogers MC, et al. *Textbook of Pediatric Intensive Care*, 3rd Edition; pp. 390,391.)

50. C Mueller maneuver is inspiration against the partially closed glottis. (Rogers MC, et al. *Textbook of Pediatric Intensive Care*, 3rd Edition; pp. 369–380.)

51. C It may increase the shunt. (Nichols DG, et al. *Critical Heart Disease in Infants and Children*, Mosby, 1995; p. 202.)

52. C Thiocyanate is removed by dialysis. (Nichols DG, et al. *Critical Heart Disease in Infants and Children*, Mosby, 1995; p. 202.)

53. B, A, A Nitroglycerin tends to decrease central venous pressure and pulmonary artery occlusion pressure without significantly lowering blood pressure. Therefore, it is the preferred drug in patients with marginal blood pressure. Sodium nitroprusside, on the other hand, is the preferred drug for patients who have a preserved blood pressure. (Nichols DG, et al. *Critical Heart Disease in Infants and Children*, Mosby, 1995; pp. 202–205.)

54–57. C, A, D, B In the United States, trauma is the leading cause of death in children beyond infancy. Shock is the major contributor to mortality in these cases. Cases of hypovolemic shock can be successfully treated with crystalloid solutions when sufficient volumes are administered. It has been shown that replacement of up to 50% of the total blood volume of the patient with crystalloids is not associated with significant expansion of the interstitial space. Fluid administration equivalent to 200% of blood volume will result in edema fluid accumulation, particularly if administered rapidly. Hetastarch is available as 6% solution in 0.9 saline. Therapeutically it is equivalent to albumin but the cost is much less. The administration should not exceed 10–20 mL/kg/day because of the concern about derangement in hemostasis. Carcillo et al. (JAMA 1991) found that fluid resuscitation rapidly in excess of 40 mL/kg in the first hour was associated with improved survival in children with septic shock. The risk of pulmonary edema was not increased. Plasma catecholamines are significantly elevated in shock states and impaired cellular metabolism occurs early with septic shock. (Carcillo JA, Davis AL, Zoritsky A. JAMA 1991; 266:1242; Martex AJ, et al. Arch Surg, 1970; 101:421; Hauser CJ, et al. Hosp Physician, 1980; 16:38.)

58. E Please *see* Rogers MC, et al. *Textbook of Pediatric Intensive Care*, 2nd Edition; pp. 585, 590,591.

59–62. D, D, D, D Fat embolism is a recognized complication of orthopedic procedures and fractures. It may also occur in sickle cell disease during painful crises. The treatment is supportive. Microscopic urine analysis may reveal fat globules. Removal of these emboli are not technically possible. Air embolism can occur in all of the clinical settings referred to in the question. (Rogers MC, et al. *Textbook of Pediatric Intensive Care*, 3rd Edition; pp. 224,225.)

63–65.   C, C, D   This is a patient with acute hemorrhagic pancreatitis. Potential complications are hypocalcemia, hyperglycemia, ARDS, and shock. Appropriate interventions would include volume resuscitation, management of the hypocalcemia, and appropriate management of the respiratory dysfunction. Surgical exploration is not indicated at this time. (Rogers MC, et al. *Textbook of Pediatric Intensive Care*, 3rd Edition; pp. 1175–1178.)

66–69.   C, B, D, E   In a patient with a pure hypovolemia and in the absence of any other complications, such as infection or myocardial dysfunction, a careful repeated physical examination and monitoring of the peripheral perfusion and urine output is usually adequate for fluid management. However, if the patient's condition becomes complicated, then central venous catheter insertion for monitoring should be a consideration. Hypokalemia and hypocalcemia may develop following vigorous correction of metabolic acidosis. (Rogers MC, et al. *Textbook of Pediatric Intensive Care*, 3rd Edition; pp. 588–597.)

70.   C   The newborn myocardium is indeed less compliant, and this leads to increased myocardial wall stress with increased myocardial oxygen consumption. (Nichols DG, et al. *Critical Heart Disease in Infants and Children*, Mosby, 1995; pp. 18–26.)

71.   D   Nerve fibers representing baroceptors located in the atrial and ventricular wall, primarily in the distribution of left coronary artery, mediate this reflux. (Rogers MC, et al. *Textbook of Pediatric Intensive Care*, 3rd Edition; p. 513.)

72, 73.   D, C   Self-explanatory.

74, 75.   B, C   Dysrhythmias are more often seen during catheter insertion into the right ventricle and include premature ventricular contractions and ventricular tachycardia.

During measurement of cardiac output by the thermal dilution technique, cardiac output is inversely proportional to the area under the curve. Prolonging the upstroke/downstroke of the curve leads to false elevation of the area under the curve, which would lead to false overestimation of the cardiac output. (Nichols DG, et al. *Critical Heart Disease in Infants and Children*, Mosby, 1995; pp. 481–488.)

76–79.   B, A, B, B   Point B is end diastolic volume. B–C is an isovolemic contraction; aortic valve opens at Point C. C–D is the period of systole; a fluid bolus increases end diastolic volume (B–B_1). Increased contractility leads to a lower end systolic volume (A–A_1). Increased afterload is associated with higher systolic pressure (C_2–D_2) but smaller stroke volume. (Nichols DG, et al. *Critical Heart Disease in Infants and Children*, Mosby, 1995; pp. 25–32.)

CHAPTER 3: CENTRAL NERVOUS SYSYTEM

1–3.   A, E, E   With central hypoventilation syndrome, apnea usually occurs during quiet sleep, however, it can happen during rapid eye movement sleep (REM). Included in questions 2 and 3 are some of the reorganized causes of central hypoventilation syndrome. (Rogers MC, et al. *Textbook of Pediatric Intensive Care*, 3rd Edition; pp. 235–238.)

4.   C, D   Both achondroplasia and Arnold-Chiari malformation give rise to a mixed type of apnea, and neither typically causes central apnea. (Canfield P, et al. Clin Pediatr, 1982; 21:684; Pauli RM, et al. J Pediatr, 1984; 104:342.)

5.   B   The absence of any chest wall movement is highly suggestive of a central apnea. (Rogers MC, et al. *Textbook of Pediatric Intensive Care*, 3rd Edition; pp. 235–238.)

6.   A   There will be some abnormalities in the respiratory function owing to the loss of abdominal muscle activity and loss of their participation in the respiratory effort. (Rogers MC, et al. *Textbook of Pediatric Intensive Care*, 3rd Edition; pp. 239–241.)

7.   E   The hypotension is typically associated with bradycardia and may be very difficult to manage.

(Rogers MC, et al. *Textbook of Pediatric Intensive Care*, 3rd Edition; pp. 239–241.)

8. C Somatosensory evoked potentials detect brain wave activities in response to peripheral nerve stimulation, and therefore, it evaluates the entire neuronal track from the cortex down to the peripheral nerve. (Rogers MC, et al. *Textbook of Pediatric Intensive Care*, 3rd Edition; pp. 693,694; Fuhrman BP. *Pediatric Critical Care*, 2nd Edition; p. 604.)

9. A Spinal cord injury without any significant radiographical abnormalities is commonly seen in the pediatric population. (Rogers MC, et al. *Textbook of Pediatric Intensive Care*, 3rd Edition; pp. 239–241.)

10–15. A, E, D, E, E, E Various portals of entry of the organism into the body are recognized. In 20% of cases, a portal of entry is not found based on history and physical examination, and therefore, absence of the portal of entry is not very rare. Also of note, is that cultures may not reveal the causative organism. Generalized seizures are not a recognized feature of tetanus; however, the so-called "respiratory convulsions" can develop and require immediate attention to opening and maintaining the airway, which often includes endotracheal intubation. The mortality resulting from tetanus is most commonly secondary to respiratory abnormalities. (Rogers MC, et al. *Textbook of Pediatric Intensive Care*, 3rd Edition; pp. 241–244.)

16. C, C, B, B Autonomic dysfunction is a recognized feature of both poliomyelitis and Guillain-Barre syndrome, and the mortality in both results from respiratory dysfunction. Poliomyelitis generally presents with asymmetric scattered weakness, as opposed to the symmetric weakness that is noted with Guillain-Barré syndrome, and the clinical progression is usually rapid with poliomyelitis. (Rogers MC, et al. *Textbook of Pediatric Intensive Care*, 3rd Edition; pp. 242–246; Fuhrman BP. *Pediatric Critical Care*, 2nd Edition; p. 638.)

17. E All of the features mentioned are correct, and this is a case of poliomyelitis, which is very rare in the United States; however, it is still seen in developing countries and can certainly be imported into the United States. (Rogers MC, et al. *Textbook of Pediatric Intensive Care*, 3rd Edition; pp. 242–244.)

18. C Syndrome of inappropriate antidiuretic hormone secretion (SIADH) occurs with both respiratory syncytial virus infection and Guillain-Barré syndrome. (Rogers MC, et al. *Textbook of Pediatric Intensive Care*, 3rd Edition; pp. 132, 244–246; Fuhrman BP. *Pediatric Critical Care*, 2nd Edition; p. 638.)

19. C Residual volume is not clinically useful in this setting. The two most commonly used parameters for monitoring of patients with neuromuscular disease who might require tracheal intubation or liberation from mechanical ventilation, are FVC and maximum or negative inspiratory force. (Rogers MC, et al. *Textbook of Pediatric Intensive Care*, 3rd Edition; pp. 245–247; Fuhrman BP. *Pediatric Critical Care*, 2nd Edition; p. 426.)

20. D In patients with neuromuscular disease, depolarizing muscle relaxants, such as succinyl choline, should be avoided because of the possibility of cardiac dysrhythmias, and sedatives should be used very cautiously. (Rogers MC, et al. *Textbook of Pediatric Intensive Care*, 3rd Edition; pp. 239–247. Fuhrman BP; *Pediatric Critical Care*, 2nd Edition; pp. 1341–1345.)

21, 22. A, A Pneumonia is a common complication in patients with Guillain-Barré syndrome. Among the options, sinus tachycardia is the most common abnormality in these patients. (Rogers MC, et al. *Textbook of Pediatric Intensive Care*, 3rd Edition; pp. 244-246; Fuhrman BP. *Pediatric Critical Care*, 2nd Edition; p. 638.)

23, 24. D, B Diaphragmatic paralysis secondary to a phrenic nerve injury most commonly follows a palliative repair of a congenital cardiac defect such as a Blalock-Taussig shunt. In infants and children, this entity is much more likely to lead to gas exchange abnormalities and could be analogous to a flail chest in an adult. This arises because of the highly compliant chest wall and poor ability of the intercostal muscle to stabilize the chest wall. (Rogers MC, et al. *Textbook of Pediatric Intensive Care*, 3rd Edition; pp. 247–249; Fuhrman BP. *Pediatric Critical Care*, 2nd Edition; pp. 360,361.)

25–29. D, B, C, E, D There are various subtypes of myasthenia gravis. Juvenile myasthenia gravis is usually seen in teenage years. Onset of symptoms often follows a viral respiratory infection and cranial nerves, particularly extraocular movements are predominantly involved. Other autoimmune diseases, such as systemic lupus erythematosus or thyroid disorders, may be associated.

Congenital myasthenia gravis has an onset a few days after birth with poor feeding and respiratory difficulty/failure. Family history is often present in a sibling, but history of myasthenia in the mother during pregnancy is absent.

Neonatal myasthenia gravis is uniformly born to mothers with myasthenia gravis; one out of five is transient in nature (as the autoantibodies resolve), and responds well to anticholinesterase medications.

Familial infantile myasthenia gravis is usually not born to mothers with myasthenia gravis even though there is often history of myasthenia gravis in a sibling. These patients develop marked respiratory depression and require tracheal intubation. The subsequent clinical course is characterized by episodes of muscle weakness in the first 2 years of life, which may progress to respiratory failure. Episodes do respond to anticholinesterase therapy.

Following general anesthesia with tracheal intubation, patients with myasthenia gravis may develop stridor with or without respiratory distress secondary to the following factors: glottic/subglottic edema owing to traumatic intubation, laryngeal muscle weakness, or vocal cord paralysis. (Rogers MC, et al. *Textbook of Pediatric Intensive Care*, 3rd Edition; pp. 249–251.)

30.   A Succinylcholine in general should be avoided in patients with neuromuscular disease. Peripheral muscle weakness does not seem to correlate well with respiratory muscle weakness. Plasmapheresis has been shown to decrease the duration of endotracheal intubation and mechanical ventilatory support postoperatively in patients with myasthenia gravis. (Rogers MC, et al. *Textbook of Pediatric Intensive Care*, 3rd Edition; pp. 249–251.)

31.   D The level of consciousness is typically preserved in patients with infantile botulism. (Rogers MC, et al. *Textbook of Pediatric Intensive Care*, 3rd Edition; pp. 251–253; Fuhrman BP. *Pediatric Critical Care*, 2nd Edition; pp. 639,640.)

32.   C Recovery of the diaphragm seems to occur prior to recovery of peripheral muscles. (Rogers MC, et al. *Textbook of Pediatric Intensive Care*, 3rd Edition; pp. 251–253.)

33.   D All of the statements regarding evoked potentials are true. (Rogers MC, et al. *Textbook of Pediatric Intensive Care*, 3rd Edition; pp. 690–696; Fuhrman BP. *Pediatric Critical Care*, 2nd Edition; pp. 604, 682.)

34.   B In severe head injury, the vasoresponsivity to changes in blood pressure is lost earlier than that in response to CO_2. (Rogers MC, et al. *Textbook of Pediatric Intensive Care*, 3rd Edition; pp. 649–652.)

35.   D In meningitis, the autoregulation to cerebral blood flow seems to be intact. (Ashwal S, et al. J Pediatr, 1990; 117:523–530.)

36.   A In a patient with head injury and coma, absence of cortical waves bilaterally with the somatosensory evoked potentials is associated with poor outcome. (Rogers MC, et al. *Textbook of Pediatric Intensive Care*, 3rd Edition; pp. 694–695. Fuhrman BP. *Pediatric Critical Care*, 2nd Edition; pp. 604, 682.)

37.   D Cerebral blood volume is an important determinant of intracranial pressure. (Rogers MC, et al. *Textbook of Pediatric Intensive Care*, 3rd Edition; pp. 648–650.)

38.   D All of the statements are true. (Rogers MC, et al. *Textbook of Pediatric Intensive Care*, 3rd Edition; pp. 648–650.)

39.   A The characteristics/pattern of cerebral ischemia is: ischemia, reactive hyperemia, followed by delayed hypoperfusion. (Rogers MC, et al. *Textbook of Pediatric Intensive Care*, 3rd Edition; p. 701; Fuhrman BP. *Pediatric Critical Care*, 2nd Edition; pp. 671–687.)

40.   E Layers CA_1 and CA_3 of the hippocampus are one of the most vulnerable areas of the brain to ischemia; others include the cerebellum and layers 3, 5, and 6 of the cerebral cortex. (Rogers MC, et al. *Textbook of Pediatric Intensive Care*, 3rd Edition; pp. 701,702; Fuhrman BP. *Pediatric Critical Care*, 2nd Edition; pp. 671–687.)

41, 42.   C / D, E   The corneal reflex tests cranial nerves 5 and 7. Midbrain lesions induce a midsize minimally reactive pupil, whereas Pontine lesions induce a pinpoint pupil. (Rogers MC, et al. *Textbook of Pediatric Intensive Care*, 3rd Edition; pp. 739–744.)

43.   D   In experimentally induced status epilepticus, which is divided into phase I and phase II, it has been shown that phase I is characterized by hypertension, lactic acidosis, hyperglycemia, and hyper- or normokalemia, whereas phase II is characterized by hypoglycemia, hyperkalemia, hyperthermia, and respiratory compromise. (Lothman E. Neurology 1990; 40:13.)

44.   C   With highly lipid soluble drugs, free brain concentration does correlate with free serum concentration of the drug. (Rogers MC, et al. *Textbook of Pediatric Intensive Care*, 3rd Edition; pp. 765–768.)

45.   D   Diazepam is one of the most lipid-soluble of anticonvulsants, and therefore, it has a very large Vd because of its high lipid solubility. The Vd of diazepam is at least five times that of lorazepam, and diazepam has significant metabolites, which tend to accumulate and contribute to the prolonged or delayed effects. (Rogers MC, et al. *Textbook of Pediatric Intensive Care*, 3rd Edition; pp. 766,767; Fuhrman BP. *Pediatric Critical Care*, 2nd Edition; pp. 629,630.)

46.   B   Phenobarbital does have a low lipid solubility, and this accounts for the very slow onset of action. The pharmacokinetics of phenytoin is nonlinear, and this accounts for a significant increase in toxicity at increasingly higher doses. Infants do have a higher elimination capacity for anticonvulsants compared with older children and adults. Lorazepam, when used repeatedly over a period of 48 hours for status epilepticus, may become progressively less effective owing to development of tolerance. (Rogers MC, et al. *Textbook of Pediatric Intensive Care*, 3rd Edition; pp. 767–769.)

47.   A   Please *see* Rogers MC, et al. *Textbook of Pediatric Intensive Care*, 3rd Edition; pp. 810,811.

48.   D   Cytotoxic edema involves primarily the cells, and therefore, is seen primarily in the gray matter. (Rogers MC, et al. *Textbook of Pediatric Intensive Care*, 3rd Edition; pp. 647,648.)

49.   D   Glutamic acid is normally found in very small concentrations in the brain interstitial fluid. When it is released from the cell in high concentrations, it is very cytotoxic to glial cells, and also contributes to increased intracranial pressure. (Rogers MC, et al. *Textbook of Pediatric Intensive Care*, 3rd Edition; pp. 705,706.)

50.   B   Initial concentration of a drug is equal to the dose administered divided by its Vd. (Rogers MC, et al. *Textbook of Pediatric Intensive Care*, 3rd Edition; pp. 766–768.)

51.   C   The majority of blood flow to the brain is committed to the gray matter, which contains the cells. Arterial oxygen tension does have a significant influence on the cerebral blood flow. Water constitutes about 65% of total brain content. (Rogers MC, et al. *Textbook of Pediatric Intensive Care*, 3rd Edition; pp. 648–650.)

52.   C, D, B, A, E, F, G   Please *see* Rogers MC, et al. *Textbook of Pediatric Intensive Care*, 3rd Edition; pp. 737–744.

53.   E   All have been recognized and associated with head injury. Other abnormalities include ST segmented T-wave changes on the echocardiogram (EKG). (Rogers MC, et al. Crit Care Med, 1980; 8:213,214.)

54.   C   Some of the initial compensatory mechanisms in response to increased intracranial volume are because of displacement of the spinal fluid from the intracranial to intraspinal space. (Rogers MC, et al. *Textbook of Pediatric Intensive Care*, 3rd Edition; pp. 646–660.)

55.   E, D, C, B, A, E   Please *see* Rogers MC, et al. *Textbook of Pediatric Intensive Care*, 3rd Edition; pp. 817–834.

56.   A   Homocystinuria is the metabolic abnormality that is most likely to be associated with the development of stroke. (Rogers MC, et al. *Textbook of Pediatric Intensive Care*, 3rd Edition; pp. 868–869.)

57.   C   This patient apparently developed communicating hydrocephalus most likely as a result of blockage of the arachnoid villi within the dural sinuses, the site of drainage for of cerebrospinal fluid back to the venous circulation. (Fuhrman BP. *Pediatric Critical Care*, 2nd Edition; p. 658.)

58. E Cerebrospinal fluid rhinorrhea is seen in approximately 7% of basilar skull fractures, and the in the vast majority of cases it resolves within a period of a few weeks. Ecchymosis in the periorbital area is referred to as racoon's eye. Corticosteroids have not been shown to be definitely beneficial in a setting of closed head injury. Cerebrospinal fluid rhinorrhea is uncommon in children less than 10 years of age because of underdevelopment of sinuses. (Rogers MC, et al. *Textbook of Pediatric Intensive Care*, 3rd Edition; pp. 816,817.)

59. A A significantly depressed skull fracture requires surgical intervention. (Rogers MC, et al. *Textbook of Pediatric Intensive Care*, 3rd Edition; p. 855.)

60. E All of the statements are true regarding cerebral circulation. (Rogers MC, et al. *Textbook of Pediatric Intensive Care*, 3rd Edition; pp. 859–872.)

61. A, B, C Please *see* Rogers MC, et al. *Textbook of Pediatric Intensive Care*, 3rd Edition; pp. 859–872.

62. A Please *see* Rogers MC, et al. *Textbook of Pediatric Intensive Care*, 3rd Edition; pp. 859–872.

63. T, F, T, F, T, T Please *see* Rogers MC, et al. *Textbook of Pediatric Intensive Care*, 3rd Edition; pp. 859–872.

64. D Please *see* Rogers MC, et al. *Textbook of Pediatric Intensive Care*, 3rd Edition; pp. 859–872.

65. T, T, T Please *see* Rogers MC, et al. *Textbook of Pediatric Intensive Care*, 3rd Edition; pp. 859–872.

CHAPTER 4: INFECTIOUS DISEASES

1. E In pediatric and newborn services, lower respiratory infections are the most common type of nosocomial infection followed by bacteremia, urinary tract, cutaneous, and surgical wound infection. *Staphylococcus aureus* predominates as the most common cause of lower respiratory infections in newborns, not *Klebsiella*. *Klebsiella* is the most common organism isolated from pediatric lower respiratory tract nosocomial infections. Other common lower respiratory pathogens include *Pseudomonas aeroginosa*, Coagulase-negative staph, and *Escherichia coli*. *E. coli* is the most common cause of pediatric, nosocomial, urinary tract infections. (Rogers MC, et al. *Textbook of Pediatric Intensive Care*, 3rd Edition; pp. 976, 997, table 30.2.)

2. A *Pneumococcus* and *Branhamella* are the most common organisms causing sinusitis in the general pediatric population younger than 10 years of age. In intensive care patients with a nasotracheal tube in place, a variety of Gram-negative organisms, including *Pseudomonas aeruginosa, Klebsiella, Proteus, E. coli, Enterobacter*, and *Serratia* are found. Often, these infections are polymicrobial. Direct aspiration and culture of the material should direct therapy. Ocular infections are often caused by *P. aeruginosa* and may

progress if left untreated. Infection from environmental contaminants also occurs. (Rogers MC, et al. *Textbook of Pediatric Intensive Care*, 3rd Edition; pp. 987,988.)

3. E Gram-negative organisms, not anerobes, are the dominant organisms that colonize the trachea in patients who are intubated. Colonization is increased in those patients receiving cimetidine or antacids. Respiratory equipment, including nebulizers, medications, and hand ventilators may also become contaminated and contribute to respiratory infections. Uncuffed endotracheal tubes contribute to the aspiration of oral secretions. (Rogers MC, et al. *Textbook of Pediatric Intensive Care*, 3rd Edition; pp. 989.)

4. C Local inflammation does not correlate with the duration of arterial catheter insertion and is not predictive of catheter tip colonization. All other responses are true. Catheters placed by surgical cutdown have twice the incidence of infection and nine-fold increase in septicemia. Disposable transducers used for 4 days had no higher risk of infection than those used for 2 days. At 8 days, the prevalence of contamination was significantly higher for the transducers (Rogers MC, et al. *Textbook of Pediatric Intensive Care*, 3rd Edition; pp. 981,982.)

5. E Approximately 30% of total parenteral infection infections are caused by fungi with *Candida albicans, Candida* sp., and *Torulopsis* being primarily responsible. All of the other statements are true. (Rogers MC, et al. *Textbook of Pediatric Intensive Care*, 3rd Edition; pp. 984.)

6. T, T, T, F, T In spite of the inherently invasive nature of extracorporeal membrane oxygenation, few reports of infectious complications have arisen. Approximately 5% of the cannulas placed for extracorporeal life support became infected. (Rogers MC, et al. *Textbook of Pediatric Intensive Care*, 3rd Edition; pp. 986,987.)

7. D Cleansing with providone-iodine or the use of antibiotic impregnated catheters have not been shown to significantly lower the incidence of urinary tract infections in the ICU. Gram-positive isolates predominate in urinary tract infections in both sexes. (Rogers MC, et al. *Textbook of Pediatric Intensive Care*, 3rd Edition; pp. 991,992.)

8. B The prophylactic use of antibiotics does not significantly decrease the incidence of infection associated with intracranial pressure monitoring devices, and therefore, use of prophylactic antibiotics in this setting is not indicated. Increasing the frequency of breaks into the system, such as obtaining samples or flushing the catheter with saline, does increase the risk of infection. However, placement of these catheters either in the ICU or the operating room has not been shown to make a substantial difference in terms of the rate of infection. The presence of blood within the ventricular system does increase the risk of infection. (Rogers MC, et al. *Textbook of Pediatric Intensive Care*, 3rd Edition; pp. 993,994.)

9. D Ampicillin and an aminoglycoside alone will not be adequate coverage for intraabdominal infection. It is necessary to cover for anerobic bacteria as well. Therefore, a combination of ampicillin, gentamycin, and clindamycin is one approach the child with abdominal sepsis. (Rogers MC, et al. *Textbook of Pediatric Intensive Care*, 3rd Edition; pp. 1012,1013.)

10. A, B, B, B Early-onset neonatal group B streptococcal infections are usually seen within the first week of birth. Early-onset disease is primarily a disease of premature infants less than 35 weeks gestation and weighing less than 2500 g at birth. Late-onset infection can be delayed up to 3 months after birth. There is a poor correlation between the late-onset group B streptococcal infection and maternal colonization, 95% of the isolates are type III, and there is a higher association with meningitis, as opposed to association with pneumonia that is seen with early-onset group B streptococcal infection. (Rogers MC, et al. *Textbook of Pediatric Intensive Care*, 3rd Edition; pp. 1016,1017.)

11. T, F, T, T, F, T, T, T The initial antibiotic therapy of the sick neonate generally consists of ampicillin and an aminoglycoside. Whereas the combination of ampicillin and gentamicin is synergistic against group B streptococcal infection, the addition of chloramphenicol to ampicillin is of no additional benefit. The immaturity of the immunological system of the newborn predisposes this group of patients to susceptibility to group B streptococcal infection. It is the deficiency in complement, antibodies, and plasma components that is thought to be responsible for the short-term outcome improvement in simple and double volume exchange transfusions. *Listeria monocytogenes* generally affects extremes of age and pregnant women, and it has a bimodal presentation similar to group B streptococcal infection (i.e., early-onset and late-onset). (Rogers MC, et al. *Textbook of Pediatric Intensive Care*, 3rd Edition; pp. 1019,1020.)

12. A, B, B, B Late-onset *L. monocytogenes* infection is usually seen in healthy, full-term infants who are born to mothers who are asymptomatic at the time. The vast majority of infections are from type 4B, and there is a higher association with meningitis. (Rogers MC, et al. *Textbook of Pediatric Intensive Care*, 3rd Edition; pp. 1020–1022.)

13. D The majority of infections in which a source is identified are related to maternal genital infections. The incubation period for neonatal herpes is usually longer than 7 days. The likelihood of the neonate contracting the disease is correlated with a prolonged rupture of membranes (>6 hours) in a mother with active genital infection. (Rogers MC, et al. *Textbook of Pediatric Intensive Care*, 3rd Edition; pp. 1023,1024.)

14. T, F, F, T, F, T Herpetic meningoencephalitis occurs in approximately 50% of neonatal diagnoses. Mothers with genital lesions need not be isolated from their babies, in contrast to mothers with oral or perioral lesions who should be preferably isolated from their newborn babies. The prognosis for babies with disseminated infection is approximately 90%. Herpes simplex virus 2 has an increased rate of pneumonitis and disseminated intravascular coagulation, which may relate to its poorer outcome when compared with herpes simplex virus 1. (Rogers MC, et al. *Textbook of Pediatric Intensive Care*, 3rd Edition; pp. 1023,1024.)

15. E *Neisseria meningitidis* is usually endemic and is commonly carried in the nasopharynx of the healthy population. The infection is more commonly in males. Influenza A and B are associated with an increased susceptibility to infection. (Rogers MC, et al. *Textbook of Pediatric Intensive Care*, 3rd Edition; pp. 1025–1027.)

16. D Several attempts at classifying meningococcal disease severity and prognosis have occurred. The characteristics that are associated with a worsened outcome represent failure of the child's organ systems to adequately compensate for the disease. A low leukocyte count in the periphery or in the cerebrospinal fluid (CSF) may represent a failure of the host's neutrophils to mount an adequate response. Similarly, the presence of shock, petechiae, and thrombocytopenia are unfavorable. The elevation of the sedimentation rate is, in part, owing to elevation of the acute phase reactants, which includes fibrinogen, and this will take at least 24 hours. A sedimentation rate of 100 mm/hour (as stated in the question) would suggest that the infection has been going on for more than several hours, and it would constitute a good prognostic feature. (Rogers MC, et al. *Textbook of Pediatric Intensive Care*, 3rd Edition; pp. 1026,1027, tables 31.13, 31.14, 31.15, 31.16, and 31.17.)

17. D The cardiovascular collapse and instability associated with meningococcal infection was originally thought to be resulting primarily from adrenal dysfunction. However, large doses of exogenous corticosteroids were not always effective in reversing the shock state, and therefore, the more recent prevailing theory is that the cardiovascular collapse is actually secondary to endotoxemia, with its effect in inducing multiple organ dysfunction syndrome. Fulminant meningococcemia has an estimated mortality rate of 85%. Petechiae are frequently present in this disease and are related to a failure of the hematopoietic system and disseminated intravascular coagulation. Corticosteroids are a promising intervention that have not been demonstrated to universally reverse the shock state. (Rogers MC, et al. *Textbook of Pediatric Intensive Care*, 3rd Edition; pp. 1026–1029.)

18. D Myocarditis, which is believed to be a form of vasculitis, generally develops 4–7 days after onset of infection, and pneumonia can be very severe and require mechanical ventilatory support. The recommendation of using Rifampin prophylaxis for household and day-care contacts is universally agreed on. Corticosteroids are a promising intervention that have not been demonstrated to universally reverse the shock state. (Rogers MC, et al. *Textbook of Pediatric Intensive Care*, 3rd Edition; pp. 1029–1032.)

19. E Petechiae and ecchymosis may be noted with any of the infections mentioned, although they are typically associated with *Neisseria* infection. (Rogers MC, et al. *Textbook of Pediatric Intensive Care*, 3rd Edition; pp. 1032–1034.)

20. E *H. influenzae* infection may mimic meningococcemia. Adrenal hemorrhage has been noted in 55% of the fatal cases of *H. influenzae* sepsis. Intractable hypotension and cardiac dysfunction usually lead to death in affected patients. Rifampin prophylaxis should be initiated immediately after diagnosis of the *H. influenzae* type B infection, in household contacts. It should be incorporated into the therapeutic antibiotic regimen of the index case in the last few days of therapy, and should not be delayed until one month after completion of antibiotic therapy. (Rogers MC, et al. *Textbook of Pediatric Intensive Care*, 3rd Edition; pp. 1032–1034.)

21. B A history of freshwater lake swimming is an important etiological risk factor for *N. meningitis*. Otitis media is often seen in association with *H. influenzae* meningitis. Meningitis in the vast majority of cases does not actually involve the parenchyma. It is limited to the three layers of the meninges. The Virchow-Robin spaces are a continuous extension of the subarachnoid space, which will allow the bacteria to gain access into the subarachnoid space, and maybe to the most superficial surface of the brain. Meningitis, when severe, is often associated with cerebral edema. (Rogers MC, et al. *Textbook of Pediatric Intensive Care*, 3rd Edition; pp. 1040–1060.)

22. D Even in the absence of an index case within the day care setting, children who attend day care centers are at higher risk of developing meningitis. Convulsions occurring within the first 24–72 hours of meningitis may represent febrile seizures, and therefore have a better prognosis. Convulsions that develop beyond this period carry a less favorable prognosis. Limitation of ocular movement may be owing to abnormalities in the 3rd cranial nerves, and does not always indicate increased intracranial pressure. When papilledema is noted on the first day of admission of meningitis, other etiologies should be sought, particularly an intracranial mass lesion, such as a brain abscess. (Rogers MC, et al. *Textbook of Pediatric Intensive Care*, 3rd Edition; pp. 1047–1060.)

23. D Limitation of ocular movements may result from irritation of cranial nerves III, IV, or VI. Convulsions do occur in at least 30% of meningitis cases. Those convulsions that are limited to the first 24–72 hours carry a better prognosis. *See* response to question 22. (Rogers MC, et al. *Textbook of Pediatric Intensive Care*, 3rd Edition; pp. 1047–1049.)

24. E Bacterial culture of the CSF is considered the gold standard. The presence of any neutrophils in the CSF in the newborn period should be treated with a high degree of suspicion. This may be one of the early manifestations of meningitis. However, in newborn infants polymorphonuclear leukocytes may comprise up to 60% of the total CSF white cell population and still be considered normal. The opening pressure in the neonate is between 90 and 110 mmH_2O, whereas in the older child and adult it may be as high as 180 mm H_2O. (Rogers MC, et al. *Textbook of Pediatric Intensive Care*, 3rd Edition; pp. 1049–1051, table 32.4.)

25. T, F, F Spinal fluid remains clear with up to 500 white blood cells/mm^3. Erythrocytes raise the CSF protein concentration by about 15 mg/dL for every 1000 red blodd cells/mm^3. A CSF lactate level of more than 14 mg% is considered abnormal. (Rogers MC, et al. *Textbook of Pediatric Intensive Care*, 3rd Edition; pp. 1049–1047.)

26. D Children who are diagnosed and admitted to the hospital for meningitis have commonly received some form of antibiotic, usually oral, prior to presentation. This form of antibiotic usually is not sufficient to treat meningitis, and therefore, it does not improve the outcome in these patients. Several hours after the administration of an appropriate antibiotic, it is certainly possible to inhibit bacterial growth in the spinal fluid. (Rogers MC, et al. *Textbook of Pediatric Intensive Care*, 3rd Edition; pp. 1051,1052.)

27. A Tuberculous meningitis, which is usually a basal form of meningitis, is more likely to present with focal neurological signs and papilledema, particularly cranial nerve palsies such as cranial nerves VII, VIII and IX. Cryptococcal meningitis may present only with behavioral changes, or it may present with symptoms of a space-occupying lesion. The opening pressure in neonates may be as high as 110 mmH_2O. (Rogers MC, et al. *Textbook of Pediatric Intensive Care*, 3rd Edition; pp. 1052–1060; American Academy of Pediatrics. In: Pickering LK, ed. *2000 Red Book: Report of the Committee on Infectious Diseases. 25th Ed.* Elk Grove Village, IL.)

28. E By day 5 of treatment with antibiotics, 85% of children with *H. influenzae* meningitis will be afebrile. SIADH has been noted in more than 50% of patients with meningitis. Under these circumstances, restriction of fluid and close monitoring of fluids and electrolytes are a necessary part of the management of these patients. Subdural effusions, which are a recognized complication of meningitis, generally resolve spontaneously and do not require surgical intervention in the vast majority of cases. Nosocomial infection is a common cause of recurrent treatment after initial treatment for meningitis. (Rogers MC, et al. *Textbook of Pediatric Intensive Care*, 3rd Edition; pp. 1052–1054.)

29. T, T, F, T The causes of fever that persists beyond the 10th day in the setting of meningitis are subdural effusions, drug fever, arthritis, brain abscess, and nosocomial infection. Thirty to fifty percent of fevers are idiopathic. Persistence of a positive CSF culture would be a poor prognostic feature in patients with bacterial meningitis. (Rogers MC, et al. *Textbook of Pediatric Intensive Care*, 3rd Edition; pp. 1053–1060.)

30. E The frequency of shunt infections varies between 2 and 30% and is influenced by a variety of factors. Children suspected of having a shunt infection or meningitis should receive coverage with antibiotics for Gram-positive organisms including the *Staphylococcus* species, as well as Gram-negative organisms. Staphylococcal species are the most common. Initial therapy should include vancomycin because the frequency of methicillin-resistant staphylococci is high. Respiratory isolation of the patient for the initial 24 hours of antimicrobial therapy is an important epidemiological consideration. The data regarding the use of dexamethasone in meningitis are controversial. (Rogers MC, et al. *Textbook of Pediatric Intensive Care*, 3rd Edition; pp. 1061,1062.)

31. T, T, F, F, T The CSF cytology in tuberculous meningitis mimics the lymphocyte predominance found in viral meningitis. CSF glucose is classically reduced and the protein level is elevated. (Rogers MC, et al. *Textbook of Pediatric Intensive Care*, 3rd Edition; pp. 1050–1061.)

32. E Aseptic meningitis is an inflammatory process of the meninges that results from a number of different etiologies. An elevated protein, a pleocytosis, and the absence of organisms on Gram stain and culture characterize it. The etiologies associated with this diagnosis are rather large and include viral, bacterial, and fungal causes. Admission of the patient to the hospital depends on the certainty of the diagnosis. To the extent that the patient is stable and the likelihood of a partially treated bacterial etiology is ruled out, outpatient management may be acceptable. (Mandell ML, et al. *Principles and Practice of Infectious Diseases*, 3rd Edition; pp. 1367–1379.)

33. E Enteroviral infections are higher in lower socioeconomic groups, have a 3- to 5-day incubation, and are typically seen in the latter part of the summer. The meningitis associated with these infections usually has a benign course. (American Academy of Pediatrics. In: Pickering LK, ed. *2000 Red Book: Report of the Committee on Infectious Diseases,* 25th Ed. Elk Grove Village, IL.)

34. T, F Please *see* Mandell ML, et al. *Principles and Practice of Infectious Diseases*, 3rd Edition; pp. 1367–1379.

35. E With HSV infection, particularly with meningoencephalitis, the electroencephalogram displays abnormalities typically in the frontal and temporal lobe area of the brain. All of the other responses are true (Rogers MC, et al. *Textbook of Pediatric Intensive Care*, 3rd Edition; pp. 1064–1066.)

36. D Arboviruses are arthropod-born viruses that are a common cause of encephalitis. These infections are usually seen in late summer and spring, and they are transmitted by arthropods. St. Louis encephalitis is the most common arbovirus infection in the United States, and is generally a mild disease. The highest mortality usually occurs with Eastern equine encephalitis. California encephalitis is usually a mild disease. (Rogers MC, et al. *Textbook of Pediatric Intensive Care*, 3rd Edition; pp. 1062–1064.)

37. B, A, C, D The St. Louis encephalitis virus is distributed throughout most of the US and causes major epidemics that peak later than other arboviruses. Most infections are asymptomatic, and less than 1% have overt neurological disease. Western equine encephalitis is the usual cause of arbovirus encephalitis and California encephalitis viruses occur in the central and eastern United States, and cause diseases with a fulminant and mild course, respectively. (Rogers MC, et al. *Textbook of Pediatric Intensive Care*, 3rd Edition; pp. 1063–1065.)

38. B Interestingly, in spite of the name, Rocky Mountain Spotted Fever occurs primarily in the eastern United States, including the Ohio Valley area. The disease is a tick-born illness. *See* Question 47. (Rogers MC, et al. *Textbook of Pediatric Intensive Care*, 3rd Edition; pp. 1106–1109.)

39. D Over the past 30 years, cyanotic congenital heart disease has replaced suppurative otitis media or mastoiditis and suppurative sinusitis as the most common predisposing factor for brain abscess. This is true for the industrial nation, but even in developing nations, it is the most likely predisposing factor. Overall, a predisposing factor can be determined in approximately 85% of all patients with brain abscess, and therefore, a meticulous evaluation for a predisposing factor is warranted in these patients. (Rogers MC, et al. *Textbook of Pediatric Intensive Care*, 3rd Edition; pp. 1071–1073.)

40. D Brain abscesses formed by hematogenous seeding tend to develop at the junction of gray and white matter and usually in the distribution of the middle cerebral artery; hence, the predominant location in the temporal and parietal lobes. Beyond the neonatal period, meningitis is a rare form of brain abscess. Seizures, when they occur, are more typically generalized. (Rogers MC, et al. *Textbook of Pediatric Intensive Care*, 3rd Edition; pp. 1071–1074.)

41. D Normal brain parenchyma is highly resistant to invasion by microorganisms and therefore, abscess formation seems to occur only in areas of the brain with focal ischemia, necrosis, or marginal perfusion. Poor vascular supply in the white matter or at the junction of the gray and white matter makes these areas the most likely to be affected by brain abscess. With the exception of the neonatal period, abscess infrequently complicates a course of bacterial meningitis. In the neonatal period, *Citrobacter diversus* and *Proteus mirabilis* are the most common etiological agents that usually cause meningitis and are subsequently complicated by brain abscess. When seizures develop in association with brain abscess, they are most commonly a generalized seizure. In up to 30% of brain abscess cases, the microbiology is polymicrobial, which could be a combination of aerobic and anaerobic organisms. Suppurative complications of otitis media or sinusitis are becoming less and less common as an etiological agent or predisposing factors for brain abscess. Because of poor penetration into the abscess cavity, aminoglycosides are not effective for treatment of brain abscess. (Rogers MC, et al. *Textbook of Pediatric Intensive Care*, 3rd Edition; pp. 1073–1075.)

42. **D** Unlike the epidural space, the subdural space is not limited by attachment of the dura to the skull sutures, allowing extension and the spread of the subdural empyema over a wide area of the cerebral hemispheres. The potential subdural space is restricted at the base of the brain, and therefore involvement of the base of the brain is rare with subdural abscesses. In infants, subdural empyema generally complicates acute meningitis, and therefore is caused by the organisms commonly implicated in causing meningitis. Because the incidence of *H. influenza* type B as a cause of meningitis in infants has decreased dramatically in the United States, this organism is becoming less and less an etiological agent for subdural empyema. The magnetic resonance imaging (MRI) is the diagnostic imaging procedure of choice for subdural empyema. Advantages of MRI over the computed tomography (CT) scan include the lack of bone artifact, the ability to detect the smaller extracranial fluid collection, and improved ability to differentiate extracranial collection of fluid from other differential diagnoses such as cerebritis, cerebral edema, and venous thrombosis. MRI can also detect the density difference from elevated protein concentration, and therefore distinguish a subdural abscess from other sterile collections, such as subdural effusions. (Rogers MC, et al. *Textbook of Pediatric Intensive Care*, 3rd Edition; pp. 1071–1077.)

43. **C, B, A** In the child and young adult, the most common organism causing localized parameningeal infections, such as a subdural empyema, are the various aerobic streptococci, such as *S. pneumoniae*, staphylococci of either the epidermidis or the aureus species. α-Hemolytic streptococci are the most frequently isolated organisms from brain abscesses in patients with cyanotic congenital heart disease. *S. aureus* is the usual organism causing spinal epidural

abscess and accounts for 80% of cases. *See* response to Question 51. (Rogers MC, et al. *Textbook of Pediatric Intensive Care*, 3rd Edition; pp. 1072–1079.)

44. **D** Proposed and simplified diagnostic criteria for toxic shock syndrome in children include: fever equal to or greater than 39°C, lymphopenia, rash, shock, diarrhea and vomiting, and irritability. The Centers for Disease Control and Prevention has not adopted these simplified criteria, however. Toxic shock syndrome can also be caused by streptococci, and is one example of severe group A streptococcal disease. (Rogers MC, et al. *Textbook of Pediatric Intensive Care*, 3rd Edition; pp. 1103–1106.)

45. **D** Staphylococcal toxic shock syndrome is caused by a coagulase positive staphylococcus that liberates an exoprotein known as TSST-1. The host does not form neutralizing antibodies to the toxin for at least 2 years after infection. This, in addition to the noninvasiveness of the organism, may help to explain the recurrent nature of disease, especially in menstrual cases. Menstrual cases are seen exclusively in the white Caucasian population. Patients who present with elevated serum creatinine, particularly when the serum creatinine is greater than 3 mg/dL tend to have a prolonged hospital course. (Rogers MC, et al. *Textbook of Pediatric Intensive Care*, 3rd Edition; pp. 1103–1106.)

46. **B** *See* response to Question 47 (Rogers MC, et al. *Textbook of Pediatric Intensive Care*, 3rd Edition; pp. 1106–1109.)

47. **B** Rocky Mountain Spotted Fever is caused by *Rickettsia rickettsii*. In the eastern regions of the United States, *Dermacentor variabilis* is the most common tick involved, whereas in the western region, the *Dermacentor andersoni* is the most common tic involved. The disease is usually prevalent in the summer months, and the highest incidence of disease among children age 5–9 years. More than half of all cases appear in persons younger than 19 years of age. The incubation period is 2–14 days, with an average of 7 days. Man is only incidentally involved when bitten by an adult tick. The initial presentation consists of headaches, malaise, and myalgias. The rash generally appears within 2–4 days after the fever, and has been noted in nearly all children with the disease. The eruptions begin as discrete macules, first observed on the ankles and feet, and shortly thereafter on the wrists and hands. Regardless of the progression of the rash, the rash is almost always most pronounced over the extremities and almost always involves the palms of the hands and the soles of the feet. Over a period of several days, the rash becomes petechial and purpuric. (Rogers MC, et al. *Textbook of Pediatric Intensive Care*, 3rd Edition; pp. 1106–1109.)

48. E Legionnaire's disease was first recognized in 1976 after an outbreak of pneumonia in Philadelphia. The organism, *L. pneumophila,* accounts for only about 15% of pneumonia in adults, but it causes acute pulmonary disease, mostly among adult males. The disease has also been noted in infants and children and the prevalence of elevated titers in children is quite high in some communities. The presenting complaints are usually fever, nonproductive cough, encephalopathy, and seizures; cerebellar signs may be markedly severe in these patients. The lung disease is usually lobar in nature; hepatic and renal abnormalities are often also noted. (Rogers MC, et al. *Textbook of Pediatric Intensive Care*, 3rd Edition; pp. 1109–1110.)

49. D Super antigens are antigens that are derived from either bacteria or viruses that interact with the major histocompatibility class II proteins and activate T-cells by binding to the variable region of the β chain of the T-cell receptor. Stimulation of the T-cell receptors leads to polyclonal T-cell activation, which results in release of massive amounts of tumor necrosis factor-α and interleukin-6. These cytokines are most likely the elements responsible for the shock and multiorgan dysfunction seen in these diseases. Super antigens differ from conventional antigens mainly in the manner in which they are processed and presented to the T-cell receptors. The polyclonal activation gener-

ally results in a reduction of the number of circulating CD4+ lymphocytes; however, this reduction is usually reversible and transient. Super antigens are potentially involved in all the three disorders mentioned in the question. (Rogers MC, et al. *Textbook of Pediatric Intensive Care*, 3rd Edition; p. 1103.)

50. B, A Some differences have been noted between children and adults with toxic shock syndrome. Whereas only a small percentage of adults have had a prominent prodromal illness, nearly all children have between 1 and 6 days of symptoms preceding the illness. These symptoms include fever, mucosal hyperemia, erythroderma, vomiting, diarrhea, dizziness, and myalgias. The vast majority of adults admitted to the hospital have hypotension at presentation. This finding is not prominent in children at the time of admission, although it may develop later during the hospitalization. (Rogers MC, et al. *Textbook of Pediatric Intensive Care*, 3rd Edition; pp. 1103–1106.)

51. D, A, B, C Brain abscesses are the most frequently encountered form of localized intracranial infection in children. Death usually occurs with rupture of the abscess and spread of the infection into the ventricular system or herniation secondary to mass effect. *Citrobacter* and *Proteus* are the most common etiological agents in the newborn period. In patients with congenital heart disease, α-hemolytic streptococci are common. Patients who have traumatic injuries are affected by *S. aureus.* Immunocompromised patients are at risk for Nocardia brain abscesses. (Rogers MC, et al. *Textbook of Pediatric Intensive Care*, 3rd Edition; pp. 1071–1076.)

CHAPTER 5: HEMATOLOGY AND ONCOLOGY

1. A Trauma is the leading cause of death in the 1- to 15-year-old population. Neoplastic disease is second. The other responses are true. (Rogers MC, et al. *Textbook of Pediatric Intensive Care*, 3rd Edition; pp. 1433–1434.)

2. D Infection is higher in patients with central lines than those without. Recent retrospective data suggests that there are no differences in infection rates between subcutaneously implanted versus externalized catheters. (Rogers, MC, et al. *Textbook of Pediatric Intensive Care*, 3rd Edition; pp. 1438.)

3. E Fifty-five to seventy percent of febrile episodes in oncology patients are of infectious origin. Blood cultures are positive in less than 50% of cases of serious disseminated fungal infections. *C. albicans* and *Aspergillus* species are the most common fungal organisms. Neutropenia is closely correlated with morbidity and mortality. Pneumocystis is unlikely in this clinical scenario; however, pneumocystis is responsible for up to 50% of nonbacterial pneumonitis in oncology patients. Chest radiographs demonstrate bilateral infiltrates radiating from the hilum. (Rogers, MC, et al. *Textbook of Pediatric Intensive Care*, 3rd Edition; pp. 1438–1445; table 42.6.)

4.   D   The half-life of transfused platelets is 7 days; with significant alloimmunization, it can be hours. All of the other statements are correct. (Rogers, MC, et al. *Textbook of Pediatric Intensive Care*, 3rd Edition; pp. 1442,1443.)

5.   D, E, C, B, F, A   Chemotherapy may promote the development of a coagulopathy associated with an increased risk of hemorrhage or thrombosis. Actinomycin D and other antibiotics decrease the vitamin K-dependent clotting factors. Anthracycline increases fibrinolysis. L-Asparaginase may cause hypofibrinogenemia. Methotrexate can cause an antithrombin III deficiency. Vincristine may cause chronic hepatic dysfunction. Glucocorticoids increase the levels of factors II, VII, VIII, and X. (Rogers, MC, et al. *Textbook of Pediatric Intensive Care*, 3rd Edition; pp. 1442–1457.)

6.   A   Primary pulmonary parenchymal involvement with leukemia is very rare. Parenchymal involvement is occasionally seen with histiocytosis X and metastatic disease (e.g., osteogenic and Ewings sarcoma, and Wilms tumor). All other statements are correct. (Rogers, MC, et al. *Textbook of Pediatric Intensive Care*, 3rd Edition; pp. 1445–1447, table 42.8.)

7.   T, T, F, T, T, F   A variety of chemotherapeutics, as well as radiotherapy, can cause cardiomyopathy. Effects appear to be dose related. Radiotherapy may cause pericarditis with a chronic effusion. Histologically, interstitial fibrosis with vascular narrowing is seen. (Rogers, MC, et al. *Textbook of Pediatric Intensive Care*, 3rd Edition; pp. 1447–1448.) The onset of *Pneumocystis carinii* infection typically occurs 3–6 months after bone marrow transplantation. Bacterial or fungal infection can occur within the first 2 weeks. Cytomegalovirus (CMV) infection occurs 6–12 weeks after bone marrow transplantation. (Rogers, MC, et al. *Textbook of Pediatric Intensive Care*, 3rd Edition; pp. 1454,1455.)

8.   B, D, A, C   The child with neoplastic disease may acquire a variety of neurological deficits related to the neoplasm, the therapy, or a combination of both. Methotrexate is associated with aseptic meningitis, arachnoiditis, demyelinization, somnolence, and chronic leukoencephalopathy. Cisplatin may cause ototoxicity, cerebral edema, and seizures. Vincristine is associated with SIADH. 5-FU may cause acute cerebellar ataxia.

(Rogers, MC, et al. *Textbook of Pediatric Intensive Care*, 3rd Edition; pp. 1449–1452; table 42.17.)

9.   B, D, A   Chemotherapy is commonly associated with renal injury. High-dose methotrexate is associated with renal tubular injury. Cisplatin may cause tubular necrosis; cyclophosphamide and ifosfamide are both associated with hemorrhagic cystitis. L-Asparaginase is not associated with renal injury. (Rogers, MC, et al. *Textbook of Pediatric Intensive Care*, 3rd Edition; pp. 1452,1453; table 42.18.)

10.   D   CMV infection occurs most commonly 6–12 weeks after bone marrow transplantation. All of the other statements are correct. (Rogers, MC, et al. *Textbook of Pediatric Intensive Care*, 3rd Edition; pp. 1454,1455.)

11.   A, D, B, C, E   Chemotherapeutic agents form the mainstay of treatment for childhood neoplasms. All agents act by disrupting some aspect of normal cell growth or division. Antimetabolites interact with various cell enzymes (e.g., methotrexate inhibits the activity of dihydrofolate reductase). Vincristine, a vinca alkaloid, inhibits microtubule function within the cell. This prevents the formation of the spindle apparatus during metaphase, thus inhibiting cell division. The anthracycline (daunorubicin and doxorubicin) and actinomycin D inhibit the synthesis of DNA in tumor cells. Alkylating agents like cyclophosphamide cause breaks in the DNA strands. The glucocorticoids are directly lymphocytotoxic to lymphoid leukemia and lymphoma cells. (Rogers, MC, et al. *Textbook of Pediatric Intensive Care*, 3rd Edition; pp. 1456–1458; tables 42.23, 42.24, 42.26, and 42.27.)

12.   E   Von Willebrand's disease is the most common inherited bleeding disorder. One percent of the population has detectable abnormalities in the von Willebrand's disease protein. All of the statements are correct. (Rogers, MC, et al. *Textbook of Pediatric Intensive Care*, 3rd Edition; pp. 1414–1416; figure 41.2.)

13.   T, F, T, T, T, F   The preferred source for factors II, VII, X, and antithrombin III is fresh frozen plasma (FFP). Vitamin K is not a stored vitamin. (Rogers, MC, et al. *Textbook of Pediatric Intensive Care*, 3rd Edition; pp. 1415,1416.)

14.   D   Antithrombin III, protein C, and protein S are the main components of the antithrombotic system. Thrombomodulin and heparin cofactor II, among others, are also included as endogenous anticoagulants. Protein B is not included among these components. (Rogers, MC, et al. *Textbook of Pediatric Intensive Care*, 3rd Edition; pp. 1421; figure 41.3.)

15.   E   When the liver itself is diseased, abnormal coagulation results. The liver synthesizes fibrinogen, prothrombin, protein C, protein S, antithrombin III, plasminogen, and factors V, VII, IX, X, XI, and XII. All of the above statements are correct. (Rogers, MC, et al. *Textbook of Pediatric Intensive Care*, 3rd Edition; pp. 1408,1409, 1415,1416.)

16.   B   ε-Aminocaproic acid prevents the breakdown of the fibrin clot by complexing with plasmin to prevent its fibrinolytic activity. Protamine is used to reverse the effects of heparin. Vitamin K deficiency generally occurs within 2–3 days following cardiopulmonary bypass. D-dimers are rarely elevated. (Rogers, MC, et al. *Textbook of Pediatric Intensive Care*, 3rd Edition; pp. 1405,1406; table 41.11; Chang, AC, et al. *Pediatric Cardiac Intensive Care*; pp. 397–399.)

17.   D   Massive transfusion is defined as the replacement of at least one blood volume; estimated as 75 mL/kg for children less than 1 year of age and burn victims, and 70 mL/kg for all others. All of the other statements are true. (Rogers, MC, et al. *Textbook of Pediatric Intensive Care*, 3rd Edition; pp. 1403–1408.)

18.   C   A variety of metabolic abnormalities can be induced by massive transfusion. 2,3-Diphosphoglycerate is decreased in transfused red cells, which increases red cell affinity for oxygen. Thus, oxygen unloading to tissues may be impaired. All other statements are correct. (Rogers MC, et al. *Textbook of Pediatric Intensive Care*, 3rd Edition; pp. 1421,1422; Gilman, AG, et al. *Goodman and Gilman's The Pharmacological Basis of Therapeutics*, 8th Edition; pp. 1316.)

19.   E   Antithrombin III primarily inhibits the vitamin K dependent procoagulant factors (II, VII, IX, and X). Deficiency will lead to recurrent thrombosis. Heparin induced antiplatelet antibodies occur in approximately 5% of patients receiving heparin therapy. Most cases are mild with platelet counts higher than 100,000/μL. All of the other statements are correct. (Rogers, MC, et al. *Textbook of Pediatric Intensive Care*, 3rd Edition; pp. 1406,1407.)

20.   D   Two forms of acute, heparin-induced thrombocytopenia occur. The mild form occurs in approximately 5% of patients, 4–15 days after initiation of full-dose heparin therapy (platelet counts higher than 100,000/μL). Severe thrombocytopenia occurs less frequently. The more severe form is associated with thrombotic complications. All of the other statements are correct. (Gilman, AG, et al. *Goodman and Gilman's The Pharmacological Basis of Therapeutics*, 8th Edition; pp. 1316.)

21.   E   Protein C activation is controlled by several different mechanisms, including by thrombomodulin. Protein C activation and thrombin generation are tightly coupled. Acquired and hereditary deficiencies are the primary cause of thrombophilia. (Nathan, DG, et al. *Nathan and Oski's Hematology of Infancy and Childhood*, 5th Edition; pp. 1545–1547.)

22.   E   In contrast to heparin, which acts as a cofactor with antithrombin III to prevent coagulation, the plasminogen activators, urokinase, streptokinase, and tissue plasminogen activator increase fibrinolysis, thereby lysing the clot. Plasminogen is cleaved into plasmin by these activators. Plasmin lyses clot directly. All of the other statements are correct. (Rogers, MC, et al. *Textbook of Pediatric Intensive Care*, 3rd Edition; pp. 1415,1416, 1423,1424.)

23.   E   Both heparin and plasminogen activators (streptokinase, tissue plasminogen activator) may be used to treat arterial thrombosis. The partial thromboplastin time should be kept 1.5–2.0 times normal during heparin therapy. *Note:* younger neonates may be resistant to thrombolytic therapy, possibly because of lower levels of plasminogen. (Rogers, MC, et al. *Textbook of Pediatric Intensive Care*, 3rd Edition; pp. 1424.)

24.   E   Disorders in children that are treated with chronic anticoagulants include cardiac disorders (prosthetic valves, Blalock-Taussig shunts, endovascular shunts), some cerebrovascular events, and Kawasaki's disease. All of the above statements are correct.

(Nathan, DG, et al. *Nathan and Oski's Hematology of Infancy and Childhood*, 5th Edition; pp. 1704.)

25.   C, D, A   Aspirin is a potent and irreversible inhibitor of cyclooxygenase and thromboxane A2. Sulfinpyrazone, like aspirin, is also a nonsteroidal anti-inflammatory agent that reversibly inhibits cyclo-oxygenase. (Gilman, AG, et al. *Goodman and Gilman's*

The Pharmacological Basis of Therapeutics, 8th Edition; pp. 652, 1524.)

26.   D   Thromboprophylaxis for prosthetic heart valves has reduced the occurrence of thromboembolic events from approximately 6% to less than 2%. The other statements are true. (Michelson AD, et al. Chest 1998; 114(5 Suppl): 748S–769S.)

CHAPTER 6: RENAL SYSTEM

1.   A   Kidneys are able to maintain renal blood flow over a wide range of systemic blood pressures by autoregulation of intrarenal vascular resistance. Therefore, hypotension with renal hypoperfusion may or may not produce ischemic renal injury. However, these autoregulatory mechanisms are not well developed in neonates. Neonates have high renin levels, which in turn, are associated with decreased glomerular filtration rate (GFR) and reduced outer cortical blood flow. The cortical glomeruli are immature and so are their corresponding tubules. This pattern of high renin and reduced outer cortical blood flow makes neonates more vulnerable to renal dysfunction as a result of hypotension of systemic pressures only slightly below the normal range. In animal studies, newborn animals have decreased production of atrial natriuretic peptide in response to saline challenge. All these factors combined make the incidence of acute renal failure in neonates, after cardiac surgery, higher than in older infants and children. (Nichols DG, et al. *Critical Heart Disease in Infants and Children*, Mosby 1995; pp. 125, 562.)

2.   C   Furosemide causes vasodilation of the cortical vasculature by direct action and through release of prostaglandins. Furosemide maintains renal blood flow and tubular blood flow when cardiac output is compromised. Mannitol is also a vasodilator of the cortical vasculature that increases renal blood flow either directly by drawing fluid from extravascular to intravascular space, thus increasing total plasma volume, or by increasing prostaglandin production. Increased plasma volume alone does not fully explain the effects of mannitol, because volume expansion with saline improves renal blood flow without improving GFR. The improvement in GFR seen with mannitol is associated with a decrease in afferent and efferent arteriolar resistance, which is probably mediated by prostaglandins. (Rogers MC, et al. *Textbook of Pedi-*

atric Intensive Care, 2nd Edition; pp. 1192–1194, 1202.)

3.   D   Clinical studies comparing prophylactic administration of mannitol (or furosemide) with maintenance of adequate intravascular volume during cardiopulmonary bypass failed to reduce the incidence of postoperative renal dysfunction. However, there are experimental studies that have shown some beneficial effects of mannitol. Mannitol has been shown to be effective in preventing deterioration of renal function before administration of Amphotericin B and Cis-Platinum. (Rogers MC, et al. *Textbook of Pediatric Intensive Care*, 2nd Edition; pp. 1194,1195; Nichols DG. *Critical Heart Disease in Infants and Children*, Mosby 1995; pp. 129,130; Olivero JJ, et al. Br Med J, 1975; 1:550; Hayes D, et al. Cancer, 1977; 39:1372.)

4.   C   Etiologies of postoperative oliguria in this patient include: (1) intra-operative blood loss; (2) third space volume loss; (3) bilateral ureteral obstruction; (4) cardiac failure; and (5) increased intra-abdominal pressure. In this patient, the latter is important to recognize (because it appears that intravascular volume has been expanded and cardiac output is normal) because prompt surgery to relieve increased intra-abdominal pressure is associated with rapid diuresis. The development of this problem is best avoided by direct measurement of intra-abdominal pressure either via the esophageal route or per gastrostomy. Data indicate that the abdominal wall should not be closed if pressure exceeds 20 mmHg. In this case, it is best to employ a silo with delayed closure to allow time for the compliance of the abdominal wall to increase. (Yaster M, et al. Anesthesiology, 1986; 65:A449.)

5.   E   Children have a lower mortality compared with adults. (Rogers MC, et al. *Textbook of Pediatric Intensive Care*, 2nd Edition; pp. 1198–1201.)

6. A An increased P–R interval is seen before changes in P-wave because the A–V node is much more sensitive to hyperkalemia than the S–A node. (Rogers MC, et al. *Textbook of Pediatric Intensive Care*, 2nd Edition; p. 1201.)

7–8. E, D All of the strategies mentioned are appropriate for oliguria in a setting of suspected renal insufficiency. With the onset of acute renal failure, hyponatremia is more commonly seen owing to the dilutional effect of intake of fluid orally, which is mostly hypotonic. (Rogers MC, et al. *Textbook of Pediatric Intensive Care*, 2nd Edition; p. 1202. Nichols DG. *Critical Heart Disease in Infants and Children*, Mosby 1995; pp. 128–138.)

9–12. B, A, D, C In the absence of significant symptoms, hypocalcemia does not need to be aggressively treated. Aggressive treatment with calcium in the presence of hyperphosphatemia, and particularly when the product of calcium and phosphorus exceeds 60, increases the risk of calcium deposition in various tissues within the body. Acidosis raises the level of ionized calcium and thus mitigates against the occurrence of symptomatic hypocalcemia. Caution must be exercised in correcting acidosis abruptly, as a rapid decline in the level of ionized calcium may precipitate tetany. Dysequilibrium syndrome is not seen with peritoneal dialysis, as the process is very slow, as compared with hemodialysis, which is done over a few hours. Such a high dose of vitamin C is unnecessary in patients with renal failure. Patients with hemolytic uremic syndrome (HUS) seem to have a better outcome with early institution of dialysis. (Rogers MC, et al. *Textbook of Pediatric Intensive Care*, 2nd Edition; pp. 1201–1205; Kaplan BS, et al. Can Med Assoc J, 1981; 124:429.)

13. A Severe hypertension with hypertensive encephalopathy is a recognized feature of rapidly progressive glomerulonephritis. (Rogers MC, et al. *Textbook of Pediatric Intensive Care*, 2nd Edition; p. 1214.)

14. A The initial concentration of a drug equals the dose administered divided by Vd: $C = D \div Vd$ (Rogers MC, et al. *Textbook of Pediatric Intensive Care*, 3rd Edition; pp. 766–768.)

15. D Saline diuresis is the most appropriate treatment for hypercalcemia. (Bilezikian J. N Engl J Med, 1992; 326:1196.)

16. A, A, A, C, D, A Please *see* Williams GH. N Engl J Med, 1988; 319:1517.

17,18. D, D High levels of urea act as an osmotic diuretic in the postoperative period. High normal intravascular volume is precisely what is desirable in the postoperative period in order to avoid the risk of thrombosis in the graft. Preoperative transfusion (with consequent hypervolemia) would increase the risk of congestive cardiac failure in the postoperative period. For cadaveric kidney transplantation, there is a positive correlation between the number of transfusions and the graft survival; the survival seems to be optimal with a transfusion from five or more different donors. With living related donors, it is unclear whether transfusion has any beneficial effects on the survival of the graft. (Rogers MC, et al. *Textbook of Pediatric Intensive Care*, 3rd Edition; pp. 1237–1240.)

19. C, A Increased platelet consumption is a feature of both HUS and disseminated intravascular coagulopathy. However, deficiency of prostaglandin I_2 activity is associated only with HUS. (Rogers MC, et al. *Textbook of Pediatric Intensive Care*, 3rd Edition; pp. 1231–1235.)

20. C Atracurium undergoes spontaneous degradation referred to as Hofmann degradation; however, some authorities believe that ester hydrolysis is the major pathway for degradation of atracurium. (Fuhrman BP. *Pediatric Critical Care*, 2nd Edition; pp. 1346,1347.)

21. E Please *see* Bennet WM. Clin Pharmacokinetics, 1988; 5:326.

22. B, C, D, A Furosemide acts at the loop of Henle, chlorothiazide at the distal tubule, spironolactone at the cortical collecting duct, and mannitol is freely filtered by the glomerulus.

23. D, A Water intoxication is characterized by absence of clinical signs of dehydration, hyponatremia, and a low urinary sodium. In SIADH, the urine osmolality continues to be high in spite of low serum sodium and osmolality. Congenital adrenal hyperplasia is associated with hyperkalemia and acidosis. Three percent salt given at an initial dose of 4 mL/kg will increase serum sodium by approximately 3–4 mEq/L and will abort the seizure. (Rogers MC. *Textbook of Pediatric Intensive Care*, 2nd Edition; Williams & Wilkins, pp. 1249–1250.)

CHAPTER 7: ENDOCRINE SYSTEM

1. D An increased anion gap (AG) is usually present with greater prerenal azotemia, and is not directly related to hyperglycemia. The shift of extracellular phosphate into the intracellular space does not occur until diabetic ketoacidosis is reversed by the administration of insulin and fluids. (Rogers MC, et al. *Textbook of Pediatric Intensive Care*, 3rd Edition; pp. 1263–1264; Adrogue H, Wilson H, Boyd A. N Engl J Med 1982; 307:1603.)

2. A In most children with a diagnosis of diabetes mellitus who develop diabetic ketoacidosis, the precipitating event is an omission of insulin, whether inadvertent or deliberate. The other causes are also possible, but not as likely. (Rogers MC, et al. *Textbook of Pediatric Intensive Care*, 3rd Edition; pp. 1261.)

3. A Hyperosmolality has also been associated with electroencephalogram (EEG) changes during diabetic ketoacidosis. The mortality in children with cerebral edema from diabetic ketoacidosis can approach 80%. An increased risk is present for children less than 5 years of age who have a new diagnosis of diabetes mellitus complicated by a prolonged untreated case of diabetic ketoacidosis. Aggressive rehydration, especially with hypotonic fluids, may acutely decrease an already hyperosmolar state in the child precipitating a picture of cerebral edema. (Rogers MC, et al. *Textbook of Pediatric Intensive Care*, 3rd Edition; pp. 1266–1267; Krane EJ, Walman JK, Walsdorf JI. N Engl J Med 1985; 316:857.)

4. E Intravenous antibiotics should be administered pending lumbar puncture. Progressive deterioration of mental status in this patient would be an indication to obtain a cranial CT scan to evaluate for cerebral edema. As stated in the rationale in Question 1 of this section, children under the age of 5 newly diagnosed with diabetes mellitus and who also have a complicated course of diabetic ketoacidosis, have an increased risk of cerebral edema. Airway and primitive reflexes should be monitored with the possibility of early intubation, if any question of those is compromised. (Rogers MC, et al. *Textbook of Pediatric Intensive Care*, 3rd Edition; pp. 1267–1269.)

5. C It is not uncommon to have hyperglycemia in association with a head-injured child. Most likely, as a result of an increase in catecholamines and corticosteroids, there is an increase in blood sugar. Hyperglycemia has already been shown to be associated with the degree of severity in brain injury. Some data suggests that ischemic brain injury may be worse in those patients who have hyperglycemia in their recovery phase as opposed to those patients who had normoglycemia. Any coagulopathy that may exacerbate an ischemic picture also may worsen the severity of brain injury. (Rogers MC, et al. *Textbook of Pediatric Intensive Care*, 3rd Edition; pp. 1271,1272. Pulsinelli W, Levy D, Sigsbee B, et al. Am J Med 1983; 74:540.)

6. E The first step in the treatment of hypoglycemia in a child is initiation of dextrose bolus followed by an infusion of 10% dextrose. All of these conditions are characterized either by the inability to release glycogen from the liver or depletion of glycogen from the liver, and therefore, glucagon is unlikely to be effective. (Rogers MC, et al. *Textbook of Pediatric Intensive Care*, 3rd Edition; pp. 1273,1274; Kogut M. Gluck L, Kone T, Dodge P, eds. *Current Problems in Pediatrics*, Chicago: Yearbook, 1974, p. 3.)

7. E The stimulus for the mechanisms which elevate blood glucose in the setting of hypoglycemia is primarily CNS hypoglycemia. The body's measures which help to remedy hypoglycemia are primarily the release of epinephrine and glucagon with their effects being additive. The neonate requires a considerable amount of glucose, especially in the perioperative period. There is a significant decline in glycogen storage within the liver within the first 3 postnatal hours. If hypoglycemia is resistant to medical therapy, a laparotomy may be indicated to determine the presence of a tumor or subtotal pancreatectomy. Ketonic hypoglycemia is the most common form in children. (Rogers MC, et al. *Textbook of Pediatric Intensive Care*, 3rd Edition; pp. 1272–1275; Mozam F, Rodgers B, Talbert J et al. Arch Surg 1982; 117:1151.)

8. B Maximum effects of arginine vasopressin result in an osmolality of 1400 mOsmol/L with a urine output of 0.5 mL/kg/hour. It is important to initiate DDAVP treatment as soon as diabetes insipidus is made as the diagnosis, to prevent large surges in fluid loss. The goal is to double the urine osmolality in comparison to the plasma, and obtain a urine output of 2 mL/kg/hour. Death can occur within 1–5 days after the presentation of diabetes insipidus with cerebral insult. Low urine osmolality (<300 mOsmol/L) and serum osmolality higher than 295 mOsmol/L is consistent with a diagnosis of diabetes insipidus without the presence of any osmotic diuretics. In the absence of ADH hormone, the urine flow will continue to increase in the range of 15–20 mL/kg/hour with a significant increase in serum osmolality. (Rogers MC, et al. *Textbook of Pediatric Intensive Care*, 3rd Edition; pp. 1275–1280.)

9. A, D, B, C Fluid overload leads to polyuria accompanied by plasma hypo-osmolality. With osmotic diuresis, the urine osmolality remains close to that of plasma. In the absence of osmotic diuretics, when the plasma osmolality is more than 295 mOsmol/L, while the urine osmolality remains 300 mOsmol/L or less, the diagnosis of diabetes insipitus is very likely. (Rogers MC, et al. *Textbook of Pediatric Intensive Care*, 3rd Edition; pp. 1275–1280.)

10. A, B, C Gastroenteritis has minimal urine sodium losses. It maintains a relatively high urine/plasma osmolality. There is a significant degree of urine sodium losses in HUS. With a high FE_{na} (>3%), a urine osmolality of approximately 300 mOsmol/L and a 1:1 urine/plasma osmolality, SIADH has the highest amount of urine sodium losses with a very high urine osmolality and 2:1 urine/plasma osmolality. (Rogers MC, et al. *Textbook of Pediatric Intensive Care*, 3rd Edition; pp. 1276–1278.)

11. B With the lack of ketonuria, a negative toxicology screen and significant hepatomegaly on exam, the diagnosis is most likely the result of a storage disease. (Rogers MC, et al. *Textbook of Pediatric Intensive Care*, 3rd Edition; pp. 1272–1275.)

12. A Blood should be collected anaerobically because CO_2 loss can alter the pH, and therefore, affect the binding of albumin. RBCs, if not removed, may cause acidosis as a result of lactate production. Some anticoagulants may attach to calcium and cause misinterpretation of calcium levels. (Rogers MC, et al. *Textbook of Pediatric Intensive Care*, 3rd Edition; p. 1281.)

13. C Lack of weightbearing is more severe in children as a result of hypercalcemia and immobility. Levels of total serum calcium more than 15 mg% may be life-threatening. Digitalis toxicity increases in the setting of hypercalcemia. Mithramycin should be avoided if surgery is anticipated because of the possibility of severe marrow suppression as a result of its administration, and therefore, complicating thrombocytopenia which could lead to significant bleeding. The product of the concentration of calcium and phosphorus should be kept below 60 when treating hypercalcemia. (Rogers MC, et al. *Textbook of Pediatric Intensive Care*, 3rd Edition; pp. 1282–1285.)

14. D For any patients admitted to the ICU with hypocalcemia, treatment should be initiated unless the hypocalcemia is borderline and without symptoms. Hypocalcemia, which is resistant to the administration of repeated doses of intravenous calcium chloride, may be an indication of hypomagnesemia, hypoparathyroidism, or vitamin D insufficiency. Magnesium sulfate should not be used because the possibility exists for a complex to be formed between magnesium sulfate and calcium. A rapid magnesium infusion leads to a peak adrenal excretion. (Rogers MC, et al. *Textbook of Pediatric Intensive Care*, 3rd Edition; pp. 1283–1285.)

15. C The daily requirement is approximately 0.3–0.4 mEq/kg/day intravenously. With a decrease in glomerular filtration rate, magnesium replacement may precipitate hypermagnesemia. Intravenous magnesium should not be given as a rapid bolus (as discussed previously). Magnesium chloride is preferable to magnesium sulphate because the sulphate can bind calcium. Rapid magnesium infusion leads to a poor clinical response because peak magnesium levels are associated with peak renal excretion. Aminoglycosides have been known to cause hypomagnesemia. (Rogers MC, et al. *Textbook of Pediatric Intensive Care*, 3rd Edition; pp. 1285–1288; Chernow B, Smith J, Rainey T, et al. Crit Care Med 1982; 10:193.)

16. E Propranolol, labetalol, lidocaine, nitroglycerine, morphine, and verapamil are not dependent on hepatic blood flow. (Rogers MC, et al. *Textbook of Pediatric Intensive Care*, 3rd Edition; pp. 1200–1205.)

17. B Dexamethasone has the least sodium retaining properties, and therefore, it is very appropriate for clinical situations where relative hypovolemia is desired. Prednisone and methylprednisolone are intermediate in terms of their salt retaining properties. Synthetic steroids are less avidly bound to protein and they undergo slower hepatic degradation, which makes them very effective in clinical practice. (Rogers MC, et al.

Textbook of Pediatric Intensive Care, 3rd Edition; pp. 1249–1252,)

18. A, A, C Pyloric stenosis usually induces metabolic alkalosis rather than metabolic acidosis, and CAH is associated with hyponatremia in the presence of hyperkalemia. (Rogers MC, et al. *Textbook of Pediatric Intensive Care*, 3rd Edition; pp. 1252–1254.)

19. D Ketoconazole, Bactrim®, and Etomidate are all known to cause adrenal suppression. (Rogers MC, et al. *Textbook of Pediatric Intensive Care*, 3rd Edition; pp. 1252–1254.)

20. D With long-term steroid use, morning administration will minimize hypothalamic–pituitary– adrenal axis suppression. Also, with prolonged use of the administration of steroids, it is best to administer the dose in the morning, because this will coincide with peak diurnal variation in the endogenous steroid levels. The 30-minute adrenocorticotropic hormone (ACTH) administration test is a reliable test for adrenal suppression. Prolonged use of 12 mg/m^2/day of cortisol does not cause clinical significant hypothalamic–pituitary– adrenal axis suppression. Methylprednisolone does not interfere with the common radioimmune assay method of cortisol administration. Dexamethasone administration will not interfere with subsequent measurement of cortisol, and therefore, it is used in the so-called dexamethasone suppression test. (Rogers MC, et al. *Textbook of Pediatric Intensive Care*, 3rd Edition; pp. 1251–1256.)

CHAPTER 8: NUTRITION AND GASTROINTESTINAL SYSTEM

1. E The fat requirement in infants is 4 g/kg/day. (Rogers MC, et al. *Textbook of Pediatric Intensive Care*, 3rd Edition; pp. 1142–1145.)

2. D The ebb phase and the flow phase are characteristic features of hypermetabolism and not features of a starvation syndrome. The ebb phase is similar to a shock stage during which the metabolic rate is slow. The flow phase is characterized by increased metabolism. Normally with aerobic glycolysis, the end product is pyruvate. Subsequently the end products enter the tricarboxylic acid cycle (kreb cycle) for production of the high-energy adenosine triphosphate. With substantial ketonemia, this process is inhibited, and therefore, utilization of glucose is impaired. (Rogers MC, et al. *Textbook of Pediatric Intensive Care*, 3rd Edition; pp. 1145–1148.)

3. B During hypermetabolism, which is characterized by an initial ebb phase followed by a flow phase, there is usually an associated hyperglycemia owing to decreased sensitivity to the effect of insulin, although the level of insulin may actually be higher than usual. (Rogers MC, et al. *Textbook of Pediatric Intensive Care*, 3rd Edition; pp. 1145–1148.)

4. B After several days of starvation, the serum glucose and insulin levels gradually decrease but eventually a plateau is reached. Levels of ketones, however, continue to rise along with an increase in the level of glucagon. With continuation of starvation, nitrogen excretion falls. There is an adaptation of the brain to use the rising level of available ketones. (Rogers MC, et al. *Textbook of Pediatric Intensive Care*, 3rd Edition; pp. 1145–1148.)

5. B, C, A These are the respiratory quotients for the various fuels. The respiratory quotient is highest for carbohydrate. Therefore, with patients who have a problem with elimination of carbon dioxide, the administration of carbohydrate should be lowered in order to minimize carbon dioxide production. (Rogers MC, et al. *Textbook of Pediatric Intensive Care*, 3rd Edition; pp. 1150,1151.)

6. E Preventive measures that are used for stress ulceration in the ICU include feeding, which by itself, acts as a protective barrier for the gastric mucosa, or the administration of H$_2$ blockers, which may be administered by continuous infusion. These would include ranitidine or famotidine. Administration of antacids has been shown to be as effective as H$_2$ blockers. Alternatives include administration of sucralfate, which has been shown to be comparable to H$_2$ blockers. Enteral feedings seem to stimulate release of the hormone gastrin. Administration of gastrin itself is not one of the measures that is clinically used in an ICU as a preventative measure against stress ulceration. (Rogers MC, et al. *Textbook of Pediatric Intensive Care*, 3rd Edition; pp. 1167,1168.)

7.   D   Administration of an elemental diet has been associated with an increased release of the hormone gastrin, which seems to be trophic for the gastric mucosa. (Choctaw W, et al. Arch Surg, 1980; 115:1073.)

8, 9.   D, A   With gastric lavage and hemodynamic support, usually most patients with gastritis and bleeding will respond. H_2 blockers have not been shown to stop gastric bleeding faster than lavage. Endoscopy should be performed to identify the site of bleeding, which if found, endoscopic therapy with electrical or laser cautery may be indicated and helpful. (Rogers MC, et al. *Textbook of Pediatric Intensive Care*, 3rd Edition; pp. 1167,1168.)

10.   D   Vasopressin, an antidiuretic hormone, appears to be released during laparotomy and contributes to the decreased motility of the small bowel. Other contributing factors are hypokalemia, particularly with potassium levels of less than 2.5 mEq/L. The colon is the portion of the bowel most dependent on neural control to achieve motility. This is the portion of the bowel that is most sensitive to anesthesia-induced inhibition of motility, and the last to recover. The role that handling or direct manipulation of the gut plays in the development of ileus is not very clear. (Livingston E, Passaro E. Dig Dis Sci, 1990; 35:121.)

11.   E   Ogilvies syndrome, which is a localized ileus of the bowel leading to pseudo-obstruction, is associated with inflammatory conditions in the intra-abdominal or para-abdominal regions. (Rogers MC, et al. *Textbook of Pediatric Intensive Care*, 3rd Edition; pp. 1168,1169.)

12.   D   Postoperative intussusception that is usually ileoileal rather than ileocecal (which is seen in late infancy) is a problem that can be overlooked in the postoperative patient, particularly in patients who are receiving analgesia for postoperative care along with nasogastric suctioning to decompress the bowel. However, this is important to recognize to avoid morbidity and mortality. (Ein H, Ferguson J. J Pediatr Surg, 1971; 6:16.)

13.   E   Please *see* the answer to Question 10.

14.   D   In the setting of postoperative ileus, if the cecum is very dilated, particularly if the diameter is greater than 12 cm, there is a very high risk of perforation even in the absence of mechanical obstruction. The only effective treatment for postoperative ileus is nasointestinal intubation to decompress the bowel and supportive measures. Neostigmine has not been shown to be a safe therapeutic intervention, and is associated with significant side effects. (Adams J. Arch Surg, 1974; 109:513; Livingston E. Dig Dis Sci, 1990; 35:121.)

15.   D   Because of the counter-current mechanism, the oxygen delivery is least to the tip of the villi. Impaired blood flow to the bowel leads to dilation of the bowel which leads to overgrowth of bacteria, and this can lead to malabsorption, including fat malabsorption. (Perman PA. In: Hokelman RA. *Principles of Pediatrics*, New York, McGraw Hill, 1978; p. 808.)

16.   C   Clostridium difficile is an important infection to recognize in the ICU, particularly where broad-spectrum antibiotics have been utilized. It presents with diarrhea, which can be bloody in nature and associated with significant volume loss. When this is diagnosed, usually by obtaining a toxin assay, oral vancomycin or intravenous metronidazole are usually effective. Stool culture for corona virus and rotavirus are important for epidemiological studies, but will not contribute to a patient's therapeutic intervention, nor do small bowel radiography or colonoscopy. (Viscidi RP. Pediatrics, 1981; 67:381.)

17.   C   Acute pancreatitis is a medical condition characterized by inflammation of the pancreas with subsequent release of the enzymes amylase and lipase. The degree of serum amylase does not seem to be proportional to the severity of acute pancreatitis. Serum lipase levels seem to be elevated for a longer period of time than serum amylase. Pancreatic trypsinogen serum levels seem to rise early in the course of pancreatitis and remain elevated for up to 5 days. In a clinical situation where amylase and lipase are normal and there is a high suspicion of pancreatitis, one could look at the level of trypsinogen. Some of the bad prognostic signs of acute pancreatitis include hyperglycemia, leukocytosis, hypocalcemia, and azotemia. (Rogers MC, et al. *Textbook of Pediatric Intensive Care*, 3rd Edition; pp. 1175–1178.)

18.   D   Reye's syndrome which has practically vanished and is very infrequently seen today, is characterized by alteration of mental status that can progress to coma in association with derangement of the liver enzymes and alteration in the coagulation profile. However, an increased level of bilirubin or jaundice is not a recognized feature of this condition. (Rogers MC, et al. *Textbook of Pediatric Intensive Care*, 3rd Edition; pp. 1178–1180.)

19. C Patients who develop fulminant hepatic failure as a result of hepatitis B virus infection (when compared with patients who do not progress to hepatic failure) tend to have earlier appearance of antibodies against hepatitis B surface antigen. Also, they have earlier appearance of antibodies against hepatitis B, E-antigen, and more rapid clearance of the hepatitis B surface antigen. (Rogers MC, et al. *Textbook of Pediatric Intensive Care*, 3rd Edition; pp. 1179–1181.)

20. D Intravenous fat emulsions may not be tolerated well in patients with significant hepatic disease because it may not be metabolized by these patients. Accumulation of fatty acids intrahepatically may further compromise the hepatic function. Furthermore, non-esterified fatty acids may compete with tryptophan for binding to albumin. This may increase the risk of encephalopathy. (Rogers MC, et al. *Textbook of Pediatric Intensive Care*, 3rd Edition; pp. 1178–1187.)

21–23. D, C, E The initial intervention for an upper gastrointestinal (GI) hemorrhage is gastric lavage and supportive measures which would include correction of any coagulopathy and use of volume expanders, either crystalloids or colloids. In patients who are hemodynamically unstable owing to upper GI hemorrhage, adequate volume expansion is crucial and this should not be withheld, even in patients who have evidence of edema. If the patient does not respond to initial intervention, an endoscopy should be performed, and if any localized area of bleeding is identified, this can be treated through endoscopy with electrical or laser cautery, or with the application of topical coagulants as indicated. (Rogers MC, et al. *Textbook of Pediatric Intensive Care*, 3rd Edition; pp. 1181,1182.)

24. D Patent foramen ovale is not a recognized cause or a contributing factor to hypoxia in patients with hepatic failure. (Rogers MC, et al. *Textbook of Pediatric Intensive Care*, 3rd Edition; p. 1182.)

25. D Ibuprofen, a nonsteroidal anti-inflammatory medication, can reduce renal plasma flow as well as glomerular filtration rate. This would result in water retention, dilutional hyponatremia, and ascites, which might be resistant to diuretic therapy. It appears that prostaglandins are important in renal vasodilation and ibuprofen may compromise this physiologically important parameter that maintains renal blood flow in patients in hepatic failure. (Rogers MC, et al. *Textbook of Pediatric Intensive Care*, 3rd Edition; p. 1183.)

26. B Hepatorenal syndrome is characterized by low urine sodium owing to the hyperaldosteronism. The associated high antidiuretic hormone levels lead to urine osmolality, which is generally greater than the serum osmolality. (Rogers MC, et al. *Textbook of Pediatric Intensive Care*, 3rd Edition; p. 1183.)

27. C Hepatorenal syndrome can develop in a setting of isovolemia. However, preventive measures that have been shown to be helpful for this clinical condition include avoiding large volume paracentesis in order to avoid intravascular volume depletion, as well as use of potent diuretics, which can also lead to intravascular volume depletion. Use of dopamine has not been shown to be effective for this clinical condition. In the early stages when this condition is suspected, expansion of intravascular volume with salt-poor albumin to raise the central venous pressure to the upper limits of normal is a helpful preventive measure. Other preventive measures include avoidance of prostaglandin antagonists, such as ibuprofen. (Rogers MC, et al. *Textbook of Pediatric Intensive Care*, 3rd Edition; p. 1183.)

28. E Arterial ammonia is preferred to venous ammonia; however, there is no positive correlation between the grade of encephalopathy and the height of the ammonia. Not all patients with hepatic encephalopathy (HE) have elevated ammonia levels. (Rogers MC, et al. *Textbook of Pediatric Intensive Care*, 3rd Edition; p. 1183.)

29. E Measures to decrease protein intake, as well as elimination of colonic bacteria by use of oral lactulose, oral antibiotics, such as neomycin, have been shown to be effective for HE. Use of hypertonic glucose to provide calories is also an important measure in the management of these patients. (Butterworth RF. Dig Dis Sci, 1992; 37: 321–327.)

30, 31. D, E In a patient with HE, there is inappropriate pathological cerebrovascular tone along with altered permeability of the blood–brain barrier that contributes to their symptomatology. In these patients, intracranial pressure monitoring along with hyperventilation to lower the PCO_2 will facilitate management. Steroids have not been shown to decrease mortality in these settings. These patients should be considered for hepatic transplantation and evaluated for this procedure in the initial stages of ICU admission because it has been shown that if the patient progresses to decorticate posturing and becomes ventilator dependent, it usually too late to initiate liver transplantation. (Zaki AEO, et al. Experientia, 1983; 39:988; Rogers MC, et al. *Textbook of Pediatric Intensive Care*, 3rd Edition; pp. 1193–1195.)

32. B, A, D, C, E Pulmonary edema is rarely associated with administration of OKT_3. Therefore, patients who are receiving OKT_3, usually in the postoperative period, are monitored in the intensive care setting. Their fluids and electrolytes are adjusted very carefully to prevent pulmonary edema. (Rogers MC, et al. *Textbook of Pediatric Intensive Care*, 3rd Edition; pp. 1202–1204.)

33. A Please *see* Rogers MC, et al. *Textbook of Pediatric Intensive Care*, 3rd Edition; pp. 1197–1199.

34. B This form of hemolytic anemia is usually self-limited and resolves spontaneously within 2–4 weeks. During this period, a serial reticulocyte count is often helpful in monitoring the progression or regression of this hematological problem. Haptoglobin may not be useful in this setting because the level of haptoglobin may be decreased owing to underlying liver disease. (Ramsey G, et al. N Engl J Med, 1984; 311:1167.)

35. A Liver disease is usually not homogenous, and therefore, drug metabolism is affected to a variable degree depending on the type of medication. It seems that the process of glucuronidation is more resistant to abnormalities in function than the process of oxidation, and therefore, in treating a patient with liver disease, preference should be given to drugs that are metabolized through this pathway. For drugs that undergo significant hepatic biotransformation clearance of these drugs tends to be proportional to the degree of liver blood flow. (Bass NM, Williams RL. Clin Pharmacokinetics, 1988; 6:396.)

36. C Branched chain amino acids have been shown to be of some use in chronic liver disease, however, they do not resolve HE on a consistent basis. (Rogers MC, et al. *Textbook of Pediatric Intensive Care*, 3rd Edition; pp. 1184–1186.)

37. A, D, C, B These are the half lives of various proteins, which can be used to evaluate the nutritional status of patients. Albumin has the longest half-life of 20–21 days. On the other hand, pre-albumin has a half-life of 2 days, and transferrin has a half-life of 8 days. Retinol-binding protein has a very short half-life of only 10 hours, and therefore, can be evaluated in patients who are suspected of having a recent onset of their nutritional deficiency. (Rogers MC, et al. *Textbook of Pediatric Intensive Care*, 3rd Edition; p. 1149.)

38. C Medium-chain triglycerides (C_6 to C_{12}) inhibit gastric emptying less than long-chain fatty acids, and are absorbed from the GI tract faster than long-chain fatty acids. Consequently, they convert into energy more rapidly than the long-chain fatty acids, or long-chain triglycerides. Medium-chain triglycerides are absorbed directly into the systemic circulation through the portal venous system, instead of being absorbed through the lymphatic lacteals and subsequently into the thoracic duct. (Fuhrman BP. *Pediatric Critical Care*, 2nd Edition; p. 907.)

39. E The presence of reducing substances in stool suggests carbohydrate malabsorption. Disaccharidases, which are located on the brush border may be diminished following acute injury and contribute to malabsorption of carbohydrates. Protein hydrolysate formulas, such as alimentum, nutramigen, and pregestimil are predigested for ease of nutrient absorption and are suitable to critically ill infants. (Rogers MC, et al. *Textbook of Pediatric Intensive Care*, 3rd Edition; pp. 1152,1153.)

40. B Stress ulcers are a recognized complication in critically ill children and are usually located high in the fundus of the stomach. (Rogers MC, et al. *Textbook of Pediatric Intensive Care*, 3rd Edition, 1996; pp. 1165–1167; Menguy R, Master YF. Gastroenterology, 1974; 66:1172.)

41. C Ranitidine (Zantac®), Famotidine, and proton pump inhibitors decrease gastric concentration. Sucralfate does not affect gastric pH or its concentration. (Rogers MC, et al. *Textbook of Pediatric Intensive Care*, 3rd Edition; pp. 1165–1168; Furhman

BP, et al. *Pediatric Critical Care*, 2nd Edition; pp. 919–932.)

42. A Iced saline lavage offers no advantages over room temperature saline lavage. A significant reduction in core body temperature is a potential complication of iced saline gastric lavage in young children. (Furhman BP, et al. *Pediatric Critical Care*, 2nd Edition; pp. 919–932; Levin D, et al. *Essentials of Pediatric Intensive Care*, 1990; pp. 565–572.)

43. C The majority of patients who die because of fulminant hepatic failure are found to have cerebral edema. Many of these patients have evidence of transtentorial herniation. Infection and sepsis are common but usually do not cause death. Gastrointestinal hemorrhage is also common, and is usually related to gastritis or ulceration. (Ware AJ. Gastroenterology, 1971; 61:877; Canalese J. Gastroenterology, 1982; 23:625.)

44. B Local complications of pancreatitis include pancreatic necrosis, pancreatic abscess, and pseudocyst formation. ARDS may occur with pancreatitis. Renal dysfunction is seen frequently in the setting of acute pancreatitis, and is related to hypoperfusion, hypotension, and volume loss. Specific renal injury, such as glomerulonephritis, has not been noted with acute pancreatitis. (Rogers MC, et al. *Textbook of Pediatric Intensive Care*, 3rd Edition, pp. 583,584. Frey CF, Bradley EL. Surg Gynecol Obs, 1988; 167: 282.)

45. D Toxic megacolon is usually a complication of ulcerative colitis but is rarely involved in patients with pseudomembranous enterocolitis, Crohn's disease or ischemic colitis. Factors involved in precipitation of toxic megacolon include barium enema, opiates, anticholinergics, antidiarrheal agents, and electrolyte derangements. (Dorudi S, Berry AR, Kettlewell MG. Br J Surg, 1992; 79:99–103; Ulshen M. *Nelson's Textbook of Pediatrics*, 15th Edition, pp. 1080–1087.)

46. D This patient has typhlitis, which is a necrotizing colitis involving the cecum. This is common among patients with immune deficiency. Typhlitis is a life-threatening condition that causes severe abdominal pain, GI bleeding, and fever. Medical management includes discontinuing oral intake, aggressive fluid management followed by total parenteral nutrition, antibiotics, and FFP to maintain adequate coagulation status. Colonoscopy would be contraindicated because of risk of perforation. (Rogers MC, et al. *Textbook of Pediatric Intensive Care*, 3rd Edition; pp. 1174,1175; Katz JA, Wagner ML. Cancer, 1990, 65: 1041–1047.)

CHAPTER 9: IMMUNOLOGY

1. E The developmental pattern of immunoglobulins (Igs) is as follows: IgG transfer across the placenta occurs as early as 8 weeks gestational age. Its level is directly proportional to gestational age, but is still less than 50% of term levels at 28 weeks gestation. The IgG levels fall during the first four months of extrauterine life reaching adult levels by 4–6 years of age. By the 10th week of gestation, the fetus is capable of producing IgM and may make large quantities in the presence of a congenital infection. IgA is not measurable until late in gestational life and is very limited in the infant, failing to reach adult values until puberty. (Rogers MC, et al. *Textbook of Pediatric Intensive Care*, 3rd Edition; p. 916.)

2. C The immunological function of the neonate undergoes maturation in both the cellular and humoral components with the child's development. The neonate's T-cells are unable to produce certain cytokines, which affects the interaction between T-cells and B-cells. In addition, there is a greater reactivity of T-suppressor cells relative to T-helper cells compared with those of the normal adult. Premature and full-term infants are deficient in all of the measurable products of complement activation. The newborn's phagocytes exhibit diminished motility, adherence, and chemotaxis. Bacterial killing by polymorphonuclear leukocytes, which depends on the generation of oxygen-derived free radicals, is intact in healthy-term and most premature newborns. (Rogers MC, et al. *Textbook of Pediatric Intensive Care*, 3rd Edition; pp. 916,917.)

3. A, B C3a is an anaphylatoxin that induces smooth muscle contraction, histamine release from basophils and mast cells, and increased vascular permeability. The C5b–C9 components are referred to as the membrane attack complex, which leads to cell lysis. (Rogers MC, et al. *Textbook of Pediatric Intensive Care*, 3rd Edition; p. 917: Table 28.2.)

4. T, F, T, T, T, F A variety of drugs and diseases can affect immune function. For example, N_2O decreases both T-cell responses to mitogen, and B-cell proliferation and activity. Halothane decreases phagocytosis, bacterial killing, and chemotaxis and has a depressant effect on reticuloendothelial phagocytic activity. The administration of thiopental and other barbiturate agents at anesthetic levels for as little as 30 minutes can produce granulocytopenia. Longer exposures to pentobarbital have resulted in an 80% decrement in the circulating granulocyte count. The major adverse effect on immunity produced by narcotics, such as morphine sulfate, is depression of leukocyte chemotaxis. A surgical wound dramatically increases the circulating neutrophil count. This is related to certain humoral effects of trauma, most notably, a strong, acute catecholamine release that is one component of the body's nonspecific response to stress. Blood levels of B-lymphocytes and T-lymphocytes decrease in response to surgical stress. (Rogers MC, et al. *Textbook of Pediatric Intensive Care*, 3rd Edition; pp. 918,919, table 28.3.)

5. B Secretory IgA appears later than serum IgA (already limited in the infant; *see* Question 1). Diseases whose defense depends primarily upon secretory IgA, such as some of the viral respiratory agents (e.g., respiratory syncytial virus) and infectious diarrheas, remain prevalent throughout infancy. The infant is at risk for encapsulated organisms and cannot localize infections well. IgM production by the non-infected newborn does not reach adult levels until 1–2 years of life. (Rogers MC, et al. *Textbook of Pediatric Intensive Care*, 3rd Edition; pp. 916,917.)

6. B A number of immune function alterations have been documented following major trauma. Many of these have also been implicated in the post-trauma sepsis syndrome. Of those listed, only the primary response to immunization does not increase. Prostaglandin E2, interleukin-6, tumor necrosis factor-α, and transforming growth factor-β all increase. (Rogers MC, et al. *Textbook of Pediatric Intensive Care*, 3rd Edition; p. 919, table 28.4.)

7. A Although the majority of infections in the post-surgical patient are nosocomial, the most likely offending organisms are *aerobic* Gram-negative bacteria (*Escherichia coli, Proteus, Pseudomonas, Klebsiella, Enterobacter,* and *Acinetobacter*). Controversy exists over the use of prophylactic antibiotics; however, prophylactic antibiotics are most beneficial in injuries involving the large and the small bowel, and in soft tissue crush and extremity avulsion injuries. In the setting of GI contamination, Gram-negative and anerobic organisms are particularly likely. (Rogers MC, et al. *Textbook of Pediatric Intensive Care*, 3rd Edition; pp. 919,920, table 28.5.)

8. E In the management of burn victims, feeding by the enteral route is preferable to parenteral nutrition, because food in the gut can decrease the rate of organism and toxin translocation across the GI tract. Burns lead to a reduction in Ig levels, chemotaxis, and T-helper lymphocytes. Colonization of the burn wound in 5–7 days postinjury is predominantly with Gram-positive bacteria. Arginine influences postburn recovery by stimulating wound-healing, potentially through its roles in the formation of nitric oxide, by enhancing growth hormone secretion from the pituitary gland and by directly modulating immune function. However, high concentrations of dietary lipids, especially of the ω-6 series, may contribute to the development of postburn sepsis by augmenting the plasma concentration of prostaglandin E2 and prostacyclin. (Rogers MC, et al. *Textbook of Pediatric Intensive Care*, 3rd Edition; p. 921.)

9. B, C, A As mentioned earlier, in the early postburn period, Gram-positive organism infections predominate. The most likely organism is *Staphylococcus aureus*, which has an insidious course, and is associated with a low mortality. Of the Gram-negative organisms that later colonize the wound, *Pseudomonas aeruginosa* and *E. coli* are the most prevalent. *Pseudomonas* infection can be particularly dangerous because it has a propensity to further devitalize intact tissue, and may convert a partial thickness burn to a full thickness one. *Candida albicans* and other *Candida* species can cause some of the most severe infections, and are associated with the highest mortality. (Rogers MC, et al. *Textbook of Pediatric Intensive Care*, 3rd Edition; pp. 921–922, tables 28.7 and 28.8.)

10. C The second most common cause of death in the pediatric trauma victim who survives the initial postinjury period is infection. In addition, infection is the major cause of death among burn victims who survive initial fluid resuscitation. (Rogers MC, et al. *Textbook of Pediatric Intensive Care*, 3rd Edition; pp. 919, 921.)

11.   T, F, T   Kwashiorkor (protein deficiency) and Marasmus (protein *and* calorie deficiency) have more significant effects on cell-mediated immunity. Children with kwashiorkor have very small thymus glands, with relative atrophy of lymph nodes and spleen. Qualitatively, this is expressed as an increased incidence of infections with viral (especially measles and disseminated herpes), fungal (*Candida*), and opportunistic organisms (*Pneumocystis carinii*). In kwashiorkor, the thymus is typically small. The B-cell system is relatively spared in children with protein calorie malnutrition. Seroconversion in response to immunization with diphtheria and tetanus toxoids, pneumococcal polysaccharide, and polio vaccines is normal even in malnourished children. (Rogers MC, et al. *Textbook of Pediatric Intensive Care*, 3rd Edition; pp. 921–924, tables 28.9 and 28.10.)

12.   A   Although steroids do not diminish serum antibody concentrations, they decrease the circulating pool of T-lymphocytes by sequestering these cells in extravascular sites. Steroids also reduce the production of IL-1 and IL-2 and adversely affect macrophage maturation. This results in diminished antigen processing and presentation to lymphocytes for antibody production. Monocytic killing of bacteria and fungi is inhibited by the administration of steroids. (Rogers MC, et al. *Textbook of Pediatric Intensive Care*, 3rd Edition; p. 923.)

13   A, B   Cyclosporine asserts its major effects by decreasing both IL-2 production, and γ-interferon. The major complications of cyclosporine include renal failure and systemic hypertension. Azathioprine inhibits purine synthesis and decreases RNA and DNA synthesis. The major complications of azathioprine include nausea, vomiting, diarrhea, and decreases in both white blood cell and platelet counts. (Rogers MC, et al. *Textbook of Pediatric Intensive Care*, 3rd Edition; p. 924, table 28.11.)

14.   D   Asplenia in children can result from a variety of conditions ranging from trauma to sickle cell disease. This makes the ability to perform randomized clinical studies of asplenia difficult. Congenital asple-

nia is most often associated with cardiac abnormalities (heterotaxy). Absence of the spleen, whether anatomic or functional, predisposes the young child to potentially fatal sepsis from encapsulated bacterial species. The most prevalent offender is the pneumococcus in 50% of cases. *Haemophilus influenzae* type B, meningococcus, and group A streptococci account for 25%. There is general agreement that immunization of asplenic patients with pneumococcal vaccine should be performed. Children who are less than 2 years of age have a poor response to pure polysaccharide vaccines, so immunization at a young age is not feasible. Although penicillin prophylaxis has become routine, others have suggested that prompt administration of antibiotics with any febrile illness will more reliably reduce the percentage of fatal episodes. (Rogers MC, et al. *Textbook of Pediatric Intensive Care*, 3rd Edition; pp. 926–927.)

15.   C   Such a communication is known as a dural fistula and may be suspected by the finding of rhinorrhea or otorrhea following closed head trauma. In adults, posttraumatic meningitis has been reported in up to 25% of those with basilar skull fractures. Organisms most frequently implicated are *Streptoccus pneumoniae* (50–90%), *Haemophilus influenzae* type b (9%), and other streptococcal species (10%), with other organisms, such as *Neisseria meningitides* (5%), *Staphyloccus aureus* (5%), *S. epidermidis* (2%), and enteric Gram-negative organisms (4%). (Rogers MC, et al. *Textbook of Pediatric Intensive Care*, 3rd Edition; p. 920.)

16.   D, C, E, B, A   Wiskott-Aldrich Syndrome is an X-linked recessive disorder manifested by eczema, thrombocytopenia, and recurrent infections with encapsulated bacteria. The disorder is related to an inability to produce antibody to polysaccharide capsule. Serum immunoglobulins show a decrease in IgM, with an increase in IgA and IgE. Ataxia-Telangiectasia is an autosomal recessive disorder involving 11q22-23. The disorder results from a defect in DNA recombination. Breakpoints involve genes that encode for T-cell receptors. Associated conditions include IgA deficiency and lymphosarcoma. Chronic granulomatous disease involves a defect in any one of the four components of the enzyme NADPH oxidase, essential for bacterial killing in the neutrophil. 65% are X-linked, and the remainder are autosomal recessive. Organisms that are catalase-positive (*S. aureus*) can produce chronic infection by preventing phagocytes from using microbial generated hydrogen peroxide. Chediak-Higashi Syndrome involves defective chemotaxis, phagocytosis, and natural-killer (NK) activity because of elevated levels of cyclic adenosine monophosphate. Abnormal giant granules formed by the fusion of lysosomes are seen in cells that contain lysosomes. The clinical characteristics include recurrent pyogenic infections, albinism, photophobia, and nystagmus. Schwachman-Diamond Syndrome is a disorder that involves deficiency of the exocrine function of the pancreas and neutropenia secondary to bone marrow failure. (Rogers MC, et al. *Textbook of Pediatric Intensive Care*, 3rd Edition; pp. 932–936.)

17. E A recurrent infection with only one source is often related to an anatomical defect rather than immunodeficiency. All others listed are characteristics that should make the intensivist suspicious of an underlying immunodeficiency. (Rogers MC, et al. *Textbook of Pediatric Intensive Care*, 3rd Edition; p. 936)

18. C Childhood sexual abuse and undetermined risk factors account for less than 1% of pediatric AIDS cases. Perinatal transmission from infected mother to infant is the most common means by which children acquire HIV infection. HIV antibody screening of all donated blood products, as well as donor self-exclusion programs, were initiated in the early 1980s has lead to a finite risk of transmission from infected blood products. Enzyme-linked immunosorbent assay (ELISA) is the primary screening test for HIV infection because of its very high degree of sensitivity, reproducibility, and low cost. (Rogers MC, et al. *Textbook of Pediatric Intensive Care*, 3rd Edition; pp. 946–949.)

19. C Although adults initially infected with HIV undergo an acute influenza like illness accompanied by a rapid fall in CD4 counts and a rise in viral antigenemia, children rarely demonstrate such clinical symptoms or viremia. (Rogers MC, et al. *Textbook of Pediatric Intensive Care*, 3rd Edition; pp. 946,947.)

20. T, T, F, T, F, F Among perinatally infected children, the earliest clinical manifestations include-lymphadenopathy, hepatosplenomegaly, hypergammaglobulinemia, and skin disease including candidal dermatitis or seborrhea. ELISA is the primary screening test for HIV infection because of its very high degree of sensitivity, reproducibility, and low cost. The ELISA detects antibodies to HIV usually within 6–12 weeks of the primary infection. Western blot is the most widely used confirmatory test for HIV. The Western blot detects viral protein antigens. In infants younger than 18 months of age, serum tests for IgG antibody to HIV do not differentiate between infant and passively acquired maternal antibody. Polymerase chain reaction permits amplification of HIV viral DNA. This process is as sensitive and specific as viral culture. Hypergammaglobulinemia, not hypogammaglobulinemia is an early clinical manifestation of HIV infection. (Rogers MC, et al. *Textbook of Pediatric Intensive Care*, 3rd Edition; pp. 946–951.)

21. E *P. carinii* pneumonia (PCP) becomes attached to the type I alveolar cells of the lung. Most normal children have serological evidence of latent infection with *P. carinii*. Therefore, this infection in older children and adults is presumably the result of reactivation of the organism. Patients with PCP typically have the tetrad of nonproductive cough, fever, dyspnea, and tachypnea. Bronchoalveolar lavage is the most widely used method for obtaining lung fluid to diagnose PCP. (Rogers MC, et al. *Textbook of Pediatric Intensive Care*, 3rd Edition; pp. 953,954.)

22. A, B, B Patient intolerance to trimethoprim–sulfamethoxazole may result in cutaneous reactions ranging from a mild rash to TEN or Steven's-Johnson syndrome. Pentamidine has a wide variety of side effects including pancreatitis, hypoglycemia, hyperglycemia, neutropenia, thrombocytopenia, and azotemia. (Rogers MC, et al. *Textbook of Pediatric Intensive Care*, 3rd Edition; pp. 954,955.)

23. C Aerosolized pentamidine, in adults has been shown to be a less effective regimen than intravenous pentamidine for PCP. All of the other statements are true. (Rogers MC, et al. *Textbook of Pediatric Intensive Care*, 3rd Edition; p. 955.)

24. B Measles is highly contagious and may have devastating effects on the lung. Measles itself may be associated with pneumonia. In addition, other viruses and bacteria may secondarily infect the lung. Herpes simplex virus, adenovirus, *S. aureus,* and Gram-negative bacilli are among the most frequent etiologies. (Rogers MC, et al. *Textbook of Pediatric Intensive Care*, 3rd Edition; p. 957.)

25. D Children with biopsy proven minimal change disease or focal glomerulosclerosis have been treated with prednisone, but no clear responsiveness has been demonstrated. Although 30–55% of infected children will develop renal disease at some point in their illness, children tend not to follow the clinical pattern of adult patients including a rapid loss of renal function and death. Children will often manifest hypernatremia and histological evidence of focal segmental glomerulosclerosis. (Rogers MC, et al. *Textbook of Pediatric Intensive Care*, 3rd Edition; pp. 961,962.)

26. F, T, T, T, T, T, T In series that include asymptomatic, mildly symptomatic, and children with advanced neurological disease, a 19.6% prevalence rate of HIV encephalopathy is reported. Although rare, primary CNS lymphomas are the most common intracranial mass lesions that develop in HIV-infected children. In a multicenter study sponsored by the National Institute of Child Health and Human Development, intravenous Ig-treated children with CD4 counts higher than 200/mm^3 had a significant decrease in both documented and suspected bacterial infections, as well as days in hospital when compared with controls. The most important mycobacterial infections in HIV-infected children are those caused by *Mycobacterium tuberculosis,* and the *Mycobacterium avium-intracellu-*

lare complex. A significant and troublesome infection among HIV-infected children is candida esophagitis. Treatment options include ketoconazole orally, fluconazole orally, or amphotericin B intravenously. The risk of acquiring HIV infection from needle stick exposure is approximately 0.5%. Epidemiological evidence suggests that blood is the single most infectious medium for HIV in the medical setting. (Rogers MC, et al. *Textbook of Pediatric Intensive Care*, 3rd Edition; pp. 958–967.)

27. E Of the total lymphocyte population, 55–75% are T-cells. B-cells are activated by antigen to secrete antibody. IgG and IgM are the only Ig classes that are capable of activating the classical complement pathway. (Rogers MC, et al. *Textbook of Pediatric Intensive Care*, 3rd Edition; pp. 568,569.)

28. E DiGeorge Syndrome includes clinical features of thymic aplasia, parathyroid aplasia, and conotruncal cardiac defects. The deficiency of cell mediated immunity in DiGeorge is a result of the thymic aplasia, and a relative absence of T-cells not B-cells. All of the other responses are true. (Rogers MC, et al. *Textbook of Pediatric Intensive Care*, 3rd Edition; pp. 931,932.)

CHAPTER 10: METABOLIC DISORDERS

1. B, C, A, D Slight elevation of ammonia is noted with organic acidemias; however, this is usually minimal compared with the significant hyperammonemia that is noted with urea cycle defects. Maple syrup urine disease (a disorder of branched chain amino: leucine, isoleucine, and valine) is characterized by metabolic acidosis and ketosis and significant hypoglycemia. The level of lactic acid will be significantly elevated with congenital lactic acidosis. (Fuhrman BP, et al. *Pediatric Critical Care*, 2nd Edition; pp. 820–825.)

2. E Urea cycle is present and is active only within the liver. In the brain there is no urea cycle that can detoxify ammonia. (Rogers MC, et al. *Textbook of Pediatric Intensive Care*, 3rd Edition; pp. 1299–1302.)

3. C In a newborn who develops significant seizures within the first 24 hours after birth, prior to having consumed a significant amount of protein in the

diet, and who does not have significant metabolic acidosis or elevation of ammonia levels, one has to think about nonketotic hyperglycinemia. Ornithine transcarbamylase deficiency is an X-linked disorder of ureacyte and is usually associated with significant elevation of blood ammonia levels. Methylmalmic acidemia, propionic acidemia, and isovolemic acidemia are organic acid disorders and are usually characterized by HAGMA. Maple syrup urine disease is discussed in Question 1, and is a disorder of branched chain amino acids caused by defective branched chain ketoacid dehydrogenase. Management of glucose and pH is most important in these patients. (Rogers MC, et al. *Textbook of Pediatric Intensive Care*, 3rd Edition; pp. 1299–1302.)

4. D All other responses are appropriate. The accepted hypotheses include:

a. The synergistic neurotoxin hypothesis which states that HE results from the synergistic accumulation of toxins, including ammonia, mercaptans, and short-chain fatty acids.

   b. The false neurotransmitter hypothesis states the octopamine acts as a false neurotransmitter and is taken up and released by neurones that normally store norepinephrine and dopamine.

   c. The neural inhibitory hypothesis implicates γ-aminobutyric acid (GABA) in the pathogenesis of HE.

(Jones, EA. Hepatology, 1984; 4:1235.)

5.   A Hypoglycemia produces selective necrosis of the superficial cortical layers sparing the non-neuronal elements (unless hypoglycemia is profound and prolonged). Infarction is usually absent even after severe hypoglycemia. In Reye's syndrome, nonspecific cytotoxic cerebral edema is seen with swelling of astrocyte foot processes. The hallmark of HE is proliferation and enlargement of the so-called Alzheimer -type astrocyte, which is basically a protoplasmic astrocyte. Long-standing heparin encephalopathy has been shown to be associated with degenervation changes in layers 5 and 6t of the cerebral cortex. (Rogers MC, et al. *Textbook of Pediatric Intensive Care*, 3rd Edition, pp. 792–794.)

6.   B, A, C, D, E These are some of the co-factors that have been shown to be helpful in the various metabolic disorders. (Batshaw M. Enzyme, 1987; 38:242; Fuhrman BP, et al. *Pediatric Critical Care*, 2nd Edition; pp. 820–825.)

7.   C With adrenocortical insufficiency, hypotension is associated with low levels of stress hormones. Thus, hypoglycemia is more of a possibility than hyperglycemia. (DiAeage AM, Levine LS. *Nelson's Textbook of Pediatrics*, 15th Edition; pp. 1613-1617; Kaplan SA. *Clinical Pediatric Endocrinology*, 1990; pp. 181–223.)

8.   C Diabetic ketoacidosis in the pediatric patient is a potentially life-threatening event. Ketosis and hyperglycemia result from an imbalance of glucagon and insulin levels with an increase in catecholamines, growth hormones, and glucocorticoids. An increase in somatostatin is not associated with diabetic ketoacidosis, but it down regulates the production and release of glucagon and growth hormones. (Rogers MC, et al. *Textbook of Pediatric Intensive Care*, 3rd Edition; pp. 1261–1270; Kaplan SA. *Clinical Pediatric Endocrinology*, 1990; pp. 127–164.)

9.   B, A, D, C Diabetic ketoacidosis or any acute metabolic acidosis state will decrease PCO_2 by 1–1.5 mmHg for each millimole change in bicarbonate concentration. In severe scoliosis, there is retraction of the chest wall causing chronic alveolar hypoventilation, with the development of chronic respiratory acidosis. A bicarbonate rise of 4 mmol will occur with a rise in 10 mmHg of PCO_2. Here both pH and bicarbonate concentrations are higher than expected for the level of PCO_2 elevation suggesting a mixed acid base disorder-metabolic acidosis superimposed or chronic respiratory acidosis. Botulism will cause rapid onset of respiratory failure causing pure respiratory acidosis. In acute respiratory acidosis, the pH will fall by approximately 0.08 U for each 10 mmHg of PCO_2. Plasma bicarbonate will increase 1 mmol/L for each increase of 10 mmHg in PCO_2. Salicylate intoxication causes acute metabolic acidosis. It also stimulates the respiratory center causing coincident respiratory alkalosis. A decrease in PCO_2 is out of proportion to the fall in plasma bicarbonate, which is suggestive of mixed acid–base disorder-metabolic acidosis and respiratory alkalosis. (Kaplan SA. *Clinical Pediatric Endocrinology*, 1990; pp. 181–234; Rogers MC, et al. *Textbook of Pediatric Intensive Care*, 3rd Edition; pp. 351–363.)

10.   D The rapid ACTH stimulation test is only a screening test that should be verified by a more definitive test when the patient's condition stabilizes. An abnormal response may be due to either primary or secondary adrenocortical insufficiency. A false-negative result has been reported in patients with early ACTH deficiency. (Kaplan SA. *Clinical Pediatric Endocrinology*, 1990; pp. 181–234; Furhman BP, et al. *Pediatric Critical Care*, 2nd Edition; pp. 826–843.)

11.   C Nearly all critically-ill patients have decreased serum levels of T3 and 50% have a decrease in the level of T4 concentration with normal or low thyroid-stimulating hormone (TSH). The reduction in T3 levels results from a decrease in deiodinase activity that occurs in critical illness. This is reflected in the increase in serum level of T3 that occurs during critical illness. This enzyme is responsible for the degradation reverse of T3, explaining the increase in serum levels of reverse T3 that occurs in critical illness. (Rogers MC, et al. *Textbook of Pediatric Intensive Care*, 3rd Edition; pp. 1290–1297; Wilson D, et al. J Ped, 1982; 101:113.)

CHAPTER 11: PAIN MANAGEMENT

1.   D   Neuroanatomical pathways are present at birth; they do not develop at 4 months of age. All of the other statements are correct. (Rogers MC, et al. *Textbook of Pediatric Intensive Care*, 3rd Edition; pp. 1548–1550.)

2.   D   The μ receptor agonists are the most commonly used opioids for analgesia. The μ_1 receptor is the subtype that provides supraspinal analgesia. The μ_2 receptor produces respiratory depression, inhibition of GI motility, and spinal analgesia. Furthermore, the μ_2 receptors cause bradycardia and sedation. Newborns may be sensitive to an age-related receptor phenomenon that leads to opiate-induced respiratory depression. (Rogers MC, et al. *Textbook of Pediatric Intensive Care*, 3rd Edition; pp. 1552–1554.)

3.   D, B, A, D, A   The μ_2 receptor inhibits GI motility. Methadone, morphine, fentanyl, and meperidine are agonists for the μ receptor. The κ receptor inhibits antidiuretic hormone release. The δ receptor produces analgesia, respiratory depression, euphoria, and physical dependence. The psychotomimetic effects that are observed with some opiates including dysphoria and hallucinations are associated with the σ receptor. Phencyclidine is an agonist for the σ receptor. (Rogers MC, et al. *Textbook of Pediatric Intensive Care*, 3rd Edition; pp. 1552–1554; tables 46.2 and 46.3.)

4.   B, C, A   Neonatal seizures can occur with the use of morphine at commonly prescribed doses. Meperidine is also associated with seizure activity. This, however, can occur in any age group and is related to the buildup of the toxic metabolite normeperidine. The serotonin syndrome occurs following the use of serotomimetic agents of which meperidine is included. When used alone or in combination with monoamine oxidase inhibitors a symptom complex characterized by myoclonus, rigidity, hyperreflexia, shivering, confusion, agitation, restlessness, coma, autonomic instability, low-grade fever, nausea, diarrhea, diaphoresis, flushing, and rarely, rhabdomyolysis and death can occur. The development of chest wall rigidity is a side effect associated with the rapid administration of fentanyl. This effect can be treated with the administration of either a neuromuscular blocker or naloxone. (Rogers MC, et al. *Textbook of*

Pediatric Intensive Care, 3rd Edition; pp. 1554–1559; Bodner RA, et al. Neurology 1995; 45:219–223.)

5.   E   All of the statements regarding the μ receptor agonist drugs are true. (Rogers MC, et al. *Textbook of Pediatric Intensive Care*, 3rd Edition; pp. 1552–1560.)

6.   B   Fentanyl is approximately 100 times more potent than morphine and is largely devoid of hypnotic or sedative activity. Sufentanil is approximately 10 times more potent than fentanyl. Alfentanil is approximately 10 times less potent than fentanyl. The α-1 acid glycoprotein is an acute phase protein that inhibits platelet aggregation and phagocytosis, and may help to regulate collagen fiber formation in healing. Fentanyl is tightly bound to α-1 glycoprotein. (Rogers MC, et al. *Textbook of Pediatric Intensive Care*, 3rd Edition; pp. 1557–1558; Fuhrman BP, *Pediatric Critical Care*, 2nd Edition; p. 807; Wilson AS, et al. Anesth Analg 1997; 84: 315–318.)

7.   B   Meperidine is 10 times less potent than morphine. It is unique among the opioids in its ability to stop shivering from amphotericin, blood products, anesthetics, and hypothermia. The metabolite normeperidine causes CNS excitation and seizures. *See* response to Question 4 from this section regarding the interaction of meperidine and monoamine oxidase inhibitors. (Rogers MC, et al. *Textbook of Pediatric Intensive Care*, 3rd Edition; pp. 1558,1559; Bodner RA, et al. Neurology 1995; 45:219–223.)

8.   D   Methadone has a half-life of approximately 19 hours. Clonidine is useful as an adjunct to treat opioid withdrawal. The bioavailability of methadone from the GI tract is excellent. It is estimated at 80–90%. (Rogers MC, et al. *Textbook of Pediatric Intensive Care*, 3rd Edition; pp. 1559.)

9.   D   Hydromorphone has a rapid onset of action with a 4- to 6-hour duration. It is 6–7 times more potent than morphine and 10 times more lipid soluble. Its half-life is 3–4 hours. Hydromorphone is far less sedating than morphine and associated with fewer systemic side effects. (Rogers MC, et al. *Textbook of Pediatric Intensive Care*, 3rd Edition; p. 1559.)

10.   D   Lipid solubility affects the transition of opioid analgesics from the aqueous side of the CSF to the lipid phase of the underlying neuraxis where the receptors are located. Hydrophilic agents, such as morphine, have a greater latency and duration of action than the more lipid soluble agent fentanyl. However, the lipid soluble agents produce more segmental analgesia associated with less rostral spread than the less lipid soluble agonists. Spinal opiates produce analgesia without altering autonomic or neuromuscular function. In addition, both light touch and proprioception are preserved. (Rogers MC, et al. *Textbook of Pediatric Intensive Care*, 3rd Edition; pp. 1561,1562.)

11. D Naloxone is a nonselective, opioid antagonist that works in small doses to alleviate the respiratory depression associated with opioids without affecting the analgesic properties. It is rapidly metabolized in the liver. Naloxone has no effect on the mental status of patients who have not received opioids. (Rogers MC, et al. *Textbook of Pediatric Intensive Care*, 3rd Edition; pp. 1562,1563.)

12. B Vertical or horizontal nystagmus heralds the onset of the loss of consciousness after ketamine administration. Ketamine is an excitatory hallucinogen that produces a coupled increase in both cerebral metabolism and blood flow. This has the effect of raising intracranial pressure. Ketamine also increases mean arterial blood pressure, heart rate, and cardiac output through an increase in plasma catecholamine levels. If a patient is catecholamine deficient, profound hypotension or death may occur. Nightmares occur as a side effect in about 10% of adult patients and 5% of pediatric patients. (Rogers MC, et al. *Textbook of Pediatric Intensive Care*, 3rd Edition; pp. 1563,1564.)

13. T, F, T, T, T, T Ketamine is a ventilatory depressant that reduces the ventilatory response to carbon dioxide. Laryngeal reflexes remain intact but this does not preclude the potential for aspiration. Ketamine increases pulmonary compliance by direct action on bronchial smooth muscle and indirectly by increasing plasma catecholamine levels. The drug is highly lipid soluble. Its redistribution rather than biotransformation or elimination is responsible for its short half-life. Reduction in liver blood flow leads to a prolongation of the serum half-life of ketamine. (Rogers MC, et al. *Textbook of Pediatric Intensive Care*, 3rd Edition; pp. 1563,1564.)

14. E The local anesthetics are of two types, amides and esters, which are both weak bases that block nerve conduction at the sodium channel when they are in their ionized form. In order to gain access to the channel, the drug must cross the membrane. It does this in its ionized form. The minimum concentration of a local anesthetic is the concentration necessary to block nerve impulse conduction. Unmyelinated nerve fibers carry nociceptive information and have a lower minimum concentration than heavily myelinated fibers. Less local anesthetic is necessary to block the transmission of pain than is necessary to produce muscle paralysis. (Rogers MC, et al. *Textbook of Pediatric Intensive Care*, 3rd Edition; pp. 1565–1567.)

15. 4, 2, 3, 5, 1 The absorption of local anesthetic is dependent on the site of the block. The order of absorption from highest to lowest is intercostal, intratracheal, > caudal/epidural > brachial plexus > distal peripheral > subcutaneous. (Rogers MC, et al. *Textbook of Pediatric Intensive Care*, 3rd Edition; p. 1566.)

16. E GABA is the major inhibitory neurotransmitter in the brain. Glycine is an inhibitory neurotransmitter in the spinal cord and brainstem. The GABA receptor has two α and two β subunits. Binding of benzodiazepines to the α subunits of the GABA receptor facilitates binding to the β-receptors and promotes membrane hyperpolarization and resistance to neuronal excitation. The benzodiazepines can blunt or abolish the respiratory responses to hypercarbia and hypoxia. They produce hypoventilation by reducing tidal volume. The benzodiazepines produce minimal cardiac affects. However, they do reduce preload and afterload. They increase, rather than decrease coronary sinus blood flow and myocardial oxygen consumption. (Rogers MC, et al. *Textbook of Pediatric Intensive Care*, 3rd Edition; pp. 1573–1574.)

17. T, F, T Midazolam is four times more potent than diazepam and can be painlessly administered. When used for continuous sedation, usually for more than a week, dependence and withdrawal may occur when the drug is stopped. (Rogers MC, et al. *Textbook of Pediatric Intensive Care*, 3rd Edition; pp. 1574–1576.)

18. B, A Recovery from the effects of thiopental and methohexital are a result of drug redistribution, and not biotransformation or elimination. Pentobarbital is used to induce sleep. It acts within 10–15 minutes of an intravenous or intramuscular injection and lasts approximately 2–6 hours. (Rogers MC, et al. *Textbook of Pediatric Intensive Care*, 3rd Edition; p. 1576.)

19. T The incidence of cardiac arrest associated with anesthesia is 1:600 for infants, 1:700 for children, and 1:2500 for adults, respectively. (Rogers MC, et al. *Textbook of Pediatric Intensive Care*, 3rd Edition; p. 1577.)

20. E, C, A, B, D The preoperative assessment of surgical risk or postoperative complications has been classified according to the American Society of Anesthesiologists. The classification ranges from class 1 to class 5. As the patient's physiological dysfunction worsens, a higher class is attained. This higher class has an increased risk of anesthetic-related complications and death. (Rogers MC, et al. *Textbook of Pediatric Intensive Care*, 3rd Edition; p. 1577; table 46.12.)

21. E All of the agents listed stimulate histamine release. (Rogers MC, et al. *Textbook of Pediatric Intensive Care*, 3rd Edition; p. 1577.)

22. T, F, T The inhalational agents mentioned are commonly used in pediatric anesthesia. The rate of delivery of the agent to the alveolus is the function of minute ventilation and inspired concentration, but the rate of removal is dependent on cardiac output and the solubility of the agent. Nitrous oxide is relatively insoluble and can achieve steady state within 5–10 minutes. Halothane requires 15–20 minutes to achieve steady state. (Rogers MC, et al. *Textbook of Pediatric Intensive Care*, 3rd Edition; pp. 1579–1583.)

23. E Hyperkalemia is associated with the administration of succinylcholine, not hypokalemia. All of the other statements are true regarding succinylcholine. (Rogers MC, et al. *Textbook of Pediatric Intensive Care*, 3rd Edition; pp. 1584–1585.)

24. E All of the statements regarding nondepolarizing neuromuscular blockers are true. (Rogers MC, et al. *Textbook of Pediatric Intensive Care*, 3rd Edition; pp. 1584–1587.)

CHAPTER 12: PHARMACOLOGY/TOXICOLOGY

1. D In this case, the lean body-weight (the 50th percentile of weight for age) is the appropriate weight to use. (Rowland M, Tozer TN. *Clinical Pharmacokinetics: Concept and Applications*. Lea & Febiger, Philadelphia; pp. 100–110.)

2. C When drug accumulation is expected, which means that the ratio of dosing interval/half-life is less than three, and when there is a need to establish a therapeutic level rapidly, then a loading dose is necessary. Loading dose = Concentration × Volume of distribution. (Kearns GL. Clin Pharmakokinet, 1989; 17[Suppl 1]:29.)

3. C First one has to calculate the creatinine clearance, which is = L × K / serum creatinine, where L is length of the child, K is a constant and it equals .45 for this age. Therefore, the creatinine clearance for this patient = $75 \times 0.45 / 1.2$. Assuming that the normal creatinine clearance is 100 mL/minute/1.73 M^2, the renal index would = 28.1 mL/minute, which is equal to 0.28 for this patient. Plugging all these numbers into the equation provided would result in 4.5 mg/kg/day as the appropriate dose. K = 0.45 for infants; 0.55 for 1–3 years; and for adolescents, 0.7 for boys and 0.55 for girls. (Bennett WM. Clin Pharmakokinet, 1988; 52:326.)

4. E Patients at risk of adrenal hypofunction who are admitted to the PICU (for nontrivial illness) require additional doses of corticosteroid coverage. The physiological dose is 12.5 mg/M^2 body surface area (BSA)/day of hydrocortisone. Patients with a febrile illness presumed to be secondary to a nontrivial infection, deserve doubling of the maintenance dose. Patients with a major trauma, major surgery, or generalized sepsis deserve 3–4 times the maintenance dose. When time allows, high-dose corticosteroids must be initiated 1–2 days prior to surgery, and weaned over a period of 5–7 days. Because the risk of undertreatment is higher than overtreatment in patients with a serious illness or trauma, it is reasonable for a clinician to administer 100–200 mg/M^2 BSA/day of hydrocortisone to these patients. Gastric acidity partially inactivates oral steroids and, therefore, higher doses are often necessary. (Migeon C. In: Collaly R, et al. *Recent Progress in Pediatric Endocrinology*, New York, Raven Press, 1981; pp. 465–522.)

5. A Adrenergic receptors comprise four subtypes: α_1, α_2, β_1, and β_2. Each of these subtypes and the family keeps growing. α_1 Receptors are typical postsynaptic receptors, mediating smooth muscle contraction in both the vascular tree (causing intense vasoconstriction) and the genitourinary system. α_2 Receptors include presynaptic and nonsynaptic sites (such as on platelets). α_2 Receptors tend to inhibit release of norepinephrine from sympathetic nerve terminals resulting in relaxation of vascular and GI tract (GIT) smooth muscles. Phenoxybenzamine, or α_1 blocking agent, is the most selective α_1 blocking agent, and is used for preoperative management of patients with pheochromocytoma. Prazosin is a potent but less selective α blocker, and its blockade of α_2 receptors (presynaptic receptors) cause uninhibited release of norepinephrine, thus counterbalancing the α_1 receptor blockade. Phentolamine is likewise not a selective α_1 blocker. Atenolol is a selective β_1 blocker. (Bravo E. N Eng J Med, 1984; 311:1298. Hoffman B. N Eng J Med, 1980; 302:1390.)

6. E Cocaine is absorbed from respiratory, GIT, and genitourinary mucosa. It is metabolized in the liver by esterases. It is metabolized by plasma pseudocholinesterase and nonenzymatic hydrolysis. The two major cocaine metabolites in urine are benzoylecgonine and ecgonine methyl ester. Most urine drug screening tests detect benzoylecgonine. There is a greater potential for toxicity in patients with pseudocholinesterase deficiency because cocaine will be less metabolized. Drug abusers ingest an organophosphate in an attempt to prolong the effects of cocaine, which also increases the risk of cocaine toxicity. (Goldfrank LR. *Goldfrank's Toxicologic Emergencies*, 6th Edition; pp. 855–856.)

7. D Deferoxamine does interfere with subsequent laboratory determination of iron level, and under these circumstances, the most accurate method of measuring serum iron is using the atomic absorption spectrophotometric method. Interestingly, deferoxamine actually potentiates the activity of *Yersinia* enterocolitis. Children usually require 24 hours or less of deferoxamine therapy. (Goldfrank LR. *Goldfrank's Toxicologic Emergencies*, 6th Edition; pp. 532–534.)

8–9. E, E Numerous substitutions of the phenylethylamine structure are possible resulting in different amphetamine-like compounds. These are referred to as amphetamines, although a more precise name, phenylethylamines, exists. The diagnosis of amphetamine overdose depends on a high degree of suspicion along with clinical judgment. Diagnosis by history alone is rarely helpful. There is no reliable blood analysis test and the quantitative urine test is not particularly useful for acute settings. One of the major differentiating features between cocaine and amphetamines is the duration of action, which lasts for about 2 hours in the case of cocaine. The half-life of amphetamines on the other hand ranges from 8 to 30 hours. Amphetamines enhance the release of, and block the reuptake of, catecholamines, resulting in excess stimulation of both α and β receptors. At higher doses, they can cause release of serotonin. The clinical manifestations are that of cardiovascular and CNS excitation. Do not neglect to obtain a rectal temperature in these patients. Hyperthermia, if not recognized and treated aggressively, may be rapidly fatal in association with delirium. These patients are often very agitated and require sedation because agitation against restraints may exacerbate the associated rhabdomyolysis. Benzodiazepines are the drug of choice because neuroleptic agents lower seizure threshold, alter temperature regulation, and may induce dystonia. Death is often from hyperthermia, dysrhythmias, or intracerebral hemorrhage. (Goldfrank LR. *Goldfrank's Toxicologic Emergencies*, 6th Edition; pp. 863–869.)

10–16. B, A, C, C, D, D, E Any child who has ingested more than 20 mg/kg body weight of elemental iron and who has not vomited spontaneously (and is awake) may be given syrup of ipecac and brought to the emergency department. If GI symptoms develop within 6 hours in these children or children who have ingested less than 20 mg/kg body weight of elemental iron and have a level of less than 500 mg/dL of serum iron, they may be discharged home because it is unlikely that children who present within 1 hour of ingestion, and who have not vomited, may benefit from ipecac (if not already given at home), as adult-strength pills are too large to be removed by lavage. Lavage may be performed if chewable forms are ingested or if pill fragments are seen in the vomitus or on the abdominal radiograph.

The properties of iron that promote its toxicity include: (1) first order or concentration dependent absorption that is seen even in the overdose setting, (2) absorbed iron cannot be rapidly excreted. Patients with massive overdose by history or clinical manifestations should be presumed to have taken a significant ingestion prior to determination of serum iron levels. The most valuable time to assess serum iron is 4–6 hours after ingestion. At this time, tablet breakdown is almost complete, but iron has not been completely distributed to tissues.

Because administration of deferoxamine (DFO) interferes with the standard calorimetric method of iron measurement, the laboratory must be informed of this fact. In this case, atomic absorption method is an accurate method and overcomes the false-negative results associated with the former test. DFO is a specific iron-binding agent that binds free inorganic iron to form ferrioxamine (which is reddish in color) that is excreted in urine. It is given intravenously because GIT absorption is poor. The efficacy of DFO is not explainable entirely on the basis of the amount of iron excreted. Therefore, it is possible that toxicity is prevented by making iron less available for cellular binding where toxicity occurs. Hb, cytochrome, and other protein-bound iron are not chelated. Activated charcoal is ineffective in the setting of iron poisoning, as are any of the lavage solutions that could theoretically bind the iron in the stomach.

(Goldfrank LR. *Goldfrank's Toxicologic Emergencies*, 6th Edition; pp. 523–530.)

17–23. A/E/A, A, B, D, A, E, C The major metabolic pathway for elimination of salicylates when therapeutic doses are used is conversion to salicyluric acid and salicylphenolic glucuronide. However, this metabolic pathway follows the Michaelis-Menten kinetics, which is a saturable form of kinetics. Therefore, in the setting of overdose, this metabolic pathway becomes completely saturated and an alternative pathway has to be available for metabolism of salicylate. This alternative pathway is option E (salicylate excretion unchanged in urine), and therefore, this route of elimination becomes of paramount importance during salicylate intoxication. Because two of the major pathways become saturated, the half-life increases from 2 to 4 hours at therapeutic doses to as long as 20 hours. Also, protein binding decreases from 90% at therapeutic levels to less than 75% at toxic levels, and Vd increases from 0.2 to 0.3 L/kg. A nomogram is of limited value and was developed to be used only 6 hours or more after a single ingestion of nonenteric coated aspirin when blood pH is known to be 7.4. Repeat testing of serum salicylate levels is mandatory every 2–4 hours after ingestion. In children, the respiratory alkalosis is transient and usually occurs with metabolic acidosis.

Respiratory acidosis with salicylate toxicity warrants an evaluation for another toxin or for pulmonary dysfunction, such as pulmonary edema, which is a rare complication of salicylate overdose. Alteration in mental status in the presence of metabolic derangements make pure acetaminophen overdose suspect, and elevation of temperature directly resulting from salicylate toxicity is an indication of severe toxicity, and often is a preterminal condition in the adult population.

Aspirin was the leading cause of child poisoning in the past; however, the incidence of poisoning resulting from aspirin has been declining over the last several years. Because acidemia tends to affect the protein binding of salicylate, hyperventilation to maintain some degree of alkalemia is clinically important in salicylate poisoning. Because salicylates are a weak acid, salicylates are ionized and less mobile in an alkaline environment, whereas with acidemia, more salicylate leaves the blood and enters the cerebral spinal fluid.

In the setting of hypokalemia, it is often difficult to achieve alkalinization because under these circumstances, there is a limitation on excretion of hydrogen ion into the tubular lumen, and one has to correct the hypokalemia in order to be able to achieve alkalinization of the urine.

(Goldfrank LR. *Goldfrank's Toxicologic Emergencies*, 6th Edition; pp. 501–510.)

24–32. D, A, D, C, E,E, C, D, E Acetaminophen (*N*-acetyl-P-aminophenol [APAP]) is rapidly absorbed from GIT and peak plasma levels almost always occur within 4 hours of ingestion. The drug is metabolized in the liver by: (1) sulfation; (2) glucuronidation, (3) p-450 oxidase system, producing the intermediate metabolite (NAPQI) thought to be responsible for the toxicity; NAPQI is normally detoxified by conjugation with reduced glutathione and excreted in urine as mercapturic acid or cysteine conjugates.

A small fraction of acetaminophen is excreted in urine unchanged. This and the product of sulfation and glucuronidation are nontoxic. In the setting of overdose, when more than 70% of glutathione is depleted, NAPQI binds covalently to hepatocytes, inducing hepatic necrosis, which is usually centrilobular with periportal sparing. Children seem to be more resistant to the toxicity of acetaminophen, presumably because of the higher activity of the sulfation pathway. One exceptional group is children on anti-convulsants, such as phenobarbital, which accelerates the p-450 mixed-function oxidase system with production of higher levels of NAPQI, which is the main metabolite responsible for toxicity. These children are a higher risk and must be treated at a lower level of serum acetaminophen.

Because APAP is so rapidly absorbed through the GIT, gastric emptying is of benefit only in the first 2 hours after ingestion. Because APAP is effectively absorbed to activated charcoal and also because binding of *N*-acetylcysteine (NAC) to charcoal is probably clinically insignificant, most physicians would use activated charcoal with NAC, with possible repeating of the loading dose of NAC. NAC is taken up by the hepatocytes and acts as a precursor for glutathione and sulfate, replenishing reduced glutathione. When given more than 24 hours after ingestion of APAP, NAC acts as an antioxidant. NAC is administered when APAP is in the toxic range based on the Rumack and Mathew nomogram. NAC is also indicated when (1) initial AST and prothrombin time are elevated, suggesting significant ingestion, (2) when there is a history of prior or present vomiting with ingestion of more than 140 mg/kg body weight, or (3) when there is a history of a large APAP ingestion at an unknown time.

The clinical manifestations of APAP toxicity is divided into four phases: Phase I is characterized by nausea, vomiting, and malaise; phase II is characterized by hepatic dysfunction; phase III is characterized by sequelae of significant hepatic dysfunction with jaundice and coagulopathy; and phase IV occurs if phase III is not reversible.

In younger children with significant toxicity, hypotension, hypothermia, and apnea may be noted. Liver enzymes (alanine aminotranferease and aspartate aminotransferase), bilirubin and prothrombin time and partial thromboplastin time should be measured every 24 hours for 4 days while therapy proceeds. It is important to recognize that APAP measured by the calorimetric method is unreliable in the presence of high salicylates, bilirubin levels, or renal failure. In these circumstances, high-pressure liquid chromatography and enzyme immunoassay may be employed. (Goldfrank LR. *Goldfrank's Toxicologic Emergencies*, 6th Edition; pp. 487–495.)

33, 34.   E, C   An acutely poisoned patient with a very high level of theophylline may be awake, alert, and merely tachycardic. If this patient does not exhibit tachycardia, the diagnosis of theophylline overdose is suspect or concurrent ingestion should be excluded.

The cardiac toxicity is owing to massive catecholamine (release of epinephrine and norepinephrine) stimulation of the myocardium and is aggravated by hypokalemia, hypercalcemia, and hypophosphatemia. β-Adrenergic stimulation is responsible for the electrolyte abnormalities, acid–base disturbances, and vasodilation. Metabolic acidosis, hypokalemia, and hyperglycemia are recognized features. The hypokalemia is from a transcellular shift (into the skeletal muscles).

The cardiovascular toxicity (dysrhythmias and hypotension) is worsened by hypoxia and co-administration of medications with b-adrenergic or anticholinergic activity. Anti-emetics with anticholinergic activity may worsen dysrhythmias, and if a pressor is used to elevate blood pressure, a pure a-adrenergic agent is preferred.

Massive theophylline toxicity can be effectively treated by hemoperfusion, and therefore, strong consideration should be given to initiating transfer of this patient to a facility with these capabilities, while the patient is still stable. At this same time, multiple dose-activated charcoal, intravenous β-blockers, and other supportive measures should be continued. The indications for initiation of hemoperfusion include a theophylline level greater than 90 mg/mL at any time; a theophylline level of more than 70 mg/mL 4 hours after ingestion of a sustained release tablet; and a theophylline level of more than 40 mg/mL with seizures, hypotension, or dysrhythmias. The author has treated a 2-year-old child with a theophylline level of 120 mg/mL without hemoperfusion. (Goldfrank LR. *Goldfrank's Toxicologic Emergencies*, 6th Edition; pp. 567–574.)

35.   C   Among the opioids in this question, morphine-6-β-glucuronide is the most potent. (Goldfrank LR. *Goldfrank's Toxicologic Emergencies*, 6th Edition; p. 776.)

36.   B   Normeperidine is a metabolic product of meperidine, and it causes CNS excitation and seizures when it accumulates. (Goldfrank LR. *Goldfrank's Toxicologic Emergencies*, 6th Edition; pp. 777–778.)

37.   A, B, C   The dose of sodium nitrite needs adjustment for Hb concentration, whereas sodium thiosulfate needs adjustment for body weight. The efficacy of both these medications is increased by the coadministration of high concentrations of oxygen. (Goldfrank LR. *Goldfrank's Toxicologic Emergencies*, 6th Edition; pp. 1195, 1228,1229.)

38. E All of the above combinations can lead to cyanide production. (Goldfrank LR. *Goldfrank's Toxicologic Emergencies*, 6th Edition; pp. 1215–1222.)

39–41. D, C, D An upper GI endoscopy is warranted to evaluate for formations of concretions and bezoars. Hypokalemia is more likely to develop because of the β-adrenergic agonist type effect of theophylline. Repeated doses of activated charcoal should be continued throughout the hemoperfusion procedure in order to minimize further absorption of theophylline into the circulatory system. (Goldfrank LR. *Goldfrank's Toxicologic Emergencies*, 6th Edition; pp. 568–574.)

42. C Intraventricular conduction defects are most commonly associated with propoxyphene overdose. Meperidine has a tendency to cause seizures, morphine causes respiratory insufficiency, and heroine has been associated with pulmonary abnormalities, such as ARDS. (Goldfrank LR. *Goldfrank's Toxicologic Emergencies*, 6th Edition; pp. 175, 198, 777.)

43. D Hypotension is multifactored in origin. (Goldfrank LR. *Goldfrank's Toxicologic Emergencies*, 6th Edition; pp. 175, 198, 777.)

44,45. A, E Propoxyphene is associated with heart block and intraventricular conduction defect abnormalities. Often, much higher doses of naloxone may be needed to reverse the toxicity resulting from propoxyphene. (Goldfrank LR. *Goldfrank's Toxicologic Emergencies*, 6th Edition; p. 198.)

46, 47. B, C Activated charcoal may be helpful in body packers. (Goldfrank LR. *Goldfrank's Toxicologic Emergencies*, 6th Edition; pp. 175, 198, 777.)

48. E 3-Methylfentanyl is an extremely potent opioid and may require higher doses of naloxone to reverse its toxicity. (Goldfrank LR. *Goldfrank's Toxicologic Emergencies*, 6th Edition; p. 30.)

49–52. B, A, C, C/D/D/A/A/B With methanol intoxication, the onset of toxic symptoms or the development of metabolic acidosis is often delayed for 24 hours, with a range of 1–72 hours from the time of ingestion. Methanol is converted to formaldehyde and then formic acid (FA). The latter is responsible for the toxicity of methanol particularly with late recognition,

with subsequent build-up of FA. Two factors that correlate best with poor outcome are: (1) delay of appearance of toxic symptoms for longer than 10 hours, and (2) elevated levels of FA. Clinically, the most characteristic clinical findings are symptoms of blurred vision (the sign of dilated pupils with sluggish response to light) and hyperemia of the optic disc. These features correlate best with metabolic acidosis.

Oxalaturia and elevated levels of glycolic acid are features of ethylene glycol (EG) poisoning. HAGMA and hyperventilation are features of both. The degree of AG or EG poisoning is the largest seen in any metabolic acidosis. However, the onset of high AG metabolic acidosis may be delayed, and therefore, if the clinical suspicion is high, ethanol therapy should be initiated promptly. Because ethanol has a greater affinity for alcohol dehydrogenase than either methanol or EG, when ethanol is administered in sufficient concentration (100–150 mg/dL), it competitively inhibits formation of toxic metabolites, allowing the primary alcohol to be eliminated in urine unchanged. An optimal blood ethanol level, 100–150 mg/dL, should be attained, either orally (using a 15–20% concentration) or intravenously using a 10% concentration. Ethanol should be continued during hemodialysis at a higher dose because ethanol itself is dialyzable.

Alkalinization with $NaHCO_3$ is also helpful because renal clearance of glycolic acid is enhanced and the amount of undissociated FA is decreased at a higher pH, thereby limiting access to the CNS.

Additional therapeutic measures EG ingestion may include 100 mg of thiamine intravenously or 50 mg of pyridoxine intravenously every 6 hours until acidosis is resolved and EG level is zero. Pyridoxine in the presence of magnesium may shunt the metabolism of EG metabolites from glycolic acid to the harmless glycine, and thiamine may reduce production of oxalic acid.

For methanol intoxication, 50–75 mg of folic acid every 4 hours for 24 hours has been suggested. Folic acid may enhance the elimination of FA.

(Goldfrank LR. *Goldfrank's Toxicologic Emergencies*, 6th Edition; pp. 827–836.)

53, 54. C, C The typical initial dose of naloxone in an adolescent is approximately 2 mg intravenously. If the first dose of naloxone fails to reverse symptoms, then 2–4 mg intravenously should be given up to a total dose of 10–20 mg. In a setting where there is no ventilatory insufficiency, it is not essential to initiate high-dose naloxone. Once the patient responds, two-thirds of the dose that reversed the respiratory depression needs to be used on an hourly basis until the patient recovers. (Goldfrank LR. *Goldfrank's Toxicologic Emergencies*, 6th Edition; pp. 26,27, 100, 422, 770–772, 784,785.)

55–59. D, E, D, C, E Cyclic antidepressants induce their toxic effects by:

   a.   Inhibition of re-uptake of neurotransmitters such as norepinephrine and Dopamine.
   b.   Membrane depressant effect by slowing sodium influx into myocardial cells during Phase 0 of depolarization.
   c.   α-Adrenergic blockade.
   d.   Inhibition of central sympathetic reflexes.
   e.   Anticholinergic and antihistamine effects.

Many of the signs noted during toxicity are caused by central and peripheral anticholinergic effects, which include agitation, confusion, hallucinations, coma, seizures (central), tachycardia, hypertension, hyperthermia, dry skin, and urinary retention (peripheral).

Cyclic antidepressants are divided into first-generation (or tricyclic) antidepressants and second-generation (or cyclic) antidepressants. These drugs have a more specific mechanism of action but their toxicity profile remains the same. Patients with antidepressant overdose often develop wide, complex dysrhythmias, hypotension, and seizures within minutes of ingestion. If a life-threatening event is going to occur, it will occur within the first 6 hours of hospitalization (most often within 2 hours of admission to the emergency department). After initial stabilization, a 12-lead EKG should be obtained and the patient placed on cardiac monitor. The finding of a small S-wave in leads I and AVL and a small R-wave in AVR along with a prolonged QT and sinus tachycardia are highly specific and sensitive for cyclic antidepressants (CAs). However, absence of these EKG changes does not exclude a cyclic antidepressant overdose (CAO). The duration of QRS has been shown to be prognostic of seizures and dysrhythmias: QRS greater than 100 msec, 30% risk of seizures; QRS more than 160 ms, 50% risk of dysrhythmias. Blood should be sent for electrolytes, glucose, and if ingestion was intentional, an acetaminophen level. It is not clinically useful or cost-effective to obtain a plasma cyclic antidepressant level because there is no good correlation between levels and symptomatology. However, with levels exceeding 1000 mg/mL, dysrhythmias and seizures are usually seen.

CAs have a membrane depressant effect on the myocardium by slowing sodium influx into the myocardium during phase 0 of depolarization. This leads to intraventricular conduction defects, dysrhythmias, decreased cardiac output, hypotension, and decreased coronary perfusion. The effects of CAs on sodium channels can be attenuated by increasing the blood pH to 7.50–7.55, either by hyperventilation or Na^+ HCO_3. At this pH, it appears that CA uncoupled from sodium channels, whereas hypotension and acidosis enhance their binding. (Lidocaine may also be effective in treating ventricular dysrhythmias.) Therefore, aggressive treatment of hypotension and metabolic acidosis is essential. If hypotension does not respond to fluid resuscitation, then depending on the underlying etiology, inotropic support or vasopressors may be used. Norepinephrine will increase the vascular tone, whereas dobutamine will increase the contractility without increasing the vascular resistance dramatically. Dopamine should be in this setting because of its arrhythmogenic potential.

Seizures that develop in the setting of CAO are usually brief and respond to lorazepam. For persistent seizures, phenobarbital is recommended. Phenytoin is not recommended because of the potential for dysrhythmias. Other drugs that must be avoided include: class IA and IC antiarrhythmias (membrane stabilizers); propanolol and verapamil (myocardial depressants); flumazenil (inhibits the chloride channel of α-adrenergic and β-adrenergic receptors similar to CA). Because of the rapid deterioration of mental status in patients with CAO, ipecac should not be used. Multiple dose charcoal does enhance elimination of CA and physostigmine has not been shown to be safe and/or effective in this setting.

(Goldfrank, LR. *Goldfrank's Toxicologic Emergencies*, 6th Edition; pp. 726–731.)

60. A, B, C, D These are the drugs/toxins that should be in the differential diagnosis of HAGMA:

   a.   Paraldehyde ingestion can be diagnosed by its distinctive pungent odor. Other findings include: gastritis, mental status changes with possible coma, tubular acidosis, azotemia, oliguria, and proteinuria.
   b.   Toluene abuse by inhalation takes two forms:

   i.   Huffers inhale from a toluene-soaked cloth.
   ii. Baggers inhale from a plastic bag containing toluene placed over the head.

They may present with HAGMA or renal tubular acidosis. Other symptoms are GI disturbances, musculoskeletal weakness, or neuropsychiatric disorders.

c. Isopropyl alcohol ingestion is characterized by hyperosmolality and ketonemia (with ketonuria) but without significant metabolic acidosis.

d. Iboniazide overdose is associated with seizures. Seizing patients should receive 1 g of pyridoxine for every gram of iboniazide ingested at a rate of 1 g every 2–3 minutes. If the seizures stop, the remainder may be given more slowly in D5W. A maximum dose of 5 g may be administered.

(Goldfrank LR. *Goldfrank's Toxicologic Emergencies*, 6th Edition; pp. 627,628.)

61. D Tachycardia may be a common feature. (Goldfrank LR. *Goldfrank's Toxicologic Emergencies*, 6th Edition; pp. 1105–1109.)

62. C Although there are authorities who believe that pralidoxime must be given within 24 hours of exposure to organophosphates, there are also reports that pralidoxime is still effective when administered beyond 24 hours after exposure. (Goldfrank LR. *Goldfrank's Toxicologic Emergencies*, 6th Edition; pp. 1117,1118.)

63. B Clinical manifestations of organophosphate poisoning are not seen until a significant portion of the cholinesterase is inhibited, and the end point for atropinization is inhibition or significant reduction in upper airway and tracheal secretions. Tachycardia is not a contraindication to atropine in this setting. (Goldfrank LR. *Goldfrank's Toxicologic Emergencies*, 6th Edition; pp. 1117,1118.)

64, 65. D, B During hemoperfusion, compounds are cleared from blood as they come in contact with an adsorbent (surface) material contained in a cartridge, within an extracorporeal circuit. The adsorbent material could be: (1) Charcoal-best for polar compounds, such as salicylates, or (2) Amberlite XAD-4-best for lipid soluble compounds, such as theophylline, phenobarbital, CAs, meprobamate, and digoxin.

Extraction of many of these compounds is almost complete and the clearance often equals the blood flow through the circuit. Many of the pharmacokinetic factors that limit the applicability of diagnosis are not significant during hemoperfusion. Thus, molecular weight, degree of protein, binding in the plasma, and water solubility are not limiting factors during hemoperfusion because of the high adsorbent area that comes in contact with the blood. The Vd remains important however. Drugs with a large Vd may be completely extracted from the blood as they pass through the adsorbent, but if only a small amount is present in the plasma compartment, only a small total amount may be removed from the body. The most frequent complications are hypotension and thrombocytopenia. Other complications are hypoglycemia, hypocalcemia and hypothermia.

(Rogers MC, et al. *Textbook of Pediatric Intensive Care*, 2nd Edition; pp. 1302–1304.)

66. E Repeated dose activated charcoal is effective for all of these medications except for iron. Activated charcoal is ineffective in a setting of iron poisoning. (Goldfrank LR. *Goldfrank's Toxicologic Emergencies*, 6th Edition; pp. 66–69.)

67. A, A, A Carbamates do not penetrate the CNS, and their effects are usually reversible and transient. Only atropine is usually needed in a setting of overdose. (Rogers MC, et al. *Textbook of Pediatric Intensive Care*, 2nd Edition; pp. 1304–1307.)

68. D P_{Ka} is an important concept in pharmacology particularly in the setting of overdose. For example, with salicylates, which have a P_{Ka} of 3.1 at a pH of 3.0, the ratio of ionized to non-ionized is 1:1. However, if the pH is increased to 7.4, the ratio of ionized to non-ionized increases to 2500:1, and this will dramatically help with elimination of the drug through the kidneys. (Goldfrank LR. *Goldfrank's Toxicologic Emergencies*, 6th Edition; pp. 503–505.)

69. D Because K^+ is exchanged with H^+ in the renal tubules, hypokalemia with total body K^+ deficit will hinder urinary alkalinization. (Goldfrank LR. *Goldfrank's Toxicologic Emergencies*, 6th Edition; pp. 503–510.)

70. E For a compound to be dialyzed efficiently, it must be poorly protein bound (<90%) and highly water soluble, have a small Vd so that the majority of the drug is in the plasma, and have a small molecular-weight; compounds with a molecular-weight higher than 500 are progressively less dialyzable. (Rogers MC, et al. *Textbook of Pediatric Intensive Care*, 2nd Edition; pp. 1302–1303.)

71. E *See* answer to Questions 64 and 65.

72. A, B, B, B Organophosphates bind irreversibly to acetylcholinesterase (the enzyme that normally hydrolyses acetylcholine). As a result, acetylcholine accumulates at the synaptic site with subsequent continuous stimulation of the neuromuscular junction. Clinical manifestations are fasciculations, weakness, and paralysis. Myoclonus is associated with the other three groups of drugs. (Rogers MC, et al. *Textbook of Pediatric Intensive Care*, 2nd Edition; pp. 1304–1306.)

73. E The pulse oximetry detects the ratio of oxy-Hb to the total Hb and is incapable of measuring the other different types of Hb, such as carboxy-Hb or met-Hb. Therefore, the saturation that is obtained may be erroneous. Under these circumstances, one has to measure the oxygen saturation using the co-oximeter. (Rogers MC, et al. *Textbook of Pediatric Intensive Care*, 2nd Edition; pp. 122,123, 321, 461.)

74. D Drugs recognized to form gastric concentrations in the setting of overdose include barbiturates, salicylates, ferrous sulfate, and slow-release theophylline preparations. In these case circumstances, attempts should be made to eliminate these concentrations from the stomach including use of endoscopy because they contribute to the toxicity of these drugs. (Rogers MC, et al. *Textbook of Pediatric Intensive Care*, 2nd Edition; pp. 1326–1339.)

75. E Activated charcoal should be administered in almost all cases of poisoning after emesis and lavage are accomplished. Exceptions are in cases of ingestion of (1) Corrosives-whether alkaline or acids, as charcoal does not absorb either one effectively and the dark charcoal may interfere with endoscopic examination; (2) Anticholinergics-overdose with ileus is an obvious situation when repeated dose-activated charcoal should not be used; (3) Enteric-coated preparations are not well-adsorbed by activated charcoal. (Rogers MC, et al. *Textbook of Pediatric Intensive Care*, 2nd Edition; pp. 1326–1339.)

76. C Hypovolemia is the most likely cause of hypotension in a patient with significant intoxication, although other etiologies must be kept in mind and should be appropriately evaluated and treated. (Goldfrank LR. *Goldfrank's Toxicologic Emergencies*, 6th Edition; pp. 726–731.)

77. C Alkalosis seems to minimize binding of CAs to sodium channels in the myocardium with resultant suppression of dysrhythmias. (Goldfrank LR. *Goldfrank's Toxicologic Emergencies*, 6th Edition; pp. 726–731.)

78. E All of the above drugs induce a state of sympathetic stimulation and therefore are likely to be associated with hypertension. (Goldfrank LR. *Goldfrank's Toxicologic Emergencies*, 6th Edition; pp. 1–100.)

79. A, B, C, D, E Detection of a distinctive odor may be a clue to diagnosis of specific poisoning. This question addresses some clinical examples. (Goldfrank LR. *Goldfrank's Toxicologic Emergencies*, 6th Edition; pp. 1–100.)

CHAPTER 13: TRAUMATOLOGY

1. D Generally, following hemorrhage in humans, a rise in osmolality is directly related to the glucose concentration in the plasma, not the result of an influx of sodium. All of the other statements are true. (Rogers MC, et al. *Textbook of Pediatric Intensive Care*, 3rd Edition; pp. 1467–1470.)

2. C Catecholamines produce hyperglycemia, hyperlipidemia, increased oxygen consumption, and hyperkalemia, and α-stimulation reduces insulin and glucagon secretion. The overall effect of catecholamines on the islet cells it to not only increase glucagon, but also decrease insulin secretion. Cortisol decreases the peripheral utilization of glucose but the increase in plasma cortisol is designed to produce an increase in osmolality in response to hemorrhage. (Rogers MC, et al. *Textbook of Pediatric Intensive Care*, 3rd Edition; p. 1470.)

3. T, T, T, F, F, T, T Angiotensin II is a powerful vasoconstrictor. Aldosterone works on the ascending loop of Henle and in the collecting ducts of the kidney to increase sodium and water absorption. (Rogers MC, et al. *Textbook of Pediatric Intensive Care*, 3rd Edition; pp. 1470–1472.)

4.   C   An attempted open-operative cricothyroidotomy may cause irreversible damage to the larynx. All of the other statements are true. (Rogers MC, et al. *Textbook of Pediatric Intensive Care*, 3rd Edition; pp. 1474–1476.)

5.   B, A, C   Hydroxyethyl starch, albumin, and lactated ringers are commonly used fluid replacement solutions. Their physical properties differ and may affect selection. (Rogers MC, et al. *Textbook of Pediatric Intensive Care*, 3rd Edition; pp. 1481,1482, table 43.5.)

6.   C   Almost all plasma coagulation factors are stable in banked blood, with the exception of factor V and VIII. With massive transfusion, defined as greater than 2 blood volumes in a child, hemostatic defects may occur as a result of dilution or a decrease in the platelet and circulating protein coagulation factors. (Rogers MC, et al. *Textbook of Pediatric Intensive Care*, 3rd Edition; pp. 1482,1483.)

7.   C   In Weil's 5-2 or 7-3 rule, the 5-2 applies to the central venous pressure (CVP), and the 7-3 rule applies to the pulmonary capillary wedge pressure (PCWP). Volume boluses are administered and the pressure response is measured. When the CVP is less than 8 or the PCWP is less than 12, 10–20 mL/kg of isotonic solution is infused over 10–15 minutes. If the CVP increases by more than 5 or the PCWP increases by more than 7, the infusion is stopped. Immediate fasciotomy is indicated when a pressure greater than 60 cm H_2O is present. Cardiac tamponade presents with paradoxical pulse and hypotension. A pulmonary hematoma takes only a few days to resolve. (Rogers MC, et al. *Textbook of Pediatric Intensive Care*, 3rd Edition; pp. 1485–1490.)

8.   F, T, T, T, F, T, F, T, T   The rupture is more likely on the left because of the presence of the liver on the right acting as a cushion to the diaphragm. Pulmonary compliance decreases with adult respiratory distress syndrome. An intravenous pyelogram is indicated for gross hematuria with clinical evidence of renal injury and unstable clinical course of blood loss

and a possible renal artery injury. (Rogers MC, et al. *Textbook of Pediatric Intensive Care*, 3rd Edition; pp. 1491–1495.)

9.   B   Loss of consciousness of 3 minutes or more is an indication for a skull film. (Rogers MC, et al. *Textbook of Pediatric Intensive Care*, 3rd Edition; p. 1495, table 43.7.)

10.   E   There is a decrease in the perfusion, which results in the initial ischemic insult to the spinal cord following trauma. All of the other statements are true (Rogers MC, et al. *Textbook of Pediatric Intensive Care*, 3rd Edition; p. 1496.)

11.   T, T, T   Please *see* Rogers MC, et al. *Textbook of Pediatric Intensive Care*, 3rd Edition; pp. 65, 1498, and table 2.10.)

12.   B   Child victims of abuse are usually younger than 2 years of age. (Rogers MC, et al. *Textbook of Pediatric Intensive Care*, 3rd Edition; p. 1498, table 43.8.)

13.   E   Hypertension is a commonly described phenomenon associated with thermal injury. The increase in plasma renin activity and aldosterone increases intravascular volume and raises blood pressure. (Rogers MC, et al. *Textbook of Pediatric Intensive Care*, 3rd Edition; p. 1522.)

14.   E   Pulmonary dysfunction after thermal injury may be secondary to inhalational injury, aspiration, shock, sepsis, congestive heart failure, or trauma. The presence of inhalational injury increases mortality by 20%, whereas pneumonia increases the risk of mortality by 40% in burn patients. In the resuscitation phase of burn injury, lung injury results from hypoxia and subsequent reoxygenation, CO and cyanide toxicity, airway edema, chest wall, and pulmonary compliance problems. Hypoproteinemia may contribute to edema formation in the postresuscitative phase. (Rogers MC, et al. *Textbook of Pediatric Intensive Care*, 3rd Edition; p. 1522.)

15.   T, T, F, F, T, T, F, T, T, T, T

16.   C, D, A, D C, C, A, B   Renal blood flow decreases immediately after injury. Later, GFR increases coinciding with the onset of the postburn hypermetabolic state. Hepatic dysfunction is commonly encountered in thermal injury, and can generally be found in more than 50% of patients. Thrombocytopenia appears first, then is followed by thrombocytosis several days later. Significant increases in fibrinogen, Factors V and VIII occur. RBC mass decreases. Hypoxia occurring in the first 48 hours was the most common cause of encephalopathy and was related to smoke and CO inhalation sustained in enclosed fires. Acalculous cholecystitis is of two types in the burn patient. The first involves bacterial seeding in septic patients and the second arises in patients with dehydration, ileus, or pancreatitis in whom the gallbladder is distended with sterile fluid. Burn-injured patients are immunocompromised. (Rogers MC, et al. *Textbook of Pediatric Intensive Care*, 3rd Edition; pp. 1522–1525.)

First-degree burns are superficial burns isolated to the epithelial cells and characterized by erythema and mild blistering. Second-degree burns involve a tissue depth into the dermis. A superficial partial-thickness burn is moist, red, and tender. It becomes pale, but dermal papillae can be visualized through the eschar within a few days. Third-degree burns extend through all layers of the skin and invade the hypodermic fat. Fourth-degree burns involve deep injury to bone, joint or muscle. (Rogers MC, et al. *Textbook of Pediatric Intensive Care*, 3rd Edition; pp. 1525–1526.)

17.   B   With the Rule of 9's, the front and back are each assigned 18% of BSA; each arm is assigned 9%; each leg is assigned 18%. Therefore, a burn that involves 9% (arm), plus 18% (leg), plus 18% (back), equals 45% total BSA burn. (Rogers MC, et al. *Textbook of Pediatric Intensive Care*, 3rd Edition; p. 1526.)

18.   B, C, A   A minor burn involves less than 5% of the BSA and no significant involvement of the hands, feet, face, or perineum. A moderate sized burn involves between 5 and 15% of the body surface area. Alternatively, any full-thickness component also qualifies. Involvement of the hands, face, feet, perineum, or the presence of a complicating factor, such as chemical or electrical injury, also constitutes a moderate burn. A severe burn is characterized by more than 15% total BSA burn or the presence of smoke inhalation or CO poisoning. (Rogers MC, et al. *Textbook of Pediatric Intensive Care*, 3rd Edition; p. 1526, figure 45.2.)

19.   B   House fires account for 84% of burn associated fatalities, the cause of which is most frequently smoke inhalation rather than tissue damage from flames. Chemical burns should be flushed with water for 20–30 minutes, not alcohol. Tetanus prophylaxis must be addressed in all burn patients. Scald burns are the most common type of pediatric burn and the home is the most common location. (Rogers MC, et al. *Textbook of Pediatric Intensive Care*, 3rd Edition; pp. 1526,1527, table 45.1.)

20.   E   The criteria for transfer to a burn center include significant underlying disease, associated inhalation injury, 10% BSA or more of partial or third-degree burns in children younger than 10 years of age or more than 20% BSA in children older than 10 years of age, third-degree burns more than 5% in any age group, electrical and chemical burns, and burns associated with major trauma. (Rogers MC, et al. *Textbook of Pediatric Intensive Care*, 3rd Edition; pp. 1527,1528.)

21.   T, F, T, T, T   Systemic blood pressure is usually maintained after thermal injury despite hypovolemia, thereby making blood pressure an insensitive measure of volume status. Generally, children with less than 5% of their BSA burned do not require intravenous fluid therapy. Children with a burn exceeding 15% BSA will require intravenous resuscitation. If the burn size exceeds 30% BSA, placement of a central venous catheter is recommended. Muscle relaxants and sedation are contraindicated in the child who has signs of upper airway obstruction up until the airway is secured. (Rogers MC, et al. *Textbook of Pediatric Intensive Care*, 3rd Edition; p. 1528.)

22.   B, A, E, B, B   Mafenide is an excellent antibacterial. It inhibits carbonic anhydrase and may lead to acidosis. It can be painful, but penetrates the eschar rapidly. It is applied twice daily. Silver sulfadiazine is a broad antibacterial agent that is painless. It penetrates fairly well through the eschar. It is contraindicated in pregnancy and has unknown absorptive properties in the fetus. Bacitracin is limited in its antibacterial action, has poor eschar penetration, but is easy to apply and cosmetically acceptable. (Rogers MC, et al. *Textbook of Pediatric Intensive Care*, 3rd Edition; p. 1530, table 45.2.)

23.   D   The Parkland formula recommends lactated Ringer's solution in the first 24 hours postburn in the amount of 4 mL/kg/% BSA burn. One half of this volume is given in the first 8 hours postburn and the remainder given over the remaining 16 hours. The resuscitation should be adjusted to maintain a urine output of 0.5–1.0 mL/kg/hour. On the second postburn day, maintenance fluid of a glucose-containing hypotonic fluid may begin. (Rogers MC, et al. *Textbook of Pediatric Intensive Care*, 3rd Edition; p. 1529.)

24. T, T, F, F, T Resistance to silver sulfadiazine is common for *Enterobacter cloacae*, *S. aureus*, and occasionally *P. aeruginosa*. All three of these organisms are usually sensitive to Mafenide. Silver nitrate can induce methemoglobinemia. Ideally surgical excision and closure of the wound should take place as soon as the child is stable enough for anesthesia. More than 105 organisms per gram of tissue constitute burn wound sepsis. Early surgical closure decreases significant blood loss. (Rogers MC, et al. *Textbook of Pediatric Intensive Care*, 3rd Edition; pp. 1530–1531, table 45.2.)

25. E An adverse effect on the immune function may occur if lipid content is more than 15% of total diet kcals particularly if it is high in the ω-6 fatty acids. Enteral feeds prevent hypermetabolism and catabolism in contrast to parenteral feeds. Positive nitrogen balance may be achieved earlier with the institution of enteral nutrition within the first 4 hours. (Rogers MC, et al. *Textbook of Pediatric Intensive Care*, 3rd Edition; pp. 1531–1532.)

26. E Thermal injury from smoke inhalation is usually limited to the supra-glottic airway. Inhalation injury accounts for more than 50% of the mortality associated with major burns. Carbon monoxide poisoning accounts for approximately 50% of the poisonings in the United States per year. The largest source of CO is generated from the incomplete combustion of carbon-containing compounds. (Rogers MC, et al. *Textbook of Pediatric Intensive Care*, 3rd Edition; pp. 1534–1536.)

27. D The oxy-Hb dissociation curve is shifted to the left in CO poisoning, thereby enhancing oxygen affinity for Hb and impeding oxygen delivery from blood to tissue. The toxic effects of CO result from its direct action on the cytochrome-oxidase system and not solely on the reduced oxygen carrying capacity of the blood. If a significant amount of time has passed since the exposure of CO poisoning, an abnormal level may not be discovered. (Rogers MC, et al. *Textbook of Pediatric Intensive Care*, 3rd Edition; pp. 1534–1536, figure 45.4.)

28. D The heart rate and coronary blood flow increase in response to CO. Pulmonary edema occurs in about 10–30% of cases, however, the mechanism for pulmonary edema remains speculative. Cerebral blood flow and edema also increase. The cherry-red skin color is not commonly seen clinically. (Rogers MC, et al. *Textbook of Pediatric Intensive Care*, 3rd Edition; pp. 1534–1536, table 45.4.)

29. T, F, F, T, T, T, T, T Muscle necrosis leads to myoglobinuria and subsequent acute renal failure. Salivary amylase is responsible for development of hyperamylasemia. A mild acidosis actually shifts the oxy-Hb dissociation curve to the right, increasing release of oxygen to the tissues and so should not be treated. The half-life of CO is 5–6 hours in room air, 1.5 hours in 100% FiO_2, and less than 30 minutes in 100% FiO_2 in 2.5 atmospheres. Hyperbaric oxygen treatment should be instituted when a patient has a CO Hb of more than 25%, signs and symptoms of CO poisoning, and a hyperbaric oxygen facility available. (Rogers MC, et al. *Textbook of Pediatric Intensive Care*, 3rd Edition; pp. 1534–1538, table 45.5, 45.6, and 45.7.)

30. C, A, B CO concentrations affect the presenting symptoms. A CO Hb concentration of more than 0.195 is rapidly fatal, a CO Hb of 0.022 is associated with disturbed judgement, and a concentration of 0.007 is associated with shortness of breath with vigorous exercise. (Rogers MC, et al. *Textbook of Pediatric Intensive Care*, 3rd Edition; p. 1537, table 45.5.)

31. E Cyanide poisoning from smoke commonly occurs and acts synergistically with CO toxicity. Smoke injury decreases ciliary function. Patients with pulmonary injury may be asymptomatic with a normal chest radiograph on presentation. Arterial blood gases may also be normal for the first 12–24 hours. (Rogers MC, et al. *Textbook of Pediatric Intensive Care*, 3rd Edition; p. 1539.)

32. D At low voltages, alternating current is more dangerous than direct current because of its ability to freeze the extremity to the electrical source. Joule's law states that power equals amperage squared times resistance ($P = I^2R$). Surface burns result from the ignition of clothing or from the heat of the current traveling close to the skin. Arc burns are produced by a current that travels external to the body, as an electric arc forms between two objects of opposite charges. (Rogers MC, et al. *Textbook of Pediatric Intensive Care*, 3rd Edition; p. 1540.)

33. F, T, T, F, F, F, T Water content and a thinner stratum corneum decrease skin resistance in children. The conducting system of the heart is particularly vulnerable and ventricular fibrillation can occur with a current of 100 mA passing through the chest. Transient arrhythmias are present in 30% of patients. Tetanic spasms of respiratory muscles occur at 30 mA. Neurological findings are common. Loss of consciousness, spinal cord lesions, deafness, seizures, and changes in mood commonly occur after electrical injury. Nearly two-thirds of people struck by lightning live. (Rogers MC, et al. *Textbook of Pediatric Intensive Care*, 3rd Edition; p. 1541.)

34. A CO_2 autoregulation is better maintained than blood pressure autoregulation.

35. D When using uncrossmatched blood, it is best to obtain at least an ABO and Rh type and partial crossmatch. This is sometimes referred to as an incomplete or partial crossmatch. The immediate phase crossmatch eliminates serious hemolytic reactions because of errors in the ABO typing. It will fail to detect only a few unexpected antibodies outside of the ABO system, most of which are clinically insignificant. If time does not permit even a preliminary screen, ABO and Rh type-specific, uncrossmatched blood is still preferable (and more abundant). Of patients never exposed to blood, fewer than 1 in 1000 will have an unexpected antibody detected in the immediate phase crossmatch. (Rogers MC, et al. *Textbook of Pediatric Intensive Care*, 3rd Edition; pp. 1482,1483.)

36. E FFP provides the equivalent clotting factors of a single unit of fresh whole blood. The administration of FFP should be considered when 200% of the calculated circulating blood volume has been replaced with crystalloids and red cell concentrates. A precipitous fall in platelet count may not be tolerated, as well as a slow decline in thrombocytopenic patients. Platelet administration begins when 100–150% of the calculated circulating blood volume has been replaced with crystalloid and red cell concentrates. The dilutional

coagulopathy is rapidly corrected once perfusion is restored, but may be exacerbated by the development or persistence of hypotension. (Rogers MC, et al. *Textbook of Pediatric Intensive Care*, 3rd Edition; p. 1483.)

37. C Bleeding and edema within an intact fascial compartment can lead to the development of increased pressure, muscle ischemia, and death. Whereas pulses may be intact distally with a compartment syndrome, one constant finding is severe pain even with passive motion. Muscle compartment pressures can be evaluated during the secondary survey of the trauma patient using an 18-gage needle and water manometer. Compartment pressures of 40 cm H_2O should cause concern, whereas pressures greater than 60 cm H_2O require fasciotomy. (Rogers MC, et al. *Textbook of Pediatric Intensive Care*, 3rd Edition; p. 1486.)

38. C In addition to measuring urine output, the bladder catheter facilitates the diagnosis of urinary tract injury and rhabdomyolysis. An oral gastric tube should be placed in all patients with abdominal trauma. This procedure removes air from the stomach and improves ventilation, empties liquid and particulate matter, decreases the likelihood of aspiration, and provides diagnostic information concerning the presence of blood in the upper GI tract. If a pelvic fracture is suspected or seen on a radiograph, a rectal examination should be performed to evaluate the possibility of bone fragment injury to pelvic structures. Pain on passive range of motion is a constant finding in compartment syndrome. See response to question 37. (Rogers MC, et al. *Textbook of Pediatric Intensive Care*, 3rd Edition; pp. 1485–1487.)

39. D Almost all deaths from thoracic injury in children occur after the victim reaches the resuscitation center, and most children can be treated successfully with prompt diagnosis and aggressive early management. Penetrating injuries to the chest are unusual in children and usually result from fractured ribs rather than from external missiles. The mediastinum of the child is more mobile and this contributes to a low incidence of major vessel and airway injury. However, serious intrathoracic injury may be present in the absence of obvious chest wall injury. (Rogers MC, et al. *Textbook of Pediatric Intensive Care*, 3rd Edition; pp. 1487,1488.)

40. A Cardiac arrest from blunt chest trauma is nearly always associated with multiple system injuries, and results from hypovolemia either from external or internal blood loss. (Rogers MC, et al. *Textbook of Pediatric Intensive Care*, 3rd Edition; pp. 1487,1488.)

41. D Flail chest injuries are rarely seen in children because high-velocity direct-chest trauma is uncommon. Additionally, rib fractures are less common in children than adults because children have very pliable ribs that are resistant to fracture. Contusions and/or penetrating injury of the lung parenchyma are frequently involved. The initial therapy should include humidified oxygen and a limitation of crystalloid resuscitation, if the remainder of the injuries permit, so that there will be a decrease in extravasation of fluid into the injured pulmonary parenchyma and a limitation of the secondary acute pulmonary edema. Definitive treatment of the flail chest takes place in the PICU by controlled ventilation and PEEP. (Rogers MC, et al. *Textbook of Pediatric Intensive Care*, 3rd Edition; pp. 1488,1489.)

42. E The least common occult and potentially serious injury to the chest of a child with multiple trauma is esophageal rupture. From most to least common, the injuries are pulmonary contusion, pulmonary laceration, pulmonary hematoma, tracheobronchial tear, myocardial contusion, diaphragmatic rupture, partial aortic or great vessel disruption, and esophageal perforation. (Rogers MC, et al. *Textbook of Pediatric Intensive Care*, 3rd Edition; p. 1489.)

43. C In the setting of pulmonary contusion, overhydration should be avoided because fluid will sequester in the damaged lung tissue and complicate the clinical condition. Radiographical evidence of a pulmonary contusion includes early consolidation of the lung parenchyma, which may be focal in nature, with resolution over 2–6 days. Empyema, or abscess formation, may occur after pulmonary contusion secondary to the extravasation of fluid and blood into the alveolar and interstitial spaces. (Rogers MC, et al. *Textbook of Pediatric Intensive Care*, 3rd Edition; pp. 1489,1490.)

44. E Drowning is the third most common cause of death by unintentional injury among persons of all ages in the United States, and the second leading cause of injury deaths in children younger than 15 years old. Males account for 78% of all deaths from drowning. Approximately 50% of the drowning deaths occur in the summer. (Rogers MC, et al. *Textbook of Pediatric Intensive Care*, 3rd Edition; pp. 875–877.)

45. E The majority of drowning accidents occur in the southern and western United States; Saturday is the most common day of the week for drowning accidents; private pools are the most common sites for submersion accidents involving children; and drowning rates are highest among the African-American population. (Rogers MC, et al. *Textbook of Pediatric Intensive Care*, 3rd Edition; pp. 875–877.)

46. T, F, T, T Drowning is death from asphyxia caused by submersion in water. Death usually occurs at the time of submersion or within 24 hours. Most human drowning victims aspirate less than 3–4 mL/kg of fluid. Fresh water causes surfactant to denature and become nonfunctional. Seawater either dilutes surfactant concentrations or washes the surfactant out of the alveolus entirely. (Rogers MC, et al. *Textbook of Pediatric Intensive Care*, 3rd Edition; pp. 875–881.)

47. E The pathophysiology of submersion injury can include the processes of asphyxia, fluid overload, pulmonary injury, and hypothermia with the diving reflex. (Rogers MC, et al. *Textbook of Pediatric Intensive Care*, 3rd Edition; pp. 878–883.)

48. D Therapeutic hypothermia has not been shown to improve outcome. A body temperature of less than 32°C causes the cessation of shivering. Resuscitation of drowning victims should continue until the core temperature is at least 32°C. Pupillary dilatation occurs at a core temperature of less than 30°C. (Rogers MC, et al. *Textbook of Pediatric Intensive Care*, 3rd Edition; pp. 882–889.)

49. T, F, T, T, T, F, F, T Chest radiographs do not correlate with clinical outcome. Steroids have not been shown to be useful in improving the outcome for ischemic or anoxic insults. Intracranial pressure monitoring has not been shown to improve outcome in submersion injury. PEEP is often useful in treating the pulmonary dysfunction that is associated with a near-drowning episode, which is unresponsive to supplemental oxygen. The drowning victim will often swallow a large amount of water, which may induce emesis and subsequent aspiration. Consciousness is then lost. (Rogers MC, et al. *Textbook of Pediatric Intensive Care*, 3rd Edition; pp. 878–889.)

50.   E   The EEG may not be reliable in very young and particularly premature infants, because there are reports of return of neuronal function and EEG activity after the demonstration of electrocerebral silence. (Rogers MC, et al. *Textbook of Pediatric Intensive Care*, 3rd Edition; pp. 896–899.)

51.   D   No corroborative testing is required in the case described. (Rogers MC, et al. *Textbook of Pediatric Intensive Care*, 3rd Edition; pp. 895–900).

52.   A   Stereotyped movement of the extremities and extensor posturing can be seen in patients who are clearly brain dead; these have been termed the Lazarus sign. Spinal and deep tendon reflexes are found on physical examination in at least 50% of brain dead patients. (Rogers MC, et al. *Textbook of Pediatric Intensive Care*, 3rd Edition; p. 902.)

53.   T, T, T, T   All of these statements are true. (Rogers MC, et al. *Textbook of Pediatric Intensive Care*, 3rd Edition; pp. 895–902.)

CHAPTER 14: STATISTICS

1.   D   Type I or α-error is more likely to occur when you have too many variables rather than too few subgroups. (Fuhrman BP, et al. *Pediatric Critical Care*, 2nd Edition; pp. 172–174.)

2.   D   The power of a study is equal to $1 - \beta$-error, which was set in this study at 0.2, and therefore the power of this study would be 0.8 or 80%. The P-value of this study was set at 0.05, and there is only a 20% chance that the authors actually missed an improvement owing to the new drug. There is an 80% chance that an improvement from the new drug was not missed. (Fuhrman BP, et al. *Pediatric Critical Care*, 2nd Edition; pp. 172–174.)

3.   A   Groups are not a factor for nominal data. (Fuhrman BP, et al. *Pediatric Critical Care*, 2nd Edition; pp. 169,170.)

4.   A   In evaluating how strong the correlation is, it is more dependent on how tightly all the points are scattered around the slope line. Correlation does not make judgments as to how one variable affects or predicts another. A regression coefficient permits prediction. (Hermansen M. *Biostatistics: Some Basic Concepts*; p. 56.)

5.   E   Relative risk (RR) refers to the risk of having complications in the presence of a risk factor compared to the absence of the factor. The range of RR is from 0 to infinity. A RR of 1-0 indicates that there is no difference in risk. Calculation of RR is explained in the answer to Question 6. (Hermansen M. *Biostatistics: Some Basic Concepts*; pp. 164–166.)

6.   B

		Infection		
		Present	*Absent*	*Total*
Risk factor				
Nurse	Present	A = 75	B = 25	100
	Absent	C = 125	D = 775	900
	Total	200	800	1000

$$\text{Relative risk} = \frac{\text{Risk of infection when risk factor present}}{\text{Risk of infection when risk factor absent}}$$

$$= \frac{A/A + B}{C/C + D} = \frac{75/100}{125/900}$$

$$= 5.4$$

(Hermansen M. *Biostatistics: Some Basic Concepts*; pp. 164–166.)

7.   C   Standard error of the mean (SEM) is a descriptive statistic, and SEM helps determine the range in which the population mean exists. SEM equals standard deviation divided by the square root of the number of variables, and therefore, SEM is always smaller than standard deviation.

$$SEM = \frac{SD}{\sqrt{n}}$$

(Hermansen M. Biostatistics: *Some Basic Concepts*; pp. 38–41.)

8.   A, B, C, E, D   Self-explanatory. (Hermansen M. *Biostatistics: Some Basic Concepts*; pp. 38–41.)

9, 10. B, A

$$CL = \frac{\text{Dose at Steady State (D}_{SS}\text{)}}{\text{Concentration at Steady State (C}_{SS}\text{)}}$$

$$= K_{el} \times Vd$$

$$K_{el} = 0.693 \div \text{Half-life}$$

$$C_{SS} = \frac{20 \times 100}{0.693 \times 1.1}$$

$$= 2.6 \text{ mg/mL}$$

It takes four times the half-life to reach a steady state concentration.

$$= 4 \times 100$$

$$= 6.7 \text{ hours}$$

(Kearns GL. Clin Pharmacol, 1988; 7:198.)

11. C Parametric methods of statistical analysis use distribution assumptions (i.e., normal distribution) of data, and the distribution is described by mean and standard deviation. Nonparametric methods are also called distribution-free. These methods are based on analysis of ranks rather than actual data, and therefore, they are sometimes called rank methods. Skewed data are commonly analyzed by nonparametric methods. Methods using ranks are especially suitable for data, which are scores rather than measurements. Examples include apgar scores and stages of disease. (Altman DG. *Practical Statistics For Medical Research*; pp. 171–173.)

CHAPTER 15: ETHICS

1. D All of the above are involved in the process of informed consent. (Fuhrman BP, et al. *Pediatric Critical Care*, 2nd Edition; pp. 10,11.)

2. E These children are referred to as emancipated minors. (Fuhrman BP, et al. *Pediatric Critical Care*, 2nd Edition; pp. 10–12.)

3. D It does not assume that the patient or the surrogate is competent. This must be assessed by the physician, as indicated in answer E. (Fuhrman BP, et al. *Pediatric Critical Care*, 2nd Edition; pp. 9–14.)

4. A It does include the ability to manipulate the information and deliberate about alternatives. (Fuhrman BP, et al. *Pediatric Critical Care*, 2nd Edition; pp. 9–14.)

5. D The best course of action is direct inquiry into their fears and guilt, which is likely to provide the best resolution for all parties. (Fuhrman BP, et al. *Pediatric Critical Care*, 2nd Edition; pp. 18–22.)

6. D In order to succeed in a claim for damage, it must meet all the above criteria. (Fuhrman BP, et al. *Pediatric Critical Care*, 2nd Edition; pp. 18–22.)

7. B As long as the reason and the date are stated, adding to medical records is not illegal. Jurisdictions vary on the essence of compliance. (Fuhrman BP, et al. *Pediatric Critical Care*, 2nd Edition; pp. 20–22.)

8. D Accidents and adverse effects are the most common causes of death in children 13–15 years of age. (Fuhrman BP, et al. *Pediatric Critical Care*, 2nd Edition; p. 4.)

9. D "Baby Doe" regulations (introduced in 1982 by the Federal government) prohibit withholding or withdrawing of beneficial medical treatment from any infant on the basis of handicap or prognosis for quality of life. The three exceptions are: (1) infant is permanently comatose; (2) treatment is inhumane; and (3) infant is immediately dying. (Fuhrman BP, et al. *Pediatric Critical Care*, 2nd Edition; p. 34.)

10, 11. C, E It is more helpful in dealing with these families to have a caring attitude rather than a defensive attitude. (Fuhrman BP, et al. *Pediatric Critical Care*, 2nd Edition; pp. 38–41.)

12. A The complete record may be needed if the case goes to trial. It is rarely helpful in the initial investigation because so much of the record pertains to investigation. (Fuhrman BP, et al. *Pediatric Critical Care*, 2nd Edition; pp. 18–23.)

Selected References

Blumer JL, *Practical Guide to Pediatric Intensive Care*, Third Edition. Mosby Yearbook, Inc., 1990.

Committee on Infectious Diseases/American Academy of Pediatrics, *1997 Red Book Report of the Committee on Infectious Disease, 24th Edition.* American Academy of Pediatrics, 1997.

Fuhrma BP, Zimmerman JJ, *Pediatric Critical Care, Second Edition.* Mosby Publishing Company, 1998.

Goldfrank LR, Flomenbaum NE, Lewin NA, Weisman RS, Howland MA, Hoffman RS, *Goldfrank's Toxicologic Emergencies, Sixth Edition.* Appleton & Lange, 1998.

Hermansen, M, *Biostatistics: Some Basic Concepts.* Caduceus Medical Publishers, Inc., 1990.

Nichols DG, Cameron DE, Greeley WJ, Lappe DG, Ungerleider RM, Wetzel RC, *Critical Heart Disease in Infants and Children.* Mosby Publishing Company, 1995.

Rogers MC, *Textbook of Pediatric Intensive Care, Third Edition.* Williams & Wilkins Publishing Company, 1996.

Shapiro BA, Peruzzi WT, Templin R, *Clinical Application of Blood Gases, Fifth Edition.* Mosby Publishing, 1994.

West JB, *Ventilation/Blood Flow and Gas Exchange, Fifth Edition.* Blackwell Scientific Publications, 1990.

From: *Pediatric Critical Care Review*
Edited by: R. A. Hasan and M. D. Pappas © Humana Press Inc., Totowa, NJ